P9-BYT-444

Readers praise Robert S. Ivker's *Sinus Survival*

"I started your sinus and candida programs and haven't had as much as a sniffle for most of the year. Thank you for the book. I found it when I thought I was at the end of my rope, and now I feel empowered about managing this seemingly uncontrollable aspect of my health."
—RONELLE C., *San Francisco*

"Thank you for saving my life. I had severe sinus problems for months and developed chronic fatigue and probably candida problems, too. Since reading your book I have been able to heal my inflamed sinuses and have not had a sinus infection for two years." —BRIAN B., *Skokie, Illinois*

"Thank you so much for your book. It completely changed my life! Within one week of starting your allergy program I noticed improvement. I have not had a migraine in two years; I breathe clearly and recover from allergy attacks quicker. I have not talked to anyone who tried the program who did not get relief from allergy suffering. It was truly a life-saver for me." —VICKI W., *Montpelier, Virginia*

"Your book was responsible for digging me out of sinus hell, and I will be eternally grateful. I haven't felt this well for twenty years. Thank you for getting me going in the right direction."
—JOHN S., *Cottonwood, California*

"I scored 180 on the candida test in the book. After being on the *Sinus Survival* treatment program for just three weeks, I feel much better and my headaches are gone. Thank you!" —KERI K., *Chicago*

SINUS SURVIVAL

SINUS SURVIVAL

THE HOLISTIC MEDICAL TREATMENT FOR SINUSITIS, ALLERGIES, AND COLDS

Fourth Edition, Revised and Updated

ROBERT S. IVKER, D.O.

Past President, American Holistic Medical Association
Co-author of *The Complete Self-Care Guide to Holistic Medicine*

Jeremy P. Tarcher/Putnam
a member of Penguin Putnam Inc.
NEW YORK

Most Tarcher/Putnam books are available at special quantity discounts for bulk purchase for sales promotions, premiums, fund-raising, and educational needs. Special books or book excerpts also can be created to fit specific needs. For details, write Putnam Special Markets, 375 Hudson Street, New York, NY 10014.

Every effort has been made to ensure that the information contained in this book is complete and accurate. However, neither the publisher nor the author is engaged in rendering professional advice or services to the individual reader. The ideas, procedures, and suggestions contained in this book are not intended as a substitute for consulting with your physician. All matters regarding your health require medical supervision. Neither the author nor the publisher shall be liable or responsible for any loss, injury, or damage allegedly arising from any information or suggestion in this book.

Jeremy P. Tarcher/Putnam
A member of
Penguin Putnam Inc.
375 Hudson Street
New York, NY 10014
www.penguinputnam.com

Copyright © 1988, 1992, 1995, and 2000 by Robert S. Ivker, D.O.

All rights reserved. This book, or parts thereof, may not
be reproduced in any form without permission.
Published simultaneously in Canada

Library of Congress Cataloging-in-Publication Data

Ivker, Robert S.
    Sinus survival : the holistic medical treatment for sinusitis, allergies, and colds / Robert S. Ivker.—4th ed., rev. and updated.
        p.   cm.
    Includes bibliographical references and index.
    ISBN 1-58542-058-1
    1. Sinusitis—Popular works.   2. Cold (Disease)—Popular works.   3. Respiratory allergy—Popular works.   4. Bronchitis—Popular works.   I. Title.
    RF425.I84   2000   00-039253
    616.2—dc21

Printed in the United States of America

30 29 28 27 26 25

Book design by Tanya Maiboroda

To all physicians and health care practitioners who began
their professional training programs envisioning
themselves becoming healers.
And to every patient who has sought healing
as well as treatment and cure.

ACKNOWLEDGMENTS

As I think about the people who have contributed to this book, I am filled with gratitude and appreciation for the privilege and the pleasure of writing this fourth and final edition of *Sinus Survival.* The two people most responsible for making it possible are Jeremy Tarcher, a publisher with vision, and his successor, Joel Fotinos. Their unwavering support has instilled in me much greater confidence as a writer, and more important, has given me the opportunity to improve quality of life for millions of people. My agent, Gail Ross, played a key role as well. She created and presented the proposal to Joel that included this book along with four of its "offspring"—a *survival guide* series. *Arthritis, Asthma, Backache,* and *Headache Survival* will follow within the next year. This commitment allowed me for the first time to feel like a full-time (well, almost) author. During the two years it will take to complete these five books I have not been seeing patients. Although I look forward to resuming my practice, I've very much enjoyed the experience of being more of a writer than a physician.

Those who have contributed most to revising and updating the content of this new edition are: Todd Nelson, N.D., who greatly improved the candida treatment program, while making the challenging candida diet far more palatable; Nancy Russell, M.D., who added several suggestions for clarifying the diagnosis of candida (she also opened the first Sinus Survival Center in the U.S. in Kansas City, Missouri, in February 2000); and Todd Bezilla, D.O., who revised the osteopathic medicine section and presented the osteopathic treatment for sinus disease. My editor, Mitch Horowitz, guided the production incisively and gracefully.

I very much appreciate the valuable input I've received from patients, letter writers, and readers. I've incorporated many of their suggestions in shaping this book, and have also attempted to respond to their greatest sources of frustration—"Is there a local doctor who knows your program?" "It's too much to do." And, "Where can I find the products that you mention?" Possibly the most significant improvement in this edition is the convenient access to the recommended products that are essential to the successful implementation of the Sinus Survival Program. For that, I have my brother-in-law Howard Goldberg to thank. At the age of 46, he left a good job and moved his family (his wife Ellen and two teenage sons, Zachary and Matthew) from New Jersey to Denver, to create Sinus Survival Products. Without any guaranty, he took the risk, launched the business, and has been successful. His commitment to Sinus Survival and the courage he and his family demonstrated have contributed tremendously to providing countless sinus sufferers the opportunity to regain their health. Thank you.

There are a number of individuals who have made contributions to this and the previous editions, all of which have been incorporated into the text of this book. Steve Morris, N.D., along with Todd Nelson, helped me create the Treatment Tables in chapters 1 and 6, which have been so valuable in helping readers to implement the Sinus Survival Program, and in educating me and my readers about naturopathic medicine. My holistic physician colleagues, Bob Anderson, M.D., Deepak Chopra, M.D., Gabriel Cousens, M.D., Sylvia Flesner, N.D., Alan Gaby, M.D., Debra Glasser-Green, M.D., Ralph Golan, M.D., Brugh Joy, M.D., Elisabeth Kübler-Ross, M.D., Lev Linkner, M.D., Evart Loomis, M.D., Bill Manahan, M.D., Ann McCombs, D.O., Joel Miller, M.D., Chris Northrup, M.D.,

Acknowledgments

Norm Shealy, M.D., Bernie Siegel, M.D., Alan Warshowsky, M.D., and Andy Weil, M.D., have all contributed significantly with their vision, support, and/or content. Bill Silvers, M.D., an allergist and collaborator with me on the first Sinus Survival Study (described on p. 349), has consistently provided me with valuable feedback and also contributed to previous editions. There are several otolaryngologists (ear, nose, and throat physicians) who have recognized the value of my holistic approach and lent their wisdom and experience to the book and the development of the Sinus Survival Program. They are: Benjamin Asher, M.D., Nikhil Bhatt, M.D., Janice Birney, M.D., Karl Diehn, M.D., Milton Ivker, M.D., Bruce Jafek, M.D., Gilbert Levitt, M.D., Reuben Setliff, M.D., and Gil Vicente, M.D. (he invited me to present the Sinus Survival Program to physicians from all over the world at the Love the Nose Conference of the International Rhinologic Society in Manila in February 1999). George Kitchie, O.M.D., helped me write the section on traditional Chinese medicine, while Ross Barrick (Rocky Mt. Air), Rex Coppum, Richard Crowther, Carl Grimes (Healthy Habitats), and Bill Lundquist (Monster Vac) assisted me in creating a healthy environment in my home and in writing about it in chapter 6. Ken Gerdes, M.D., who practices environmental medicine in Denver, helped me to more fully appreciate the link between the environment and chronic disease.

There are a number of patients whose commitment to their health not only taught me a great deal about holistically treating sinus disease, but continually reinforced my belief that anything is possible. Working with them has helped to strengthen my passion for the practice of medicine. Their success has contributed significantly to the development of the Sinus Survival Program, and their stories have been an inspiration to me, my patients, seminar attendees, and readers. I am most grateful and would like to thank the following individuals for their effort, perseverance, and courage: Kathy Cuddy, Jackie Culp, Dee Gielissen, Bob Gorham, Cab Grayson, Lynn Hawthorne, Syd Henry, Dave Hofmockel, Steve McDonald, Tari SG Mitchell, Claude and Debbie Selitrennikoff, Dorothy Scott Seymour, Doug

Shapiro, Gloria Shell, John Snider, Jamie Starner, Marion Steeples, Bethany Ward, John Warner, Pat Warren, Rene Weidel, and Claire Zimmerman.

Since 1988, with the self-publishing of the first (70-page) edition, this book has mirrored my evolution from family physician to healer, and from sinus survivor to thriver. I would not have been able to make this journey without the help of my healers, teachers, spiritual guides, and friends: Carl Flaxer, Jaison Kayn, Apisai Lailai, Myron McClellan, my parents Thelma and Morris Ivker, and my in-laws Doris and Irv Goldberg. But it was the support, encouragement, trust, and love of my daughters Julie and Carin and my wife, Harriet, that kept me in the game for the duration. I love you.

Chronic sinusitis has totally transformed my life. Thank you, God, for such a wonderful gift. And thanks even more for allowing me to return it!

CONTENTS

SINUS SURVIVAL

INTRODUCTION:
THE SINUS SURVIVAL STORY

"Only when we are sick of our sickness shall we cease to be sick."

LAO-TZU, FROM THE TAO TE CHING

Since I began writing the first edition of *Sinus Survival* in 1987, this book has been a chronicle of my transformation from physician to healer as well as my quest to cure chronic sinusitis for myself, my patients, and millions of fellow sufferers. It presents much of what I've learned about healing during my thirty-two years of training and practice. Now, after more than twenty years of evolution, I am thrilled to report that the Sinus Survival Program has proven to be even more successful than I had originally hoped it would be. Not only has it helped to heal sick sinuses, noses, and lungs, but for myself and many others it has also been a life-changing process providing a greater degree of health and happiness than we've ever known.

This book will enlighten and educate you: You'll learn why you've felt so miserable for so long, and what you can do to improve that condition. But for the Sinus Survival Program to truly make a difference in your life, you'll need to give yourself a gentle but firm push to get moving in the direction of optimal health—a condition of physical, environmental, mental, emotional, spiritual, and social well-being. The critical ingredients for your success are a heightened **awareness** of your needs and desires (What do you want your life to be like?), a **commit-**

ment to providing them for yourself, the **time** required to incorporate new healthy habits into your life, and the **discipline** to stay on your course in spite of pain and setbacks. These are the essential factors in learning to love and nurture yourself, and especially your nose and sinuses. That is the primary objective of this holistic medical treatment program.

My "sinus story" began as a child with hay fever. I had two courses of allergy shots during late childhood and early adolescence. The condition improved to some extent, although I still had a few weeks each spring and early September when I wished the shots had been more effective. During those uncomfortable times, my only relief came from antihistamines, which made me feel drugged and drowsy.

Shortly after moving to Denver in 1972 to begin a three-year family practice residency, I experienced my first sinus infection. Wow—what a jolt that was! And I thought *allergies* were bad! The infections continued throughout the 1970s with increasing frequency and severity. The otolaryngologist (ENT—ear, nose, and throat physician) with whom I consulted could only recommend continued antibiotics or possibly even surgery. However, neither option provided me a guaranteed cure. He told me, "Rob, you're just going to have to learn to live with it." I was both shocked and depressed with his dismal prognosis. Although sinusitis is not a terminal disease, I felt as if I'd just been handed a death sentence.

In retrospect, today I'm able to see this affliction as a gift. It provided the impetus I needed to move beyond the limitations imposed by my training in modern medicine and find new therapeutic options. I was in my early thirties and was determined not to accept such a diminished quality of life for another fifty-plus years. This low point marked the beginning of the twenty-year evolution of the Sinus Survival Program. And it allowed me the opportunity to learn the true meaning of Hippocrates's sage advice, "Physician heal thyself."

It wasn't long before I began experimenting with dietary

changes (eliminating dairy, especially ice cream, had an immediate impact), taking vitamins and supplements to strengthen my immune system, and using a saline nasal spray. I remembered the holistic philosophy I learned during my first year at the Philadelphia College of Osteopathic Medicine. I was taught that to understand why a person develops an illness, you must address not only the physical but the mental and spiritual aspects of his or her life as well. Even my allopathic (conventional medical) family practice training was directed toward treating the **whole person.** The problem was that the reality of a busy practice did not allow me enough time to do much more than focus on a patient's chief complaint, perform a brief physical exam of the dysfunctional part of the body, and write a prescription. But now I had become the patient, and I was determined to rid myself of sinusitis by eliminating all of the causes of my "dis-ease."

Along with diet, I began to change my beliefs and attitudes: "No, I don't have to live with this. I can cure chronic sinusitis." I wasn't sure how I'd do it, but at least I believed it was possible. I also became more aware of my feelings and the harmful physical effects of painful emotions, especially anger, on my sinuses. I spent more quality time with my wife and daughters, and tried to figure out what in the world was meant by the term "spiritual health."

During those early years I did a lot of trial-and-error experimentation, and whatever worked for me, I then tried with my patients. By 1981, acute sinusitis had become the most frequent diagnosis in my practice, while that same year the National Center for Health Statistics ranked chronic sinusitis as the most common chronic illness in America. By the mid-1980s the Sinus Survival Program had reached new heights. It was during that period of time that I began working with Doug Shapiro, a two-time Olympian and one of the top bicycle racers in the United States. Chronic sinusitis was threatening to end his cycling career. Doug was desperate to try anything that might help him to continue racing. I couldn't have asked for a better test subject. During his almost daily hundred-plus–mile rides, his air filter (nose and sinuses) was continually assaulted with heavily polluted, extremely dry, or cold air. Whatever we found that kept his sinuses healthy, I thought would surely work for most other people, including me. And that's precisely what happened. By 1987, Doug and I were both free of chronic sinusitis. He went on to race successfully as a professional for another three years, and I began a crusade for healthier respiratory tracts and optimal well-being that has gained tremendous strength during the past fourteen years.

I could hardly wait to get the word out and tell as many sinus sufferers as possible, "No, you don't have to live with this misery. Chronic sinusitis is curable." I sold my family practice, Columbine Medical Center in Littleton, Colorado, to a local hospital. Since they would not permit me to do so in their "new" center, I began practicing holistic medicine out of my home. By 1988, I had joined the American Holistic Medical Association and written and self-published the first edition of *Sinus Survival*. Within three years the book had sold 40,000 copies and attracted the attention of a publisher with vision. Jeremy Tarcher published holistic health and paradigm-shifting books, so I felt very much at home. My mission was (and still is) to help transform health care in America, and I believed that presenting a highly therapeutic nonsurgical and unconventional approach for treating our most common disease might be an effective way to do so.

Amazingly enough, it seems to be working. During the past decade, public awareness of sinusitis has risen dramatically. In addition, there has been much greater attention given this condition from the medical community as well as from the insurance and pharmaceutical industries. I've had several hundred radio interviews and numerous television appearances, and the Sinus Survival Program has been the focus of many magazine articles. Both before and throughout my term as President of the American Holistic Medical Association (1996–99), I taught a number of Sinus Survival Seminars and Workshops to both physicians and the public.

As we enter the new millennium, the Program is gaining far greater acceptance from my conventional medical colleagues. In

February 1999, I was invited to speak at the International Rhinologic Society conference in Manila. The theme of the conference was *"Love the Nose,"* and the opening remarks were made by Eugene Kern, M.D., a professor of rhinology (diseases of the nose and sinuses) at the Mayo Clinic. Dr. Kern inspired his predominantly surgical brethren from all over the world to begin looking at chronic sinusitis as more than simply a bacteriological and/or anatomical problem, but as a dysfunction of the immune system triggered by a fungus. (The study upon which his remarks were based was published and widely publicized in September 1999.) I was surprised but pleased to hear what he was saying. The treatment of *Candida albicans,* a fungus, has been an integral part of the Sinus Survival Program since 1994 and, along with the concomitant focus on strengthening the immune system, has made a dramatic difference in the therapeutic outcomes of my patients. Following my presentation of the Sinus Survival Program I was enthusiastically accepted by these physicians as a rhinologist. I have also been invited to present the Program at the Annual Conference of the American Academy of Otolaryngology in September 2000. The results of the first scientific study on the therapeutic benefits of the Sinus Survival Program, performed in collaboration with William Silvers, M.D., former president of the Colorado Allergy Society, will be presented at that conference. The study will have a significant impact on the willingness of physicians to offer this holistic approach as an acceptable option to those patients who choose to avoid taking antibiotics, undergo surgery, or have failed to improve with either of these conventional treatments. During 1999 and 2000, I've been invited to speak at nearly twenty medical schools on the subjects of holistic medicine and *Sinus Survival.* Coupled with the meteoric rise in interest in alternative medicine (about 50 percent of Americans currently use some form of alternative medicine and spend nearly $30 billion doing so), we're beginning to see holistic medicine emerge as the foundation for primary care in America in the twenty-first century. To some extent *Sinus Survival* has contributed to this profound change in health care.

The book is currently a best-seller, exceeding 300,000 copies in sales. From the time it was first published, *Sinus Survival* attracted the most challenging sinus patients I'd ever treated. They came from all over the country, but their stories were remarkably similar. (You'll read some of them in the new chapter entitled "Sinus Survival Success Stories.") Thanks to these courageous people with such a strong commitment to their health, the Sinus Survival Program continued to evolve through the second (1992), third (1995), and now fourth and final edition of the book.

What originally took me about ten years to accomplish, now takes most of my patients a matter of months. Although curing chronic sinusitis may have been their primary goal when they began (just as it was for me), for most people who have been willing to make the commitment, the Program has also empowered them to heal their lives. As they addressed the multiple causes of their sinus dis-ease, they also discovered a dimension of health they never knew existed—one infused with high energy and vitality, peace of mind, and self-acceptance. Although many of them still have an occasional sinus infection (I've had three over the past twelve years), they are no longer chronically ill. More importantly, they now understand why they got the infection and have the tools to treat it quickly and avoid being sick for a prolonged period. But most significant in their healing process is that they almost always learn or re-learn a valuable lesson through their illness that helps to **prevent** subsequent infections.

The truth is that Sinus Survival is far more an intensive course in self-care and optimal health than it is a medical treatment or preventive medicine program. This fourth edition, revised and updated, is the textbook for that course. Unlike the third edition, which contained a wealth of new information, e.g., the "*Candida*" chapter, **this book is focused upon the successful implementation of the Sinus Survival Program.**

After hearing that I'm the author of a book about the holistic treatment for sinus problems, many people have then asked me, "What do you recommend for treating sinusitis?" They're expecting me to respond with one or two remedies—an herb, a homeopathic, a vitamin, a dietary change, or even acupuncture—that quickly and efficiently do the job. They don't really want to hear that "I've written over two hundred pages on what I recommend for holistically treating chronic sinusitis." And I've realized that for many this is a deterrent for them to even attempt to read the book or implement the Program. Although I've clarified and distilled this book down to the essence of the healing process, and made it more user-friendly, I've left the Program largely intact. However, I have prioritized components of the physical and environmental aspects of health to make it much less overwhelming for people who are just beginning. The "Success Stories" in Chapter 9 are about people who were very sick with chronic sinusitis, some nearly incapacitated. The inspiring stories of their return to excellent health include suggestions on how you, too, can be free of sinusitis and healthier than you've ever been.

Although optimal health requires a commitment to a lifelong healing **process,** we live in an age of the quick fix. We've grown up believing that there's a fast and effortless solution to any of life's hardships. And if there isn't such a miracle available today, it won't be long before science and technology provides it. I no longer have allergies or sinusitis. But to heal your diseased nose and sinuses and create a balance of optimal well-being throughout every dimension of your life, it requires a commitment to the Sinus Survival Program comparable to one you'd make if you'd just started a new job. **Healing yourself is the most important work you'll ever do, and the greatest gift you'll ever receive.**

It may also help to think of this commitment as if you had just one year to live, and during this final year of your life you're going to treat yourself as you've always wanted to be treated. In the past there's usually been something or someone that's prevented you from having what you wanted. Now there are no obstacles to living the life of your dreams. It's your choice to make.

Remember that the primary objective of your work on the

Sinus Survival Program is not about treating or "surviving" sinus disease and allergies. The title is, in fact, a misnomer. The book is actually focused far more on **thriving**—restoring balance to the dis-ease in your life and simply learning **to love and nurture your body (especially your nose and sinuses), mind, and spirit.** In meeting your greatest needs and desires, you will have become much more attuned to the heart of the healer within you.

After one month of making a commitment to this Program, you will be "surviving" quite well. If you can maintain and strengthen that commitment to yourself, within six months you will be healthier than you've been in years, and within one year you'll be experiencing a state of well-being you've never known before. The most important advice I can give you is to take your time, be gentle and accepting of yourself, and know that there are no mistakes—only lessons. Study diligently, listen attentively, be willing to take risks, and have fun while you're at it. Sure it's a challenge, but the rewards are unimaginable!

Rob Ivker
May 2000

Chapter 1

THE "QUICK FIX" FOR SINUSITIS, ALLERGIES, AND COLDS

After just describing the Sinus Survival Program in the Introduction as a *healing process* and not a *quick fix,* you may be wondering about the title of this chapter. After working with thousands of individuals suffering from chronic sinusitis in my practice, seminars, and workshops, and responding to countless callers and questioners via phone, letter, Web site, and radio call-ins, it's clear to me that most people need an easier way to get started on the Program. It may be the time, the expense, fear of stopping antibiotics or cortisone or of an allergic reaction to the vitamins or supplements, or simply that you don't like to take so many pills. Rather than trying to do everything at once, which for many can also be a bit overwhelming, this chapter will offer you different options for more *gradually* introducing this holistic approach into your life while experiencing rapid symptom improvement.

The primary objective of the Sinus Survival Program and the holistic treatment for any chronic disease is to heal the specific part of the body that is not functioning properly. The method for correcting this physical dysfunction is for you to nurture not only the diseased part but your entire body along with your mind and spirit.

This healing process usually begins on the physical level because the body provides the most immediate feedback: telling you what feels good and what makes you feel worse. But if you're feeling some degree of misery all the time, it's very difficult to determine what one intervention—an herb, vitamin, or air cleaner—is doing for you. It has usually taken many months or years to produce the conditions creating your ongoing sinus or allergy problem. To speed the process of correcting this imbalance in your life, I have developed the initial **Physical** and **Environmental Health** Component of the Sinus Survival Program, which is summarized in this first chapter. There's still a lot for you to do, and I apologize for that. But if you're committed to healing and curing your sinus disease, this is the most effective way to begin. This will enable you to feel better as quickly as possible. Chapters 2 through 6 will help you to understand *why* all of these recommendations are included and better appreciate how they are helping to maintain and enhance your health.

I've found that if you stay on this complete regimen for four to eight weeks, you will usually be able to at least partially restore the physical imbalance and experience considerable and often dramatic improvement. If after four weeks you've noticed no change, then consider the possibility of candida as a significant cause of your chronic sinusitis. You should then take the Candida Questionnaire and Score Sheet in Chapter 6 and follow the candida treatment aspect of the Program outlined in that chapter along with the Physical and Environmental Health recommendations in this chapter. The improvement in your physical condition will usually provide the motivation to make a deeper commitment to the rest of the Program while addressing all of the causes of your illness.

If you choose to take your time and more gradually implement this first phase, perhaps taking two months to do so, you will still feel better, albeit more slowly. Once you're on the entire regimen, then give it at least one to two months for a fair trial. To fully benefit from the Mind and Spirit Components of the Program, you should begin with the Body. By improving physically at the outset, you'll become much more aware of what you can do to heighten this feeling of well-being and what behaviors—what you're eating, too little or too much exercise, not enough sleep, stress—make you feel worse.

The practice of holistic medicine is based upon loving yourself physically, environmentally, mentally, emotionally, spiritually, and socially. There is no quick fix in this lifetime process of experiencing optimal health. Since each of us is a unique individual, our prescription for *healing is based upon self-awareness*. However you can give yourself a jump start by closely following these initial recommendations, which work quite well for almost anyone.

In the tables that follow, I have placed **one asterisk** in the left margin next to the recommendations, vitamins, and supplements that should be started at the outset—**stage one. Two asterisks** denote the **second stage,** which you can begin three weeks later. The **third stage,** marked by **three asterisks,** begins after another three weeks. You always have the option of doing and taking everything right from the beginning or at any time of your choosing, and simply following the instructions in the table. The only risk that I'm aware of in starting out with the entire program is that it could feel a bit overwhelming and may be more challenging to *maintain* the new daily practices than if you gradually ease into it.

Each of the different therapeutic options presented in these tables will contribute some benefit. There is no single remedy or magic potion that I'm aware of that will quickly cure chronic sinusitis or allergies, and I've been searching for over twenty years. However, most people who are interested in this Program have been uncomfortable for many months, if not years. For them, taking one to two months to feel better than they have in a long time can be described as a *quick fix*.

After about two months of incorporating most of the physical and environmental health recommendations into your daily routine, you can begin the mental and emotional health components of the Program, followed in another one to two months by spiritual and social health. These facets of the Program will be described in chapters 7 and 8. With each component you will be uncovering factors that have contributed to causing your sinus condition or allergies, or have triggered most of your colds. The more often you are experiencing a sense of physical well-being, the more acutely aware you'll become of what makes you feel good and what makes you feel sick. You'll also understand why you developed the sinus infection, got a cold, or had a sudden episode of sneezing. This information initially will allow you to make healthier choices regarding what you're breathing, where and how you exercise, and what you eat and drink. And although your diet can make a significant difference, you'll find that what you eat is far less important than what's eating you. You'll soon realize that the latter four aspects of health—comprising *mind* and *spirit*—require far less of your time but a deeper commitment and greater awareness than the recommendations for the *body.* However, the more you can work on these less tangible but potentially more immune-suppressing and -enhancing factors, you will be able to effectively *prevent* colds, sinus infections, and even allergy attacks.

Before you begin implementing the physical and environmental health components, please take the Wellness Self-Test in Chapter 2 and the Candida Questionnaire and Score Sheet in Chapter 6. Your Wellness score will help you to see where your life is unbalanced and what aspects will require the most attention. If your Candida score is above 180 (woman) or 140 (man), then I would recommend adding the *Candida* Treatment Program (Table 1.5) right from the start to the following recommendations. If it's lower, then I'd wait four weeks and see how you feel after practicing the rest of the Program. I would also suggest reading chapter 6, "Healing Your Body," to have a better understanding of why these therapies are used.

Many of the products included in these tables that are not readily available at most health food stores, can be obtained by referring to the Product Index at the end of the book.

Table 1.1

The Physical and Environmental Health Components of the *Sinus Survival Program* for Preventing and Treating *Sinusitis,* and Preventing *Allergies* and *Colds*

	PREVENTIVE MAINTENANCE FOR SINUSITIS, ALLERGIES, AND COLDS	TREATING A SINUS INFECTION
★ Sleep	7–9 hrs/day; no alarm clock	8–10+ hrs/day
★ Negative ions or air cleaner	Continuous operation; use ions especially with air-conditioning.	Continuous operation
★★ Room humidifier, warm mist; and	Use during dry conditions, especially in winter if heat is on and	Continuous operation
★★★ central humidifier	in summer if air conditioner is on.	
★ Saline nasal spray (SS spray) (p. 135)	Use daily, especially with dirty and/or dry air.	Use daily, every 2–3 hrs.
★ Steam Inhaler (p. 134)	Use as needed with dirty and/or dry air.	Use daily, 2–4×/day add V-VAX (eucalyptus oil).
★ Nasal Irrigation (p. 136)	Use as needed with dirty and/or dry air.	Use daily, 2–4×/day after steam.
★ Water, bottled or filtered (p. 131)	Drink 1/2 oz./lb. body weight; with exercise, drink 2/3 oz/lb.	1/2 to 2/3 oz/lb of body weight
★ Diet (p. 140)	↑ Fresh fruit, vegetables, whole grains, fiber ↓ sugar, dairy, caffeine, alcohol	No sugar, dairy
★ Exercise, preferably aerobic	Minimum 20–30 min, 3–5×/week; avoid outdoors if high pollution and/or pollen, and extremely cold temperatures.	No aerobic; moderate walking OK. Avoid outdoors if high pollution and/or pollen, and cold temperatures.

Table 1.2

Vitamins and Supplements for Preventing and Treating *Sinusitis,* and Preventing *Allergies* and *Colds*

	ADULTS		CHILDREN (Over 3 Yrs of Age)		PREGNANCY	
	(*1) PREVENTIVE MAINTENANCE FOR SINUSITIS, ALLERGIES, AND COLDS	TREATING A SINUS INFECTION	PREVENTION	TREATING A SINUS INFECTION	PREVENTION	TREATING A SINUS INFECTION
* Vitamin C (polyascorbate or ester C)	1,000–2,000 mg 3×/day	3,000–5,000 mg 3×/day	100–200 mg 3×/day	500–1,000 mg 3×/day	1,000 mg 2×/day	1,000 mg 4×/day
** Beta carotene	25,000 IU 1 or 2×/d	(*2)25,000 IU 3×/d	5,000 IU 1 or 2×/d	10,000 IU 2×/d	25,000 IU 1×/d	25,000 IU 2×/d
* Vitamin E	400 IU 1 or 2×/d	400 IU 2×/d	50 IU 1 or 2×/d	200 IU 2×/d	200 IU 1×/d	200 IU 2×/d
* Proanthocyanidin (grape-seed extract)	100 mg 1 or 2×/d (on an empty stomach)	100 mg 3×/d (on an empty stomach)	—	100 mg 1×/d	—	100 mg 1×/d
*** Vitamin B₆	50 mg 2×/d	200 mg 2×/d	10 mg 1×/d	25 mg 1×/d	25 mg 1×/d	25 mg 2×/d
(*3) Multivitamin	1 to 3×/d	1 to 3×/d	Pediatric multivitamin		Prenatal multivitamin with 800 mg folic acid	
** Selenium	100–200 mcg/d	200 mcg/d	—	100 mcg/d	25 mcg/d	100 mcg 2×/d
** Zinc picolinate	20–40 mg/d	40–60 mg/d	10 mg/d	10 mg 2×/d	25 mg/d	40 mg/d
** Magnesium citrate, aspartate, or glycinate	500 mg/d	500 mg/d	150–250 mg/d	300 mg/d	500 mg/d	500 mg/d
** Calcium (citrate or hydroxyapatite)	1,000 mg/d; menopause: 1,500 mg/d	1,000 mg/d; menopause: 1,500 mg/d	600–800 mg/d from diet		1,200 mg/d	1,200 mg/d

	ADULTS		CHILDREN (Over 3 Yrs of Age)		PREGNANCY	
	*1 PREVENTIVE MAINTENANCE FOR SINUSITIS, ALLERGIES, AND COLDS	TREATING A SINUS INFECTION	PREVENTION	TREATING A SINUS INFECTION	PREVENTION	TREATING A SINUS INFECTION
*** Chromium picolinate	200 mcg/day	200 mcg/day	—	—	in prenatal multi-vitamin	
* Garlic	1,200 mg/d	1,200–2,000 mg 3×/d	—	1,000 mg 3×/d	—	1,200 mg 3×/d
* Echinacea	200 mg 2×/d or 25 drops 2–3×/d (allergy prevention)	200 mg 3×/d or 25 drops 4–5×/d	—	100 mg 3×/d or 7–10 drops 3×/d	—	200mcg 3×/d or 25 drops 4×/d
** Berberis or ⊛⁴goldenseal	—	200 mg 3×/d or 20 drops 4–5×/d	—	100 mg 3×/d or 7–10 drops 3×/d	—	—
*** Bee propolis	—	500 mg 3×/d	—	200 mg 3×/d or 500 mg 1×/d	—	500 mg 3×/d
* Grapefruit (citrus) seed extract	—	100 mg 3×/d or 10 drops in water 3×/d	—	4 drops in water 2×/d	—	100 mg 3×/d or 10 drops in water 3×/d
*** Flaxseed oil (or Omega-3 fatty acids in fish oil)	2 tbsp/d	2 tbsp/d	1 tbsp/d	1 tbsp/d	2 tbsp/d	2 tbsp/d
⊛⁵Antibiotics						

Key to Tables 1.1 and 1.2

*[1]Use the higher dosage on days of higher stress, less sleep, and increased air pollution.

*[2]Use this dosage for a maximum of 1 month.

*[3]Dosage depends on brand.

*[4]Avoid with ragweed allergy.

*[5]Antibiotics—an option for sinusitis if taken infrequently, i.e., 1 or 2×/year, or if no improvement with this Program after 2 weeks.

* Stage One—begin the Program with these.

** Stage Two—take these after 3 weeks into the Program, or earlier if you choose.

*** Stage Three—start these 6 weeks into the Program, or sooner if you're comfortable with doing so.

Table 1.3

Allergy Treatment

These recommendations should be followed *in addition* to those listed in tables 1.1 and 1.2 in the *preventive maintenance* column.

	ADULTS	CHILDREN (Over 3 Yrs of Age)	PREGNANCY
★ Grape seed (empty stomach)	(★¹)100 to 200 mg 3×/day	50 mg 3×/day	100 mg 2×/day
★ Nettles, freeze-dried	300 mg 1–3×/d	—	—
★ Quercetin + Bromelain (empty stomach)	1,000–2,000 mg/day (into 3–6 doses/d)	250–500 mg 1–2×/d	—
★ Echinacea	200 mg 3×/d or 25 drops 3–4×/d	—	—
★(★²)Ephedra or Ma huang	12.5–25 mg 2 or 3×/d	5 mg 2×/d	—
★★(★³)Licorice (Glycyrrhiza glabra)	(★⁴)10–20 drops 3×/d	5–10 drops 2–3×/d	—
★★ Pantothenic acid	500 mg 3×/d (after meals)	50 mg 2–3×/d	—
★★ Hydrochloric acid	1 or 2 after protein-based meals	—	—
(★⁵)Antihistamines	OTC or Rx	OTC or Rx	OTC or Rx
(★⁵)Corticosteroid nasal spray	Rx	Rx	Rx
Allergy desensitization injections	Physician supervised		

Key to Table 1.3
★¹ Use the higher dosage of grape seed (200 mg 3×/day) only during the peak of your pollen allergy season.
★² Use only if nasal congestion is a primary symptom, but do not use with high blood pressure.
★³ Do not use with high blood pressure or an enlarged prostate.
★⁴ Watch for low potassium with long-term use.
★⁵ OK to use both antihistamines and steroid nasal spray at the outset of allergy treatment program, or wait and see outcome of taking the supplements. They can safely be taken along with the supplements.
★Stage One—begin allergy treatment with these.
★★Stage Two—if after 4 or 5 days you still have uncomfortable allergy symptoms, then begin taking these.

Table 1.4

Cold Treatment Program★

- Rest and get more sleep.
- Take vitamin C (in the form of ester C), between 15 and 20,000 mg in the first 24 hours; either 5,000 mg 3 or 4×/day or 2,000 mg every 2 hours, or 1000 mg every waking hour; very gradually taper this dose over the next 3–5 days.
- Take vitamin A (kills viruses), 150,000 IU daily for 2–3 days; you can take 50,000 IU three times, then gradually taper over the next 2–3 days.
- Take Yin Chiao, a Chinese herb, 5 tablets 4 or 5×/day in the first 48 hours.
- Take garlic, eaten raw (one or two cloves a day) or in liquid or capsule form, 4000 mcg (of allicin) per day.
- Take echinacea, or EchinOsha Blend ® (combination of echinacea with osha root and other herbs), 1 dropperful in water 3–5×/day for 3–5 days; or 900 mg 4×/day. Do not take echinacea if you have an autoimmune disease like lupus, MS, or HIV.
- Take zinc gluconate lozenges, containing at least 13 mg, every 2 hours.
- Gargle with salt water.
- Use a saline nasal spray hourly, preferably the Sinus Survival Spray containing antiviral herbs.
- Take lots of warm or hot liquids; take ginger root or peppermint tea; you can include ginger, honey, lemon, cayenne, cinnamon, and a teaspoon of brandy.
- Take a hot bath and inhale steam, adding a few drops of eucalyptus, peppermint, and/or tea tree oil.
- Take the "homeopathic vitamin Cs," *Aconitum* (monkshood) and *ferrum* phos (iron phosphate).
- Use acupuncture and acupressure, especially points 3, 4, and 8 (see diagram on p. 200).
- Eliminate dairy products and sugar and eat lighter foods; eat less protein; also include warm soups, steamed vegetables, and generous amounts of garlic, ginger, and onions.

★ This treatment program is highly effective for diminishing both the duration and intensity of a cold, and works best the more quickly you respond to the first symptoms of a cold. They are usually a sore throat, fatigue, feeling weak or achy, mucus drainage, and possibly some sneezing.

Table 1.5

Candida Treatment Program ⍟¹

- Candida diet—refer to Chapter 6.
- Antifungal medication (Rx)—Diflucan, Sporanox, Lamisil, or Nizoral.⍟²
- Antifungal homeopathic—Mycocan Combo, Aqua Flora, Candida-Away, and several others—an alternative to antifungal Rx.
- Latero-Flora (found in health food stores as Flora Balance)—2 capsules 20 min before breakfast.⍟³
- *Acidophilus* (*Lactobacillus acidophilus* and *bifidus*)—½ teaspoon or 2 caps 3×/day for adults and during pregnancy; ¼ teaspoon 3×/day for children over 3.⍟⁴
- Intestinalis—1 tablet 3×/day.⍟⁵
- Colon hydrotherapy (colonic) treatments.⍟⁶

Key to Candida Treatment Program

⍟¹ To determine if you are a candidate for candida treatment, first take the Candida Questionnaire and Score Sheet in Chapter 6. If your total score is in the "Probably Yeast-Connected" range or higher (above 60 for women and 40 for men), then consider committing to the candida treatment if there is no improvement after one month on the Sinus Survival Program outlined in the preceding tables.

⍟² Antifungal medication needs to be prescribed and monitored by a physician. If you are unable to find a physician willing to prescribe this, you can either find a holistic physician or consider taking an antifungal homeopathic. The higher your Candida Score the more important it is to include an Rx or homeopathic in your treatment program. Expect some "die-off" effect with possible worsening of your symptoms within the first 2 weeks after beginning this medication. Recommended dosage is 200 mg daily for 4 to 6 weeks, then every other day for 3 to 4 weeks.

⍟³ A beneficial bacteria that is effective in killing candida. Usual dosage is 2 capsules daily for 2 or 3 months, then 1 capsule 20 min before breakfast for an additional 2–3 months.

⍟⁴ Begin taking acidophilus after completing the course of antifungal medication, about 6 weeks into the program.

⍟⁵ A combination of about 20 herbs that helps to kill harmful bacteria in the intestine, along with parasites and excessive candida. Recommended dosage is 1 tablet 3×/day for the first 4 to 6 weeks, then 1 tablet 2×/day for another 6 weeks, tapering to 1 daily for another 2 months. It also works well in preventing traveler's diarrhea with a dosage of 1 tablet daily.

⍟⁶ Not absolutely necessary, but can speed your progress especially during the first month of treatment. To find a colon hydrotherapist, call the office of a holistic (M.D. or D.O.) or naturopathic (N.D.) physician, or a chiropractor.

Table 1.6

Natural Quick-Fix Symptom Treatment

Cough
Gargle, then drink lemon juice and honey (1:1) with a tablespoon of
   vodka or a pinch of cayenne pepper.
Ginger tea
Wild cherry bark syrup
Bronchial drops (a homeopathic)
Sinus Survival Cough Syrup (with elderberry)

Fatigue
Ginseng
Antioxidants, especially vitamin C
Folic acid
Vitamin B_{12} 500 mcg 2×/day
Vitamin B_6 75 to 100 mg/day
Pantothenic acid 500 mg 1 or 2×/day
Meditation
Exercise
Sleep
Pace yourself between activity and rest.
Rule out anemia.

Headache
Adequate water intake
Negative air ions
Steam
Eucalyptus oil
Acupressure/reflexology points
Hydrotherapy—alternate hot and cold shower
Garlic or horseradish (chew it)
Calcium/magnesium
Quercetin, 2 caps 3×/day
Fenu/Thyme (Nature's Way), 2 caps 3×/day
Ginkgo biloba, 40 mg 3×/day
Feverfew avena, 20 drops 3×/day

Runny Nose
Adequate water intake
Saline spray every 1 to 2 hours

Ephedra (not with high blood pressure)

Nettles, 1 cap 3×/day

Quercetin, 1000 mg, 2 tabs 3×/day (on an empty stomach)—take with bromelain

Vitamin C, 6,000 to 10,000 mg/day or higher—take as ascorbate or Ester C

Sneezing

Adequate water intake

Acupressure/reflexology points

Nettles, 2 caps 2–3×/day

Quercetin, 1000 mg, 2 tabs 3×/day (on an empty stomach)—take with bromelain

Sore Throat

Gargle with lemon juice and honey (1:1).

Gargle with pinch of cayenne + 1 tsp salt in 8 oz water.

Licorice-based tea (Long Life, Traditional Medicinals, or Throat Coat)

Lozenges (Zand Eucalyptus, Holistic brand Propolis)

Zinc picolinate, 30 mg 3×/day—begin with zinc gluconate lozenges for three days, then switch to picolinate

Garlic, 2 caps 3×/day

Zand Throat Spray

Stuffy Nose

Adequate water intake

Hot tea with lemon

Hot chicken soup

Steam

Hydrotherapy (hot water from shower) or hot compresses

Eucalyptus oil

Horseradish

Anger release, especially punching

Acupressure/reflexology points

Massage

Orgasm

Exercise

Garlic

Onions

Cayenne pepper

Breathe Right™—External Nasal Dilator

No ice-cold drinks
No dairy
No gluten (wheat, rye, oats, barley)
Ephedra, 20 to 30 drops 4×/day for 2–3 days (max.)
Rule out allergies.
Papaya enzyme, 1 or 2 tablets 4×/day (dissolved in mouth)—use also
    for ear congestion, sinus congestion, and sinus pain
Sinupret, or Quanterra Sinus Defense (a combination of five herbs)

Chapter 2

HOLISTIC MEDICINE AND THE WELLNESS SELF-TEST

"The only thing I know that truly heals people is unconditional love."

ELISABETH KÜBLER-ROSS, M.D.

Most people who read this book have sinus and allergy problems and don't consider themselves to be particularly healthy. But **what is health?** The conditioning that the majority of us have grown up with has taught us to define health as the absence of illness. We may respond to the question "Are you healthy?" by thinking, *I'm not sick, so I must be healthy.* Yet the words *health, heal,* and *holy,* are all derived from the same Anglo-Saxon word, *haelen,* which means, **to make whole.** Viewed from this perspective, two questions that more directly and accurately address the issue of health are "Do you love your life?" or "Are you happy to be alive?" For health is far more than simply a matter of not feeling ill: It is the daily experience of *wholeness and balance—a state of being fully alive in body, mind, and spirit.* Such a condition could also be called optimal, or holistic health, or wellness. I like to call it *thriving.* Whatever term you choose, helping you to achieve this state of total well-being is the primary objective of this book (along with improving your sinus condition), as well as the essence of the practice of holistic medicine.

"Holistic medicine is the art and science of healing that addresses the whole person—body, mind, and spirit. The practice of holistic medicine integrates conventional and alternative therapies to prevent and treat disease, and, most importantly, to promote optimal health."

Definition of holistic medicine, established by the American Holistic Medical Association.

HALLMARKS OF OPTIMAL HEALTH

Optimal health results from harmony and balance in the physical, environmental, mental, emotional, spiritual, and social aspects of our lives. When this harmonious balance is present, we experience the *unlimited and unimpeded free flow of life force energy throughout our body, mind, and spirit.* Around the world, this energy is known by many names. The Chinese call it *qi* ("chee"), the Japanese refer to it as *ki,* in India it is known as *prana,* and in Hebrew it is *chai.* But in the western world, the phrase that comes closest to capturing the feeling generated by this energy is *unconditional love,* regarded by holistic physicians as *our most powerful medicine.*

Though each of us has the capacity to nurture and to heal ourselves, most of us have yet to tap into this wellspring of loving life energy. Yet, there is no one who can better administer this life-enhancing elixir to you than yourself. As you uncover the root causes (other than genetics) of your chronic dis-ease—sinusitis, allergies, or any other condition—you will be directed by your illness in the art of self-care. The improvement with each of your symptoms will give you the necessary feedback to know if you're on the right track. By committing to caring for yourself in the manner recommended in chapters 6, 7, and 8, you will in essence be learning how to better *give and receive love*—to yourself and others. As a result, you will be enhancing the flow of life force energy throughout every aspect of your life. This holistic healing process will also provide you with the opportunity to safely and effectively treat any physical, mental, or spiritual conditions that may be restricting the flow of life force energy, i.e., love.

Living a holistically healthy lifestyle can facilitate the realization of your ideal life vision in accordance with both your personal and professional goals. But since the majority of us are only aware of health as a condition of not being sick, a mental image of what living holistically means is usually needed in order to achieve it. Briefly, let's examine this state of optimal well-being to give you a glimpse of what it looks and feels like.

A list of the six components of health follows; the first italicized item in each category encompasses the essence of that component. For example, physical health can be simply described as a condition of *high energy and vitality,* while mental health is a state of *peace of mind and contentment.* The italicized items can also serve as a health gauge you can use to measure your progress in each area.

PHYSICAL HEALTH
High energy and vitality
Freedom from, or high adaptability to, pain, dysfunction, and disability
A strong immune system
A body that feels light, balanced, strong, flexible, and has good aerobic capacity
Ability to meet physical challenges
Full capacity of all five senses and a healthy libido

ENVIRONMENTAL HEALTH
Harmony with your environment (neither harming nor being harmed)
Awareness of your connectedness with nature
Feeling grounded
Respect and appreciation for your home, the Earth, and all of her inhabitants
Contact with the Earth; breathing healthy air; drinking pure water; eating uncontaminated food; exposure to the sun, fire, or candlelight; immersion in warm water (all on a daily basis)

MENTAL HEALTH
Peace of mind and contentment
- A job that you love doing
- Optimism
- A sense of humor
- Financial well-being
- Living your life vision
- The ability to express your creativity and talents
- The capacity to make healthy decisions

EMOTIONAL HEALTH
Self-acceptance and high self-esteem
- Capacity to identify, express, experience, and accept all of your feelings, both painful and joyful
- Awareness of the intimate connection between your physical and emotional bodies
- The ability to confront your greatest fears
- The fulfillment of your capacity to play
- Peak experiences on a regular basis

SPIRITUAL HEALTH
Experience of unconditional love/absence of fear
- Soul awareness and a personal relationship with God or Spirit
- Trust in your intuition and a willingness to change
- Gratitude
- Creating a sacred space on a regular basis through prayer, meditation, walking in nature, observing a Sabbath day, or other rituals
- Sense of purpose
- Being present in every moment

SOCIAL HEALTH
Intimacy with a spouse, partner, relative, or close friend
- Effective communication
- Forgiveness
- Sense of belonging to a support group or community
- Touch and/or physical intimacy on a daily basis
- Selflessness and altruism

The Wellness Self-Test

Now that you understand the six categories that comprise optimal health, it's time to measure how close you are to *thriving* in each area. The following questionnaire is designed to provide you with a much clearer idea of the status of your health in all six areas. You can use the results of the test to guide you through this book (chapters 6 through 9), and it can become a blueprint for restructuring your life. You can also measure your progress by taking the test again every two or three months.

Answer the questions in each section and total your score. Each response will be a number from 0 to 5. Please refer to the frequency described within the parentheses (e.g., "2 to 3 times/week") when answering questions about an activity, for example, "Do you maintain a healthy diet?" However, when the question refers to an *attitude* or an *emotion* (most of the mind and spirit questions), for example, "Do you have a sense of humor?" the response is more subjective, less exact, and refers to the terms describing frequency, such as *often* or *daily,* but not to the numbered frequencies in parentheses.

0 = Never or almost never (once a year or less)
1 = Seldom (2 to 12 times/year)
2 = Occasionally (2 to 4 times/month)
3 = Often (2 to 3 times/week)
4 = Regularly (4 to 6 times/week)
5 = Daily (every day)

BODY: PHYSICAL AND ENVIRONMENTAL HEALTH

_____ 1. Do you maintain a healthy diet (very low in fat, sugar, caffeine, and alcohol; high in organic fruits and vegetables, whole grains, and protein)?

_____ 2. Is your water intake adequate (at least one-half ounce per pound of body weight; 160 lbs. = 80 ounces)?

_____ 3. Are you within 20 percent of your ideal body weight?

_____ 4. Do you feel physically attractive?

_____ 5. Do you fall asleep easily and sleep soundly?

_____ 6. Do you awaken in the morning feeling well rested?

_____ 7. Do you have more than enough energy to meet your daily responsibilities?

_____ 8. Are your five senses acute?

_____ 9. Do you take time to experience sensual pleasure?

_____ 10. Do you schedule regular massage or deep-tissue body work?

_____ 11. Does your sexual relationship feel gratifying?

_____ 12. Do you engage in regular physical workouts (lasting at least 20 minutes)?

_____ 13. Do you have good endurance or aerobic capacity?

_____ 14. Do you breathe abdominally for at least a few minutes?

_____ 15. Do you maintain physically challenging goals?

_____ 16. Are you physically strong?

_____ 17. Do you do some stretching exercises?

_____ 18. Are you free of chronic aches, pains, ailments, and diseases?

_____ 19. Do you have regular effortless bowel movements?

_____ 20. Do you understand the causes of your chronic physical problems?

_____ 21. Are you free of any drug (including caffeine and nicotine) or alcohol dependency?

_____ 22. Do you live and work in a healthy environment with respect to clean air, water, and indoor pollution?

_____ 23. Do you feel energized or empowered by nature?

_____ 24. Do you feel a strong connection with and appreciation for your body, your home, and your environment?

_____ 25. Do you have an awareness of life force energy or *qi*?

TOTAL BODY SCORE: _____

MIND: MENTAL AND EMOTIONAL HEALTH

_____ 1. Do you have specific goals in your personal and professional life?

_____ 2. Do you have the ability to concentrate for extended periods of time?

_____ 3. Do you use visualization or mental imagery to help you attain your goals or enhance your performance?

_____ 4. Do you believe it is possible to change?

_____ 5. Can you meet your financial needs and desires?

_____ 6. Is your outlook basically optimistic?

_____ 7. Do you give yourself more supportive messages than critical messages?

_____ 8. Does your job utilize all of your greatest talents?

_____ 9. Is your job enjoyable and fulfilling?

_____ 10. Are you willing to take risks or make mistakes in order to succeed?

_____ 11. Are you able to adjust beliefs and attitudes as a result of learning from painful experiences?

_____ 12. Do you have a sense of humor?

_____ 13. Do you maintain peace of mind and tranquillity?

_____ 14. Are you free from a strong need for control or the need to be right?

_____ 15. Are you able to fully experience (feel) your painful feelings such as fear, anger, sadness, and hopelessness?

_____ 16. Are you aware of and able to safely express fear?

_____ 17. Are you aware of and able to safely express anger?

_____ 18. Are you aware of and able to safely express sadness or cry?

_____ 19. Are you accepting of all your feelings?

_____ 20. Do you engage in meditation, contemplation, or psychotherapy to better understand your feelings?

_____ 21. Is your sleep free from disturbing dreams?

_____ 22. Do you explore the symbolism and emotional content of your dreams?

_____ 23. Do you take the time to let down and relax, or make time for activities that constitute the abandon or absorption of play?

_____ 24. Do you experience feelings of exhilaration?

_____ 25. Do you enjoy high self-esteem?

TOTAL MIND SCORE: _____

SPIRIT: SPIRITUAL AND SOCIAL HEALTH

_____ 1. Do you actively commit time to your spiritual life?

_____ 2. Do you take time for prayer, meditation, or reflection?

_____ 3. Do you listen to and act upon your intuition?

_____ 4. Are creative activities a part of your work or leisure time?

_____ 5. Do you take risks or exceed previous limits?

_____ 6. Do you have faith in a God, spirit guides, or angels?

_____ 7. Are you free from anger toward God?

_____ 8. Are you grateful for the blessings in your life?

_____ 9. Do you take walks, garden, or have contact with nature?

_____ 10. Are you able to let go of your attachment to specific outcomes and embrace uncertainty?

_____ 11. Do you observe a day of rest completely away from work, dedicated to nurturing yourself and your family?

_____ 12. Can you let go of self-interest in deciding the best course of action for a given situation?

_____ 13. Do you feel a sense of purpose?

_____ 14. Do you make time to connect with young children, either your own or someone else's?

_____ 15. Are playfulness and humor important to you in your daily life?

_____ 16. Do you have the ability to forgive yourself and others?

_____ 17. Have you demonstrated the willingness to commit to a marriage or comparable long-term relationship?

_____ 18. Do you experience intimacy, besides sex, in your committed relationships?

_____ 19. Do you confide in or speak openly with one or more close friends?

_____ 20. Do you or did you feel close to your parents?

_____ 21. Do you feel close to your children?

_____ 22. If you have experienced the loss of a loved one, have you fully grieved that loss?

_____ 23. Has your experience of pain enabled you to grow spiritually?

_____ 24. Do you go out of your way or give your time to help others?

_____ 25. Do you feel a sense of belonging to a group or community?

_____ 26. Do you experience unconditional love?

TOTAL SPIRIT SCORE: _____

TOTAL BODY, MIND, SPIRIT SCORE: _____

HEALTH SCALE:

325–375	Optimal Health: **THRIVING**
275–324	Excellent Health
225–274	Good Health
175–224	Fair Health
125–174	Below Average Health
75–124	Poor Health
Less than 75	Extremely Unhealthy: **SURVIVING**

Once you have completed this questionnaire, pay attention to which categories you need to make the most improvements in, and start to implement the tools and suggestions that are outlined in chapters 6, 7, and 8. Chapter 6 gives you a blueprint for improving your overall physical and environmental health with a specific focus on healing your mucous membranes and strengthening your immune system. Chapter 7 outlines a holistic approach for mental and emotional health, while Chapter 8 will help you enhance your spiritual and social health. Begin where you are most comfortable and take your time. You are committing to a life-changing process, one that requires patience and discipline, so proceed at your own pace. Remember, too, that everyone is unique and no two of us will follow the exact same healing path. While the Sinus Survival Program and the science of holistic medicine provides a universal foundation and structure, its art lies in the writing of your own personal prescription for optimal health, so feel free to adapt the techniques in those chapters to tailor-make the holistic self-care program that is most ideally suited for you. While practicing these healthy options you will become more aware of what feels good and what doesn't, and you will learn to make choices that are life-enhancing. You are, in essence, learning to love yourself in body, mind, and spirit, and in so doing you will be better able to give and receive love from others. This Program is based upon the belief that *unconditional love is life's most healing medicine.* Your heart will be your primary guide on this odyssey of realizing your full potential as a human being.

Chapter 3

WHAT ARE SINUSES AND WHY ARE THEY SICK?

Most people probably assume that the word *sinus* means "nose." They would be close, both anatomically and physiologically, but although the nose and sinuses are connected, they are separate parts of the body. The sinuses are air-filled cavities located behind and around the nose and eyes. In anatomy texts they are called air sinuses or paranasal sinuses. There are usually four sets, roughly divided in half for each side of the head. The halves can be asymmetrical in size and shape.

The sinuses are identified as frontal, maxillary, sphenoid, and ethmoid (Fig. 3.1). The frontal sinuses lie above the eyes, just above the nose and behind the forehead. The maxillaries, the largest of the sinuses, are pyramid-shaped cavities located inside each cheekbone. The ethmoids, multicompartmental sinuses behind the maxillaries and between the bony orbits of the eyes, are complex labyrinths of small air pockets. The sphenoids are situated deep in the skull behind the nose, slightly below the ethmoids. The ethmoidal, sphenoidal, and maxillary sinuses are all present at birth, although the latter do not reach full development until a person is sixteen to twenty-one years of age. The frontal sinuses are not present until the age of eight.

To make mucus drainage and air exchange possible, each sinus is connected to the nasal passage by a thin duct about the size of pencil lead. The openings of the ducts are called ostia,

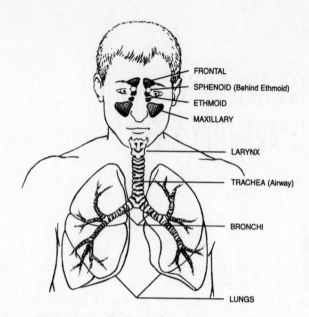

FIGURE 3.1. *Sinuses and respiratory tract.*

and they average about two millimeters in diameter. The ducts of the maxillaries are located at the top of the sinus, making drainage difficult and blockage easy. A series of small ducts in the nasal wall drain the ethmoid sinuses; these openings are also easily blocked. Although most of the human body seems to have been created perfectly, the maxillary sinuses are a distinct exception. They appear to be better suited to four-legged animals, particularly with regard to the position of the ostia. As upright posture evolved, ease of sinus drainage diminished.

The outer-most lining of the entire respiratory tract (Fig. 3.1) is one continuous tissue, called the *respiratory epithelium,* that extends from just inside the nostrils to the alveolar sacs in the lungs. The outer layer of this tissue is called the mucous membrane or mucosa. Like an extension of the skin covering the external surface of your entire body, this membrane is a connected porous protective shield for the air portal of your body. It serves as your first line of defense against bacteria, viruses, pollen, animal dan-

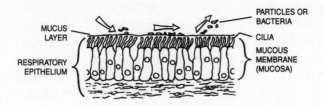

FIGURE 3.2. *The sinus lining, healthy.*

der, cigarette smoke, dust, chemicals, automobile exhaust, and any other potentially harmful air pollutants. With a protective capability and breathability far beyond that of Gore-Tex or any similar high-tech material, this membrane also has the job of humidifying dry air and warming cold or cooling hot air. The bulk of the job of filtering, humidifying, and regulating temperature occurs in the nose and sinuses—the entrance and vestibule of the respiratory tract. If the mucous membrane breaks down, the immediate consequence might be a cold or sinus infection. Since the lungs are the site of oxygen/carbon dioxide exchange, they need the protection provided by the nose and sinuses to do their best in carrying out this vital life-giving function. Unfortunately, the frontline nose/sinus defense is losing the battle to the massive assault by a barrage of air pollutants.

Since this is a continuous mucous membrane lining the sinuses, ducts, and nasal passages, anything that causes a swelling in the nose can similarly affect the sinuses. On the surface of this membrane are cilia, microscopic hairlike filaments that maintain a constant sweeping motion to remove the watery discharge called mucus (Fig. 3.2). The mucous membrane and its cilia provide a good defensive mechanism against infections. The entire mucus covering of the maxillary sinus, for example, is normally cleared every ten minutes. The mucous membrane lining the entire respiratory tract produces between a pint and a quart of mucus daily. The mucus traps particles that enter the nasal passage, and the cilia sweep them toward the back of the nose, after which they are swallowed and broken down by stomach acids.

No one has definitively established the exact function of the sinuses, although there is agreement that they lighten the weight of the skull. By virtue of the sinuses' location and structure and the microanatomy and function of the mucous membrane, most physiologists would agree with the following conclusions.

The sinuses, along with the nose, as the upper part of the respiratory tract, serve as the body's chief protector of the lungs. They do this by acting as a *filter,* defending against bacteria and viruses, dirt and dust particles, pollen, and anything airborne that would harm the lungs; as a *humidifier,* by moistening dry air that would irritate the lungs; and as a *temperature regulator,* by cooling excessively hot air and warming extremely cold air that would shock the lungs. Humans inhale about 23,000 times a day, moving the equivalent of about two gallons of air per minute—almost 3,000 gallons per day or one pint of air per breath. The nose and sinuses are always at work, shielding the lungs from harm. Our lungs are the vehicle through which our bodies obtain oxygen, which is vital to life itself.

The sinuses are the lungs' leading defenders against injury and illness, but their importance has been neglected by both doctors and patients. Think about a quarterback on the football field whose offensive line is weak and beginning to break down. He might not be killed, literally, but what about his health and his ability to perform optimally? Our nose and sinuses are being assaulted and are beginning to deteriorate. The condition of our lungs is already being affected, and ultimately the health of our bodies is at stake. A primary objective of the Sinus Survival Program is to heal the mucous membrane lining our entire respiratory tract. This is the key to curing chronic sinusitis and allergies, preventing colds, and providing a strong foundation for optimal health.

THE PREVALENCE AND CAUSES OF SINUS DISEASE AND ALLERGIES

Today and since 1981, sinusitis has been the most common chronic condition in the United States. According to the most recent survey from the National Center for Health Statistics, about 40 million Americans suffer from this ailment. It was the primary reason for 11.9 million physician office visits in 1995. Allergies or hay fever, medically known as allergic rhinitis, is ranked fourth with 27 million people afflicted. If we add asthma and bronchitis, ranked eighth and ninth, we currently have over 90 million people, about one out of every three, suffering with a chronic respiratory condition. Unfortunately, this dismal statistic is similar to most other developed countries throughout the world. Respiratory disease has become our planet's first environmental epidemic. The plague of air pollution may have already begun to destroy our species.

Since the nose and sinuses are the body's primary air filter and are positioned at the entryway to the respiratory tract, they have been most adversely affected by unhealthy air. Breathing pollutant-laden air can be a chronic irritant that can create hypersensitive mucous membranes and predispose one to develop nasal allergies. It is estimated that allergies are a primary cause of chronic sinusitis in about one-half of the sinus sufferers, especially children. The remainder of this chapter will focus on the factors that trigger sinus infections. In addition to air pollution (both indoor and outdoor) and allergies, these are: the common cold, cigarettes and other sources of smoke, dry air, cold air, fumes, occupational hazards, dental problems, immunodeficiency, malformations, and emotional stress. These factors have the potential to adversely affect even the healthiest sinus. However, a person who has had previous sinus infections, or whose sinuses (mucous membranes) have been weakened for any of the aforementioned reasons, is at especially high risk for developing further infection. The disease-fighting white blood cells, the body's immune response to infection, can themselves damage the mucous membrane lining the sinus cavity as they kill the bacteria causing the sinus infection.

THE COMMON COLD

The story of what has become a lifetime of sinus problems usually begins with the common cold. Normally air and mucus flow freely through the ducts connecting the nose and sinuses. Trouble starts when the system becomes obstructed, often by a cold. The nasal mucous membrane becomes inflamed and swollen and the cold virus inactivates the cilia of the nasal membrane, causing the mucus in the nose to stagnate rather than flow (Fig. 3.3). As a result, the mucus being produced in the sinuses cannot drain properly, and the sinuses become a breeding ground for bacteria. This pooling of stagnant mucus can easily result in a sinus infection, especially in individuals who have had previous infections.

Through the early and mid-1970s, I treated many patients who had nothing more than a bad cold. By the late seventies, and certainly by the early eighties, patients with the common cold became less frequent visitors to my office. They were being replaced by patients who greeted me with complaints such as "Doctor, I've had this cold for the past two weeks now" (or three weeks, or several months, or in a few cases a year or more). These people almost always had sinusitis, and not until they had completed a course of antibiotics were they able to rid themselves of their "colds." It also became quite apparent that those who had never before had a sinus infection were now frequently returning with the same problem.

In 1993, Jack Gwaltney, M.D., at the University of Virginia at Charlottesville, performed a landmark study. He studied col-

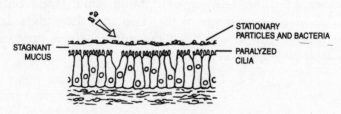

FIGURE 3.3. *The sinus lining, sinusitis.*

lege students and employees who thought they had the common cold. Following CT or "cat" scans, the most definitive diagnostic test to evaluate sinuses, 87 percent of these people were found to have sinus infections. What I began observing in my family practice almost twenty years ago had now been scientifically documented: The vast majority of people who think they have a simple cold actually have a sinus infection, called acute sinusitis, as an integral part of the cold. After a first bout with sinusitis, the mucous membrane, especially its cilia, is left in a somewhat damaged and weakened state. For many, the membrane never completely recovers, especially in an environment that is harsh on the sinuses. What I was seeing, increasingly, was that one or two "bad colds" could result in a permanently weak sinus. This impaired sinus then becomes much more susceptible to additional infections, whether from a cold or any of the other risk factors that follow.

CIGARETTES AND OTHER SOURCES OF SMOKE

Whenever a patient with a sinus infection returned to my office after completing a two-week, or longer, course of antibiotics and complained, "Doctor, I'm not any better," my first response was always a question: "Have you been smoking?" The patient often answered yes. It is extremely difficult to have healthy sinuses if you smoke cigarettes. Nicotine paralyzes the cilia. I would be hard-pressed to name anything more harmful to the body's air filter than smoke of any kind. Cigarette smoke is most often involved, but cigar, pipe, campfire, and cooking smoke are also frequent villains. Marijuana and cocaine (whether smoked or snorted) are also quite harmful to the nasal mucous membrane.

If you are curious about what smoke does to the sinuses, take a look at the accumulation of tar and smoke particles that discolor a used cigarette filter, turning it brown or black. This will give you some idea of what is happening not only to the sinuses but also to the lungs. At the tissue level, smoke causes irritation of the mucous membrane. The weaker the sinus, usually one that has been infected previously, the greater the level of irritation. The greater the irritation, the more inflamed the mucous membrane becomes. Inflammation of the mucous membrane results in swelling, increased mucus secretion, and damage to the cilia. This swelling may obstruct the sinuses, producing a condition very similar to that created by the common cold.

When fluids or secretions are unable to drain normally, the potential for infection is high. This principle holds true for almost any part of the human body, whether it is the bladder, bowel, lung, kidney, or middle-ear space. The theory that smoking can cause sinus infections has not yet been proven. It is currently beyond the scope of science to observe what is happening to the mucous membrane in someone's sinus as it is being suffocated with smoke. However, as with the speculation on the function of the sinuses, this theory, too, has strong support among most physicians.

Those of you who are sinus sufferers but do not smoke are not necessarily immune to the problems caused by cigarette and other types of smoke. Studies have shown that nonsmokers who live or work with smokers are also adversely affected. Laws that prohibit cigarette smoking in public places are helping, but we have a long way to go.

In 1992 a Harvard research team reported the first direct medical evidence that secondhand smoke can damage the lungs of nonsmokers. The study reported that secondhand smoke:

- Kills at least 4,000 people annually from lung cancer
- Increases the risk of respiratory infections in children
- Aggravates the symptoms of asthma in children

The American Heart Association estimates that, in addition to its effects on lungs, secondhand smoke could be a contributing factor in the heart-disease deaths of 40,000 nonsmoking Americans every year. The association also estimates that 50 million nonsmoking adults over the age of thirty-five are exposed to secondhand smoke and about 50 percent of all American children live in families with one or more smokers.

As yet, there is no direct scientific data on what secondhand smoke is doing to our nose and sinuses. But with this recent evidence documenting its devastating effects on our lungs and hearts, it's obviously not too speculative to assume that secondhand smoke is also causing significant damage to the body's air filter.

AIR POLLUTION: OUTDOOR

I was struck by a comment made many years ago by one of the *Apollo* astronauts. He said that the most disturbing part of his flight was seeing a grayish haze over almost every land mass on earth. What was this ugly blanket covering our beautiful planet?

Having lived in Denver since 1972, I had a good clue. The Mile-High City, one of this country's most polluted metropolitan areas, is often covered by a thick, brownish-gray pall of smog, known locally as the brown cloud. Most cities in the world are similarly afflicted, but especially those situated in valleys where temperature inversions are frequent; in cities where diesel fuel is used extensively, especially in Europe; in heavily industrialized regions; and in most areas where there are coal-fired power plants. Almost every country in the world is now familiar with this rapidly growing dilemma; it has reached such immense proportions that it is visible from space. The question is, What is this filthy air doing to the human beings who created the problem?

In Denver the incidence of acute sinusitis has risen dramatically since the early 1970s. From 1981 it was consistently the most common illness in my medical practice. Air pollution is most acute from mid-November to mid-January, when temperature inversions—warm air aloft trapping cold air and pollutants near the ground—are most common. This also happens to be the time of year when Denver's doctors see the greatest number of patients with sinus infections. Many people who work in the center of the city or in other highly polluted areas are aware of the connection between their sinus congestion and sinus headaches on days with particularly bad air quality.

There is scientific evidence to implicate carbon monoxide as the most dangerous element of air pollution. Why? Because, in high enough concentrations, it is capable of killing people with weak hearts and lungs. It is also the component of air pollution most often measured, and we know that about 25 percent of it comes from vehicle emissions. It is therefore not surprising that Los Angeles is the metropolitan area with the highest levels of carbon monoxide. But carbon monoxide is an odorless and colorless gas. What is that stuff that we can see—the brown cloud—and what is it doing to our sinuses when we breathe it?

Visible pollution consists primarily of the following elements: particulates, oxides of sulfur, oxides of nitrogen, hydrocarbons, and ozone. *Particulates* are tiny particles of dust, sand, cinders, soot, smoke, and liquid droplets found in the atmosphere. They come from a variety of sources, including roads, farm fields, construction sites, factories, power plants, fireplaces, wood-burning stoves, windblown dust, and diesel and car exhaust. When inhaled, larger particles (those greater than 10 microns in diameter; a human hair is about 75 microns in diameter) are known to lodge in the nose and sinuses. After all, what is a filter for? While the large particles seem to have the greatest adverse impact on the nose and sinuses, those smaller than 10 microns are doing the most damage to the lungs.

In 1993, calculations derived from studies at the Environmental Protection Agency and the Harvard School of Public Health estimated that 50,000 to 60,000 deaths a year are caused by particulate pollution. This number far surpasses that of any other pollutant and is one that rivals the death toll from some cancers. The most harmful particles are small—less than 10 microns in diameter—and are produced chiefly from industrial plants and to a lesser extent from the exhaust of diesel vehicles.

The federal government's current standard for these small particulates, called PM-10, doesn't consider air hazardous until it reaches 150 micrograms of these particles per cubic meter.

Yet, a study conducted in the Utah Valley found that hospital admissions for respiratory-related illnesses such as pneumonia and asthma jumped 50 to 90 percent during the times particulate pollution was above only 50 micrograms of breathable particles for each cubic meter of air.

Although our nation spends about $35 billion a year on scrubbers, catalytic converters, and other air-pollution control efforts, only one third of that money is aimed at removing particulates, and just a fraction of that goes toward the small PM-10 particles. Most regulatory efforts have been focused more on other types of pollutants, such as ozone and sulphur dioxide, that have been shown to damage health; it is uncertain whether they cause death. Aside from particulates, the EPA believes that, of all pollutants, indoor pollution, especially secondhand cigarette smoke, and radon cause the greatest health damage.

Scientists, unfortunately, are reluctant to establish conclusively a cause-and-effect relationship between particulates and respiratory disease until they have detailed biological studies of the effect of the PM–10 particles on the respiratory mucous membranes themselves. Particulates, with their adverse health effects, however, have been around for a long time. Such pollution has been recorded as early as the seventeenth century in England. Today the effects may be more subtle but just as devastating. Deaths from particulates occur primarily among children with respiratory problems (mostly asthma), people of all ages with asthma, and the elderly with illnesses such as bronchitis, emphysema, and pneumonia. A comment from C. Arden Pope, Ph.D., one of the researchers in the Harvard particulate study (officially called the "Harvard Six Cities Study"), was most revealing. He said, "People who live in highly polluted cities die earlier. It's just that simple."

One of the largest studies of air quality and health ever carried out was published in the March 1995 issue of the *American Journal of Respiratory and Critical Care Medicine*. Performed by researchers from the Harvard School of Public Health and Brigham Young University, the study tracked the health records of 552,138 people in 151 cities between 1982 and 1989. The findings showed that fine particles, smaller than 2.5 microns, can increase the risk of death by 15 percent in cities with the dirtiest air, compared with the cleanest cities. This study bolsters the earlier Harvard study that showed particulates are costing tens of thousands of lives each year in the United States.

The act of breathing in those cities highest in particulates, such as Riverside and San Bernardino in the LA basin, might be comparable to rubbing a piece of very fine sandpaper (particles larger than 10 microns constitute a coarser piece) against the delicate and sensitive mucous membranes of the entire respiratory tract, 23,000 times a day, day in and day out. The larger particulates, not usually measured by the EPA, take more of a toll on the "gatekeeper filter"—the nose and sinuses—while the smaller ones, less than 2.5 microns, are most devastating to the lungs.

Oxides of sulfur, especially *sulfur dioxide* (a colorless gas with a rotten-egg odor), are typically transformed into smaller, finer particulates, less than ten microns in diameter. Emitted mainly by coal- and oil-fired power plants, refineries, pulp and paper mills, and nonferrous smelters, they are a major contributor to acid rain, and are also filtered through the sinuses. Unfortunately there is a price to be paid for protecting the lungs from this toxic substance. Sulfur oxide particles easily penetrate the mucosal lining. Studies have shown that they have an intensely irritating effect on the bronchial mucosa, resulting in damage to the cilia and initiation of bronchitis. If sulfur oxides can cause bronchitis in the lungs, would it be a far-fetched assumption that they can also cause sinusitis? Cities with high levels of sulfur dioxide include: Steubenville, Ohio; Weirton, West Virginia; Pittsburgh, Pennsylvania; and Billings, Montana.

Nitrogen oxides are the most obvious components of smog, providing color to the noxious cloud of air pollution. Their principal constituent is *nitrogen dioxide,* a yellowish-brown, highly reactive gas. Nitrogen oxides form when fuel is burned at high temperatures. The two major emission sources are internal combustion engines—motor vehicles and aircraft—and stationary fuel combustion sources such as electric utilities and industrial boilers. Like sulfur oxides, nitrogen oxides can irritate the lungs, causing ciliary paralysis, bronchitis, and pneumonia. They are also capable of impairing the body's immune defenses against bacterial and viral infection. Los Angeles has, by far, the highest nitrogen dioxide levels of any American city.

Hydrocarbons are evaporated or incompletely burned organic compounds. The largest sources of hydrocarbons in the atmosphere include internal combustion engines; certain industrial processes, such as coke ovens in steel mills; and evaporation of liquids, such as gasoline in fuel transfers, and industrial and household solvents. Hydrocarbons are known to be highly irritating to the mucous membrane.

Prior to the recent findings about particulates, *ozone* was believed to be the most dangerous component of smog. It is produced when sunlight acts upon nitrogen oxides and hydrocarbons. The many sources of both of these substances have already been mentioned. Ozone in the lower, breathable part of the atmosphere (within 1,000 feet of the earth's surface) is harmful to human and animal health, crops, and forests. In the upper atmosphere, ozone is beneficial, absorbing the harmful rays (ultraviolet-B) of sunlight. The continuing depletion of the upper ozone layer has become a serious health concern. Unfortunately, harmful ozone in the lower air does not move up to replenish the deteriorating ozone layer in the higher reaches of our atmosphere.

Ozone in the lower atmosphere is one of our greatest environmental challenges. Few, if any, urban areas are free of it. Four broad geographic regions are seriously affected: southern California (by far the worst), the Northeast especially the New York City area), the Texas Gulf Coast (Houston), and the Chicago–Milwaukee area.

A growing body of scientific data indicates that ozone is a significant risk to human health, affecting not only those with impaired respiratory systems, such as asthmatics, but many with healthy lungs, both children and adults. Ozone can cause shortness of breath and coughing during exercise in healthy adults and more serious effects in the young, old, and infirm. Almost all of the research on ozone's effects has been done on lungs. There has not been any direct research on ozone and the sinuses. At the Air Pollution Health Effects Laboratory at the University of California, Irvine, however, its effects on the nasal cavities of rats have been studied. The findings lend substantial support to the connection between ozone and sinus disease. The researchers found significant damage to the mucous membrane surrounding the opening to the maxillary sinuses as a result of inhaling ozone. This could easily lead to the obstruction of the sinuses and subsequent infection. Robert Phalen, Ph.D., director of the laboratory, has also affirmed that "exposure to particulate pollution over a lifetime can be associated with increased infection and more exposure to diseases."

(Although not a part of the respiratory tract, the exposed surface of our eyes is covered by another mucous membrane called the conjunctiva. Eye irritation, burning, and tearing resulting from air pollution afflicts millions of people. Widely observed by eye doctors in the Los Angeles area, these symptoms are directly attributed to ozone. Although probably not quite as severe, particulates and the other pollutants can also cause similar symptoms. Dry air in combination with pollution can aggravate this condition even more.)

In 1997 the EPA adopted tough new clean-air standards for ozone, which will not be enforced until 2004. In preliminary tests performed in May 1998, thirty states failed to meet these new limits for ozone. These findings were particularly disturbing since they occurred two months before the peak summer smog season. By late 1998 the EPA reported significant decreases in emissions from 1970 to 1997 of every major pollutant except nitrogen oxides, the principal contributor to ozone.

Nowhere in the United States is the problem of air pollution more acute than in Los Angeles. A study on a group of that city's ten- and eleven-year-olds revealed that their lung capacity is already diminished by 17 percent compared to the normal range for that age. A pathologist at the University of Southern California, in performing autopsies on Los Angeles children killed accidentally, has found a disturbing frequency of emphysematous changes previously seen only in adult lungs. And the respiratory tract is not the only part of the body affected. The EPA announced on March 1, 1999, the results of a study that warns of the "carcinogenic dangers of breathing." The study found that the risk of cancer in Los Angeles is 426 times higher than the most basic standards established by the 1990 Clean Air Act.

But Los Angeles is not unique. Other areas of the country are well on their way to matching that city's severity of pollution and its damaging effects on the lungs, sinuses, and the rest of the body. There are also many agricultural communities that claim to be sinus "capitals" as a result of the pesticides and fertilizers that fill the air. I've heard from people in South Dakota, southern Minnesota, Iowa, North Carolina, and California's San Joaquin Valley, all reporting that "everyone has sinus problems." The residents of Dayton, Ohio, refer to their city as "Sinus Valley."

Most physicians would probably rate air pollution as the primary cause of the dramatic increase in the incidence of asthma, emphysema, chronic bronchitis (all have increased by 50 percent since 1981), and lung cancer. Americans are certainly not alone in suffering with this plague of pollution. According to the World Health Organization, residents of New Delhi, India; Seoul, Korea; Manila, Philippines; and Mexico City breathe far worse air than that in Los Angeles. The air quality in many cities in China and in eastern Europe is atrocious. Dying forests across Central Europe are a testament to the air pollution of that heavily industrialized continent. Huge demonstrations demanding a cleanup of air pollution have been reported in many cities throughout the countries that formerly made up the Soviet Union.

There are solutions, of course, but most entail a change in lifestyle. In 1950 there were 50 million cars worldwide, 75 percent of them in the United States. This number doubled by 1960, redoubled by 1970, and doubled again by 1990—an eightfold increase to 400 million cars. American drivers now own only one third of the world's total, but half of us have two cars in our garages. We have created a monster and it is killing us and the planet we live on. Automobiles, trucks, and buses are the chief sources of our air pollution. And as we enter the new millennium we are confronted with a new challenge. By 1998, sales of sport utility vehicles (SUVs) exceeded those of passenger cars. The problem with SUVs is that they can legally emit *twice* the pollution of cars. The EPA has responded to the SUV pollution problem by proposing that SUVs be held to the same emissions-control standards as cars. This proposal was officially endorsed by President Clinton in December 1999 and will begin in 2004.

The availability and use of alternative fuels—ethanol, methanol, hydrogen, solar, and natural gas—or the electric car would also make a profound difference. These fuels are domestic, cheaper, and more plentiful than gasoline. One sign of progress will be the EPA's new standards for gasoline, which will reduce sulfur levels by 90 percent. Sulfur emissions damage vehicles' air pollution-control systems—known as catalytic converters—diminishing their ability to reduce carbon monoxide, hydrocarbons, and nitrogen oxides released into the air. This new standard for cleaner gasoline will be in effect by 2004. Greater enforcement of engine emission tests, development of mass transit systems, participation in carpooling, and construction of bicycle paths—along with the conversion of power plants from coal to natural gas, the development of solar energy, and a reduction in wood burning—would have an immediate impact on cleaning our air.

Many of us are already suffering the ill effects of breathing unhealthy air. If the EPA is correct in concluding that air pollution is responsible for approximately 60,000 deaths a year, that would make it one of the leading causes of death in the United States. In a landmark eleven-year study completed in 1991 by the UCLA School of Medicine, it was proven that irreversible lung deterioration can result from chronic exposure to polluted air. According to the American Lung Association, annual medical costs associated with human exposure to all outdoor air pollutants from all sources range from $40 billion to $50 billion. If each of us will do at least one thing to decrease air pollution, collectively we can cure this plague of unhealthy air.

AIR POLLUTION: INDOOR

Unfortunately, we cannot escape dirty air by remaining indoors. In 1988 the EPA reported that indoor air can in some instances be as much as 100 times more polluted than outdoor air, noting that Americans spend 90 percent of their time indoors. All of the indoor air pollutants listed in Table 3.1 have been proven harmful to the respiratory tract. Some of these pollutants originate in outdoor air.

Sick-building syndrome is an unscientific term used to describe a pattern of disease symptoms linked to poor indoor air quality in workplaces, schools, homes, and other buildings. A sick building is one in which at least 20 percent of the occupants experience discomfort that is suspected to be caused by contaminated indoor air. It need not be proven. The World Health Organization estimates that 30 percent of new or remodeled commercial buildings generate unusually high health and comfort complaints, and could be considered "sick buildings." Nationwide, as many as 80 million buildings may be of this type. Nearly a fifth of the workforce in the United States has reported indoor air pollution ailments, ranging from headaches and fatigue to colds, influenza, and chronic respiratory illnesses (e.g., chronic sinusitis and chronic bronchitis). One million hospital visits a year are attributed to poor indoor air quality. According to John Sturdivant, president of the 700,000-member American Federation of Government Employees, "threats to health as a result of poor indoor air quality in the workplace have long been speculated. But as more and more of us experience sinus or nasal congestion, shortness of breath, and other symptoms, a pattern seems to be developing."

The EPA's own building in Washington, DC, ironically, serves as an excellent example of sick-building syndrome. Following renovations made to the building between 1987 and 1989, more than a thousand of the 5,500 employees at EPA headquarters complained of headaches, rashes, nausea, fatigue, blurred vision, chills, sneezing, fever, irritability, forgetfulness, hoarseness, dizziness, and burning sensations in their throats, ears, eyes, and chests. One employee commented, "I was afraid I was going to die in the place." Several of these symptoms can be attributed to sick sinuses and chronically inflamed respiratory tracts.

Table 3.1

Indoor Air Pollutants

Automotive Fumes
From outdoor traffic, outdoor parking lots, and outdoor loading and
    unloading spaces, as well as indoor garages

Chemicals and Chemical Solutions (Chemicals that affect indoor air
    quality are those associated with architecture, the interior,
    artifacts, and maintenance.)
Fungicides and pesticides in carpet-cleaning residues and sprays;
    formaldehyde, used in the manufacture of insulation, plywood,
    fiberboard, furniture, and wood paneling; toxic solvents in oil-
    based paints, finishes, and wall sealants; aerosol sprays; office
    equipment chemicals, especially photocopiers and computers

Combustion Products
Tobacco smoke★
Coal- or wood-burning fireplaces and stoves
Fuel combustion gases from gas-fired appliances such as ranges,
    clothes dryers, water heaters, and fireplaces (they produce nitro-
    gen dioxide, carbon monoxide, nitrous oxides, sulfur oxides, hy-
    drocarbons, and formaldehyde)

Ion Depletion or Imbalance
Too few negative ions
Excess of positive ions over negative ions

Microorganisms (primarily from humidifiers, air conditioners, and
  any other building components affected by excessive moisture)
Bacteria
Viruses
Molds
Dust mites (usually found in more humid areas)

Particulates
Dust
Pollen
Animal dander
Particles (frayed materials)
Asbestos

Radionuclides
Radon, a radioactive gas emitted from the earth that enters homes
  primarily through basements, crawl spaces, and water supply, especially from wells (it can attach to the particulates of cigarette
  smoke, dust particles, and natural aerosols)

★From all of the available scientific data, tobacco smoke is the most unhealthy
indoor air pollutant.

A major explanation for sick-building syndrome, experts say,
is the nationwide campaign, which emerged during the energy
crisis of the mid-1970s, to conserve energy by sealing and insu-
lating buildings. The tight, energy-efficient homes and buildings
that evolved have a relatively low energy demand but a correspondingly low ventilation rate. The demise of the operable-
window building and the replacement of natural ventilation
with mechanical ventilation have diminished the flow of fresh
air, trapping pollutants inside. Furthermore, the fresh air in most
cities is anything but fresh. There has also been an increase in the
use of energy efficient heating and air-conditioning systems,
which has often led to increased circulation of polluted indoor
air. Another factor in the deterioration of indoor air quality is
the type of materials used to construct and furnish buildings.
Building materials and furniture made of petrochemical-based
products and materials that can emit harmful chemical vapors

over long periods of time are used in place of nonpolluting natural materials and fibers.

A fascinating aspect of this problem was revealed when several sick buildings were tested for the amount and type of ions present in the air. Areas having a high rate of employee complaints were found to have one of two ion conditions: (1) an abnormally low level of negative ions, or (2) an excess of positive ions compared to negative ions. When a more natural level of negative ions was reestablished through the use of negative-ion generators, the high complaint rate decreased dramatically. In energy-efficient buildings the constant recirculating of room air leads to a depletion of beneficial negative ions and often an increase in detrimental positive ions. The EPA spent hundreds of thousands of dollars trying to solve the problem of its sick headquarters, but the symptoms continued. On December 23, 1993, in Superior Court in the District of Columbia, five EPA employees were awarded $950,000 for ailments they said were related to unhealthy indoor air. There is a great deal that can be done to improve indoor air quality. Chapter 6 will offer many suggestions.

DRY AIR

An important function of the sinuses is to humidify the air we breathe; a person with weak sinuses may therefore have a problem in especially dry air. Moist air, that between 40 and 60 percent humidity, is very helpful for the proper functioning of the mucous membrane, especially the cilia. Dry air is usually found in conjunction with:

- Arid or semiarid climate
- Forced-air heating systems (they not only dry, but give the sinuses more to filter, and also deplete the air of negative ions)
- Air-conditioning, especially in cars
- Oxygen therapy for various respiratory conditions
- Wind

- Mountains (the higher the elevation, the drier the air)
- Wood-burning stoves

Dry air is hard on sinuses, but excessively moist air can also cause problems. Many microorganisms, such as bacteria, viruses, and molds, thrive when the humidity exceeds 60 percent.

COLD AIR

Although the moisture content of cold air is generally much higher than that of dry air, the shock of cold temperatures to the mucous membrane of an impaired nose and sinus can cause significant irritation and ciliary injury, and often results in at least a runny nose. Many of us are familiar with the constant mucus drip associated with cold weather activities such as ice skating, skiing, and snowmobiling. If you have chronic sinusitis or another respiratory condition, it is wise to take some precautions to protect your mucous membranes from cold air. In the early 1990s it was reported that many members of the Swedish cross-country ski team developed adult-onset asthma due to their strenuous exercise in cold, dry air. The least stressful air temperatures on the respiratory tract are between 65° and 85°F.

Air-conditioning, which creates negative-ion depletion, has also recently been shown to be a respiratory health hazard. In 1997, researchers from France found that workers in air-conditioned environments are twice as likely to have respiratory problems than people who work outside or indoors without air-conditioning. Among the conditions reportedly caused by the cooled circulated air are asthma, colds, runny noses, sore throats, and tightness in the chest. Dr. Dan Teculescu, a member of the European Respiratory Society, revealed the results of his study of office workers in Britain, Italy, and Scandinavia. The research indicates that seven out of eight respiratory conditions are linked to air-conditioning, and that air circulated through air-conditioned environments "can carry airborne bacteria and fungi."

ALLERGIES

Those with asthma and *nasal allergies* or hay fever, are very susceptible to sinus infections. (About one half of the people with chronic sinusitis also suffer from allergies.) Their nasal and sinus mucosae are extremely sensitive and often hyperactive and potentially hypersecretory. When an allergic reaction to pollen or mold takes place, substances known as IgEs flood the nasal lining, along with eonsinophils (a type of white blood cell) and a tremendous release of inflammatory substances such as histamine, prostaglandins, and leukotrienes. This dramatic response results in the swelling of the mucosa and obstruction of the sinuses. Although the theory is untested, I strongly believe that chronic breathing of polluted air heightens the sensitivity of the nasal mucosa, creating an increasing number of new allergy sufferers and worsening the allergic condition of many others. As yet, I haven't heard any other scientific explanation for the significant increase over the past decade in the number of people with allergies.

Many people claim that they are "allergic" to cigarette smoke, or dust, or some other irritant in the air. Most of the time they are not really describing an allergy but rather a hypersensitivity caused by extreme irritation of the mucous membrane. This sensitivity causes a similar end result, nasal stuffiness and mucus drainage (and often a headache), but the process is a bit different. Actual nasal allergies are usually caused by airborne pollen from grass, trees, weeds, and flowers; molds; and dander from cats, dogs, horses, or other animals. In many areas of the United States, especially in parts of California and Florida where there is something pollinating year-round, allergies are the major contributors to sinus problems. Be aware, however, that if you are complaining of a year-round allergy problem, you may have chronic sinusitis.

In recent years an increasing number of physicians are recognizing that *food allergies* are also a factor in chronic sinusitis. The foods most often implicated are wheat, cow's milk and all other dairy products, chocolate, oranges, eggs, and artificial food coloring.

OCCUPATIONAL HAZARDS

A job performed in dirty, dry, and extremely hot or cold air should be considered a high risk to the sinuses. In recent years I have added high levels of positive ions as an additional risk factor. This applies especially to pilots and flight attendants, because of the high level of positive ions in aircraft cabin air, and to people who work in front of computer screens all day. In my experience, those at highest risk include:

- Auto mechanics
- Construction workers (especially carpenters, who are America's highest-risk group for ethmoid sinus cancer)
- Painters
- Beauticians
- Airport and airline personnel (mechanics, maintenance workers, baggage handlers, flight attendants, and pilots)
- White-collar workers in offices where there are one or more smokers, and who spend most of their time working with computers
- Policemen
- Firemen
- Parking garage attendants
- Professional cyclists (the highest-risk group; they have more air to filter and are exposed to extremely cold, dry, and often dirty air)

When I worked as the team physician for the 7-Eleven cycling team during the 1986 Coors International Bicycle Classic, a total of five riders in the competition, including Olympic gold medalist Eric Heiden of 7-Eleven, had to drop out because of sinus infections—this in spite of the fact that professional cyclists are the most physically fit human beings I have ever known.

DENTAL PROBLEMS

The roots of the upper teeth and the maxillary sinus are in close proximity; they are separated only by paper-thin bone or sinus mucosa. Because of this proximity, dental infections of the upper teeth can extend into the sinus cavity and cause maxillary sinusitis. It is also why toothache is a common symptom associated with maxillary sinusitis. Minor trauma or injury, dental instrumentation, extraction, or displacement of a chronically inflamed tooth can lead to perforation of the sinus cavity. The incidence of dental-related sinusitis in children is unknown but probably significant, particularly in adolescents. In adults, possibly 10 percent of maxillary sinus infections are thought to be of dental origin.

IMMUNODEFICIENCY

The immune system is the body's natural defense against infection, cancer, or inflammation—indeed, any form of illness. Sometimes, for reasons medical science has been unable to explain, the immune system does not function normally. Vital components of this system are infection-fighting proteins called immunoglobulins. In immunodeficiency there is a decrease in the amount of one or two of these proteins. This condition can be diagnosed by a blood test. People who have a hereditary predisposition to it, who are on a course of chemotherapy, or who are taking cortisone long-term for a chronic condition are likely to have impaired immune systems. Most often, however, there is no known cause.

Other than air pollution, what may eventually prove to be the most significant cause of the epidemic of chronic sinusitis is the depressed immunity resulting from the overuse (long-term or repeated courses) of broad-spectrum antibiotics. This problem will be discussed in depth in Chapter 5.

MALFORMATIONS

Malformations include any physical problem that would result in the obstruction of the tiny sinus openings, the ostia. The most common malformations are a deviated septum (the wall that divides the two sides of the nose), enlarged adenoids (especially in young children), and polyps, cysts, or turbinate hypertrophy (swelling of the mucosal lining covering the internal nasal ridges).

A deviated septum is most often diagnosed by ear, nose, and throat surgeons as the primary cause of repeated sinus infections. In most instances, however, I strongly believe that this is not the case. The obstruction of the ostia by the deviated septum is usually a result of the *swollen mucosa* covering the septum and the turbinates of the opposite side of the nostril. If the cause of this swelling and inflammation is treated, then the surgery so often recommended by these surgeons becomes unnecessary. Remember, too, that most deviated septa have been present since birth. Sinus problems usually have not.

EMOTIONAL STRESS

Emotional stress is probably the single most important determinant in whether someone develops a sinus infection. All of the other factors described in this chapter have the potential to adversely affect the sinuses, but what is it that triggers that potential? Why is it that a person with weak sinuses can be exposed to the same "risky" conditions many times but only occasionally develop a sinus infection? I am convinced that the answer is usually stress.

During the past twenty years the science of psychoneuroimmunology has legitimized the old notion that thoughts and emotions can both cause and combat disease. Recent research has provided a wealth of information on the profound impact our thoughts, beliefs, feelings, and attitudes have on our immune system and on our health. This knowledge is not new to holistic medicine. You will find its application to the treatment of sinus disease in chapters 7 and 8.

Chapter 4

DIAGNOSING SINUSITIS, ALLERGIES, AND COLDS

Throughout this book I use the term *sinusitis* to refer to sinus problems in general. This word actually means "inflammation of a sinus" and encompasses two distinctly different medical diagnoses: acute sinusitis and chronic sinusitis. The criteria for these diagnoses, as they are presented in this chapter, have been jointly established by myself and Bruce Jafek, M.D., former chairman of the Department of Otolaryngology at the University of Colorado School of Medicine.

ACUTE SINUSITIS

Acute sinusitis is another way of saying **sinus infection.** This is the problem that usually requires medical attention. The common cold is most often the cause of a sinus infection, so let's look at this a bit more closely, along with the other primary symptoms of acute sinusitis: head congestion, headache and facial pain, fatigue, and yellow-green mucus.

The Common Cold

A person who has had negligible or no sinus problems previously will notice that after seven to ten days a cold still won't quit, or that the cold symptoms have actually gotten much worse, or that the cold was almost gone for one or two weeks and now it's back again. Close questioning reveals that the "cold" never really went away.

Each of these scenarios is becoming much more commonplace. As I have previously mentioned, one study has revealed that 87 percent of those people who thought they just had a cold actually had an infected sinus as revealed by a CT scan, the most diagnostic test for sinusitis.

Just what is a cold? It is a viral infection of the nasal and usually sinus mucous membranes that is often immediately preceded by a sore throat. The primary symptoms are a stuffy and runny nose with thin clear or white mucus, fatigue, and mild muscle aching. Secondary symptoms might include headache, persistent sore throat, cough, and a low-grade fever. The average cold lasts from four to seven days. (see Table 4.1.)

In people whose sinuses have been weakened by previous infections, the common cold causes problems more quickly. These patients might notice the symptoms of a sinus infection within two or three days of the onset of the cold. The underlying condition of the sinuses will usually determine how soon the symptoms appear. Keep in mind that *a common cold very often precedes the onset of acute sinusitis.* Its appearance in the history of one's illness will help in the diagnosis of acute sinusitis. The most common symptoms follow. Note that the symptoms may differ for children under age twelve.

Head Congestion

Most people describe this symptom as fullness or a stuffy head. The nose may be stuffy as well. This symptom is most obvious in the morning upon arising from bed. It is often relieved, although not eliminated, by a hot shower. Voice, smell, and taste may be altered. These symptoms, however, are more subtle than the primary one of head congestion. There is a very definite awareness of a fullness in the head or a dull ache behind or above the eyes. *Dizziness* and *light-headedness* are other words that may be used to describe this symptom.

Headache and Facial Pain

I have combined these two symptoms because it is often difficult to differentiate between them. With acute sinusitis, pain, and sometimes swelling, will occur in the region of the affected sinus (Fig. 4.1). This usually results from air, pus, and mucus being trapped within the obstructed sinus. An infected maxillary sinus will cause pain, and sometimes swelling, in the cheek. Pain may occur under the eye and in the upper teeth, particularly the molars. At times, the *toothache* can be so severe as to prompt a visit to the dentist. When air is prevented from entering a sinus by a swollen mucous membrane at its opening, a vacuum can be created, also resulting in severe pain in the affected sinus. This is why many sinus sufferers experience pain with the barometric

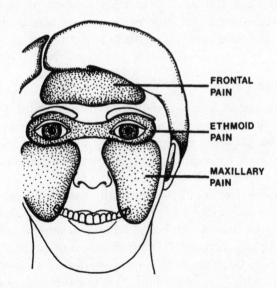

FIGURE 4.1. *Location of sinus pain in acute sinusitis.*

pressure changes related to weather systems (low pressure) and while descending (prior to landing) in an airplane.

Infected ethmoid sinuses produce pain between and behind the eyes, and tenderness when pressure is applied to the sides of the nose. Infected frontals cause pain in the forehead and over the eyes. Infected sphenoids produce a generalized pain, deep in the head, which becomes aggravated whenever your head is jarred. Sphenoid pain is often perceived as a headache in the back of the head at the base of the skull.

Children may experience facial pain accompanied by swelling of the orbit of the eye that involves the upper eyelid. Gradual in onset, the swelling is most obvious in the early morning, shortly after rising. The swelling might decrease or even disappear during the day, only to reappear the following day. Children may also experience photophobia, which is an unwillingness to open their eyes in bright light.

Some of the most incapacitating headaches I have treated resulted from infected frontal sinuses. Sinus headaches tend to worsen when you bend your head forward or lie down, and tend to be worse in the morning (after you have been in bed for hours), and then ease somewhat later in the day.

Extreme Fatigue

There is scarcely a sinus patient I can think of who doesn't complain of some degree of fatigue. Most people, even if they are not ill, would admit to being tired for some part of the day. The word *extreme* in regard to fatigue means a definite change in normal energy level.

In addition to inquiring about the nasal and head symptoms that are usually mentioned by the patient, I always ask the questions "Does your whole body feel sick in some way?" and "Do you feel especially tired?" The answer to these questions is frequently yes because acute sinusitis is usually a systemic illness, one that affects the entire body. These patients are sick all over. The medical term that best describes this phenomenon is *malaise,* meaning a feeling of general discomfort. It is often accompanied by significant irritability. People with sinus infections usually sleep more at night than they normally would, have some difficulty getting through a full day at work, and perhaps even take unaccustomed naps. In people who exercise regularly, the drop in energy level is even more evident.

At times, fatigue is the chief complaint. The bad cold someone had was as long ago as two or three months, and they say, "I just haven't been myself since." These people do not come in complaining of the cold they still have; most of the time they think they are finished with it. If asked, however, they will admit to a stuffy head in the morning and occasional yellow mucus they have to spit out. These patients pose a tough diagnostic challenge to the physician, as some of them have been tired for so long they have no recollection of any previous illness. Others have been misdiagnosed with anything from depression to menopause. However, if they are treated for sinusitis, it can do what months of estrogen or an antidepressant were unable to do.

Yellow Mucus

The question that seems to make patients most uncomfortable is "What color is your mucus?" The usual response, accompanied by a grimace, is "Eww, I never look at it!" The classic presentation of acute sinusitis in children, less frequently seen in an adult, is yellow (actually a yellow-green) mucus coming from one nostril. If it's not (no pun intended), the diagnosis may be difficult. Most kids are not great nose-blowers, but sniffing actually makes matters worse, since it tends to suck bacteria up into the sinuses. I usually try to have young patients blow their noses in the examination room. If you are checking your child at home, please remember to use white tissues; yellow won't help at all. Sinusitis is often missed in children. An article several years ago in a pediatric journal stated that almost 25 percent of all diagnosed upper respiratory tract infections (the common cold) in kids were actually cases of acute sinusitis. In light of the recent study revealing 87 percent of adults with "colds" were, in fact, suffering from sinus infections, I would speculate that there is a similar high percentage in children as well.

In adults, yellow mucus from the nose will help make the diagnosis. However, in many cases the mucus is either clear or white, or there is none at all from the nose. It seems that in most adult cases of acute sinusitis the infected or yellow mucus drains down the back of the throat. People are most aware of this in the morning, when they get out of bed and spit into the sink some of the mucus their sinuses have produced during the night. This morning yellow mucus is helpful in making the diagnosis but it can also be present in the absence of acute sinusitis. Therefore, the most important question I ask an adult is "Are you spitting out yellow mucus during the rest of the day, other than first thing in the morning?" (It is the consistent, all-day colored mucus that is most definitive in making the diagnosis.) Unfortunately, most people will respond with "I swallow it," or "It's not convenient to spit it out," or the old standby, "I never look at it!" If I still suspect a sinus infection, I will ask if they are even aware of mucus dripping down the back of the throat. If they're not aware of this occurring during the day, I then ask, "How about when you wake up in the morning?" Often I see patients who aren't aware of mucus drainage, but when I look at their throats, there is a thick yellow band of mucus running down from their sinuses.

I've spent a lot of time on the topic of mucus not because I enjoy discussing "gross" subjects, as my daughter Julie would say, but because it is extremely helpful in making the diagnosis. There are very few objective, or visible, signs of acute sinusitis, but this one is consistently present.

Refining the Diagnosis

Most ear, nose, and throat (ENT) specialists would find yellow mucus too indefinite a finding with which to make a diagnosis. Until about 1986 they usually attempted to confirm the diagnosis with a sinus X ray. However, this is unreliable. Some pa-

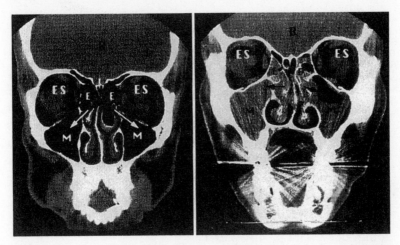

FIGURE 4.2. *CT ("CAT") SCAN Severely diseased sinuses (markedly thickened lining) are seen on the right with normal sinus computed tomogram (CT) X ray on the left for comparison. The maxillary (cheek: labeled M) and ethmoid (between eye sockets: E) sinuses are seen here with the brain (B) and eye sockets (ES) for anatomical reference. The arrows on the right clearly show the blockage of the outflow (osteomeatal complex) of the ethmoid and maxillary sinuses on the right with a clear opening on the patient on the left.*

tients will have every symptom of a sinus infection although an X ray shows a normal sinus.

Since then, new technology has made the definitive diagnosis of acute sinusitis much more feasible. The CT ("cat") scan, a computerized tomographic X-ray technique, can show areas of the sinuses never clearly visible with conventional X rays. As a result, the diagnosis of sinus disease and, correspondingly, the statistics on its incidence have risen dramatically. Unfortunately, the average sinus CT scan is costly and not very convenient.

To help reduce medical costs—as well as to assist primary care physicians, allergists, and ENT specialists in treating sinus infections—it would be a great advantage to have a generally accepted clinical diagnosis of acute sinusitis. Together with Dr. Jafek, this is what we are offering here: a list of signs and symptoms that are so often present with sinus infections that they will preclude the need for X rays and other expensive diagnostic procedures.

The picture presented by acute sinusitis can vary greatly; some people are very sick, others minimally uncomfortable. However, you can usually depend on most of these elements to make a definitive clinical diagnosis in an adult: *a preceding cold, head congestion, headache, extreme fatigue, and postnasal yellow mucus.* In a child the most common symptoms are nasal yellow mucus, fever, foul-smelling breath, and cough.

More Diagnostic Clues

The following symptoms are not quite as consistent as the foregoing, but are frequently present.

Fever   A high temperature accompanying sinusitis is much more common in children than in adults. When fever is present in an adult, it is usually less than 101°F. It is not uncommon to see kids run high fevers (as high as 103° to 105°F) with acute sinusitis. Fever often appears early in the course of the infection, when other symptoms are not yet obvious—making the diagnosis difficult. Because fever accompanies so many different infections, it can't be considered an important diagnostic symptom. However, if I suspect sinusitis, fever, along with the other symptoms, can be a helpful sign in confirming the diagnosis.

Nasal congestion and rhinorrhea   A stuffy and runny nose (rhinorrhea) is a primary symptom of the common cold that usually precedes acute sinusitis. The two infections very often overlap. The important thing to remember in adult sinusitis is that stuffiness is more common than a runny nose and is often present on only one side of the nose. In children with sinusitis, the yellow nasal discharge can be copious. With a cold, draining mucus is usually clear or white and thin or watery. With sinusitis it is usually thick and yellow.

Sore throat   A sore throat is probably the most common complaint in any family doctor's office. The underlying problem is not always sinusitis, but a substantial number of sore throats do result from mouth breathing and from postnasal mucus drainage down the back of the throat. A sore throat from sinusitis is usually not consistent throughout the day; it is much worse in the morning upon awakening. In fact, the soreness, caused by constant postnasal mucus drainage, a stuffy nose, and mouth breathing, can keep people from sleeping through the night. The dry air most of us breathe in our bedrooms can be irritating too. Once I have established that a patient's sore throat is much worse first thing in the morning, I ask if the patient is aware of mucus draining down the back of the throat. (In children, this drainage often results in bad breath.) After that, I merely have to run through a checklist of the other sinus symptoms—mucus color, recent cold, fatigue, fever, and so on—to decide if this is sinusitis or something else. Most of these questions would be asked as part of a thorough investigation of any sore throat.

Laryngitis   Laryngitis, or hoarseness, is another common symptom of sinus infection. It results from the same factors that cause sore throat, primarily postnasal mucus draining down into the larynx, causing irritation, inflammation, and swelling of the vocal cords and the arytenoid cartilages in the larynx.

Cough   For most of the patients who come to a family doctor's office with a sinus infection, cough and sore throat are the symptoms that have resulted in the greatest discomfort and the most loss of sleep. Unfortunately they are also the symptoms that have resulted in the highest number of misdiagnoses. A cough may be mistaken for bronchitis. Why? Because the cough of a sinusitis patient comes from yellow mucus draining down the back of the throat and continuing into the trachea or upper airway. Most physicians are aware that a productive cough that brings up a purulent or yellow mucus is often bronchitis. It isn't unusual to make that diagnosis in spite of hearing clear lungs with the stethoscope. It is easy to understand this common mistake, but it is just as easy to ask a few simple questions to rule out bronchitis and rule in acute sinusitis.

The cough from a sinus infection in adults isn't usually too bad during the day, when they are upright, but often worsens as soon as they lie down in bed at night. In children, the cough tends to be persistent throughout the day, just as it is in adults with bronchitis. Adults usually swallow the postnasal mucus drainage unconsciously, while up and about. This gets the mucus away from the trachea and into the stomach. (Swallowing the mucus can result in another not uncommon symptom that accompanies sinus infections: gastrointestinal upset, i.e., abdominal discomfort and loose bowels. There may be two or three loose movements a day—not quite diarrhea, but a definite change in bowel pattern. However, this isn't nearly as common as other symptoms I've mentioned, so I apologize for getting off the tract—respiratory, that is. Now, back to the cough.)

After asking about the timing of the cough, I usually want to know, "Does the cough feel like it's deep in your chest or does it feel more like a tickle in the back of your throat?" The latter, a dry cough, is much more typical of sinusitis, whereas the former, a wet, mucusy cough, is more indicative of bronchitis. In the past few years I have noticed a definite increase in the number of patients who are infected simultaneously in the sinuses and lungs. This is called sinobronchitis. If the antibiotic treatments for sinusitis and bronchitis were the same, there would be no need to differentiate between the two. However, this is not the case, and I believe it is valuable to be as specific as possible in a treatment program.

I began this chapter by describing acute sinusitis as an infection usually requiring medical attention. A visit to the doctor has a twofold purpose: to diagnose the problem and to begin treating it. Ideally there should also be a third objective: education and prevention—that is, teaching the patient how to care for his sinuses so that future office visits for the same problem will be unnecessary.

Again, the recognition of acute sinusitis is not a simple matter, even for physicians. Because the condition can manifest itself differently from one time to the next, this chapter and the next should be referred to frequently.

CHRONIC SINUSITIS

According to the most recent National Health Interview Survey, administered jointly by the Centers for Disease Control and Prevention and the National Center for Health Statistics, *chronic sinusitis is the most common chronic disease in the United States.* For all ages, it afflicts nearly 15 percent, or one out of every seven people in this country. That's approximately 40 million people. When the same study was performed in 1989, just less than 14 percent of all Americans had the problem. For some reason it is more common in women than men, reaching its peak incidence among middle-aged women. Twenty-two percent of all women between the ages of forty-five and sixty-four have chronic sinusitis (15 percent of men in this age group have it), about equal with the incidence of high blood pressure (hypertension). This makes it second only to arthritis among the most common chronic diseases for women this age. In men of this age group, it ranks fourth, behind high blood pressure, hearing impairment, and arthritis.

Although sinus disease has reached epidemic proportions, most people who have chronic sinusitis couldn't tell you they do. Their situation is similar to that of the hundreds of thousands of people who are unaware they have hypertension or diabetes, two other common chronic conditions. They may be experiencing some of the symptoms of these ailments but are unable to attach a label or diagnosis to their problem. However, what the vast majority of these sinus sufferers are very familiar with are tissues and handkerchiefs, postnasal drip, congestion, headaches, fatigue, irritability, halitosis, a weak sense of smell and taste, and, to an increasing extent, frequent courses of antibiotics and even sinus surgery.

Chronic sinusitis can be either:

Type 1: a persistent low-grade infection with periodic flare-ups of acute sinusitis These people are always sick to some degree. It may have been many months, and in most cases years, since they've been healthy, or completely normal. Their chronic illness takes the form of an ongoing sinus infection with any or all of the symptoms I've previously described for acute sinusitis. Extreme fatigue, headaches, and persistent yellow-green postnasal mucus drainage top the list of a multitude of systemic (total body) symptoms usually present in these sinus sufferers. They have taken multiple ten-day or two-week courses of powerful broad-spectrum antibiotics, and have often undergone multiple sinus surgeries, with minimal to moderate improvement in their symptoms. But the sinus infection never totally clears up. (One sure sign of a lingering infection is persistent yellow-green mucus drainage.) Some of these Type 1 people have been on continuous antibiotics for months, and in some cases a year or more. I know of one woman who has had fourteen sinus surgeries. These people constitute the majority of the patients I've treated during the past seven years. They are often frustrated, angry, and depressed, and they feel chronically ill. Their physicians share their exasperation. Conventional medicine has done all it can do for them, and to no avail.

Type 2: recurrent or repeated sinus infections (acute sinusitis)
These people suffer at least three or more infections within a six-month period. They usually have most of the symptoms I've already described for each episode of acute sinusitis. However, they often do not have a cold before their sinus infection begins. What might have started out as a cold in someone with healthier mucous membranes becomes, in most Type 2 people, an almost immediate sinus infection with an accompanying prescription for an antibiotic. Following the course of antibiotic treatment and between infections, these people usually feel okay or almost "normal." Their normal condition, however, may now include frequent sinus headaches, a stuffy nose and head, a somewhat diminished energy level, chronic postnasal drip (white or clear mucus), and increased irritability.

Type 3: chronic inflammation with little or no infection These people are not nearly as sick or uncomfortable as those with types

1 and 2. They have chronic inflammation of the mucous membranes lining their nose and sinuses with infrequent (one or two per year) or no infections at all. Inflammation involves pain, swelling, and increased secretions from the mucous membrane, but without the causative agents of bacteria, viruses, or fungi that are present with infection. Most of the Type 3 people do not realize they have a treatable disease called chronic sinusitis, and usually do not seek medical attention. For those who have, many have heard from their doctors "There's nothing that can be done for you." A more accurate statement would have been "There's nothing that I can do for you."

As a result, the majority of chronic sinus sufferers have learned to accept their condition and have adjusted to a compromised quality of life that includes head and nasal congestion, headaches, a runny nose and/or postnasal drip, increased irritability, halitosis, and possibly a diminished sense of smell and taste. These sufferers usually have an increased sensitivity to the factors mentioned in Chapter 3, such as cigarette smoke, pollution, dryness, cold, and fumes. The more they are exposed to any one of these irritants, the more pronounced the symptoms will be, and the more often they are likely to develop sinus infections. Although most of these symptoms are similar for all three groups of chronic sinusitis, they are usually less severe with Type 3. The majority of the members of the first two groups of chronic sinus sufferers began with Type 3. After a gradual weakening of their mucous membrane due to chronic inflammation, and a corresponding decrease in their natural resistance to infection (a normal mucosa protects against infection), colds become more frequent. These are often followed by sinus infections, and the cycle escalates to weaker membranes and more infections, more antibiotics, and a subsequently weaker immune system. The common cold becomes a rare occurrence and almost every illness, whether it begins as influenza, strep throat, or stomach flu, eventually seems to end up as a sinus infection. Unless the cycle can be broken, the immune system remains depressed and the sinuses are left in a permanently weak and damaged state.

Almost everyone who has made at least a two-month commitment to practicing the "quick-fix" component of the Sinus Survival Program (including candida treatment if applicable), described in chapters 1 and 6, has either dramatically improved their condition, returned to Type 3, or cured their chronic sinusitis. For many of these "sinus survivors," their ongoing or chronic symptoms may be so negligible that it is difficult to make a distinction between being cured and being a Type 3. They may not be aware of any symptoms at all unless they have developed a sinus infection. Just as with types 1 and 2, there is a spectrum of severity of symptoms and degrees of discomfort. Usually the longer a person adheres to the entire Sinus Survival Program, including the components of Mind and Spirit (chapters 7 and 8), the more mild a Type 3 they become. If there are *no persistent symptoms* but the individual still has one or two episodes of acute sinusitis during the year, I would consider that person to be *cured* of chronic sinusitis.

There are other methods of classification. Some physicians label anyone who has had an infection of the sinuses lasting three months or more as suffering from chronic sinusitis. But I believe that this is too limited a definition to account for the 40 million chronic sinus sufferers identified by the National Health Interview Survey.

ALLERGIC RHINITIS

Human beings, along with most other mammals, are meant to breathe through our noses. When a stuffy nose prevents us from doing so, it can be very unpleasant and uncomfortable. Nasal congestion is the most frequent and possibly the most troublesome symptom of allergies or hay fever. It results from the swelling and inflammation of the nasal mucous membrane. This inflammation is the key factor in causing hyperreactivity of the nasal mucosa, resulting in the other common nasal allergy symptoms of sneezing and itching. The sneezing usually occurs in a rapid, multiple sequence, and the itching may include the eyes as well. A thin, clear mucus drainage is also usually present with allergies (refer to Table 4.1, pp. 74–75).

It has nothing to do with hay and rarely produces a fever, but hay fever still makes about 27 million Americans miserable on an annual basis. Most people with allergies are sensitive to *pollen*—either tree, grass, or ragweed—and they make up the largest group of allergy sufferers. (North America is host to seventeen species of ragweed.) Their symptoms are **seasonal,** with tree pollen usually most plentiful from March to May, grasses from May to July, and ragweed from August to October. These seasons vary according to your locale and weather conditions. If the highly allergic person also has asthma, then the same pollen or allergens that trigger the nasal symptoms can also precipitate an asthmatic attack.

In addition to pollen, there are many other substances that can cause allergic rhinitis on a **perennial** or year-round basis, but these are more challenging to identify. To help make a diagnosis, ask yourself the following questions:

(1) Do you or does anyone in your family have a history of hay fever, asthma, or eczema?
(2) Do your symptoms tend to worsen during certain times of the year or day?
(3) Do you or does anyone else in your home smoke?
(4) Do you have any pets?
(5) What type of heating system is in your house?
(6) What types of occupational and leisure activities are you involved in that may trigger symptoms?
(7) What have you tried thus far to treat your allergies and how well has it worked?

Among the most difficult allergens to avoid are *dust mites,* microscopic insects that thrive by the millions wherever dust collects in a house. They live on shed human skin cells and leave droppings that are about the size of pollen grains, and just as easy to inhale. The mites prefer the warm, humid climates of coastal cities—New Orleans is high on the list of offenders in the United States—but they are very rare in cities above 6,000 feet, where the air is dry.

Mold spores can be found on food, leather, furniture, and especially in dark, damp areas such as bathrooms, basements, refrigerators, and air conditioners. Outdoors, they can grow on crops, grass, and dead leaves. There can be hundreds of thousands of mold spores per cubic meter of air, and we inhale about 10 to 12 cubic meters of air each day. Unfortunately these spores cause significant allergic reactions in millions of people.

About 25 percent of allergy sufferers are allergic to *cats*. The offending substance is the cat's saliva, which is left on their fur during preening. Homes with cats can be so full of cat hair and dander that it can take up to six months after the cat is removed before it can be considered safe for someone who is allergic to cats.

There are a multitude of *foods* that can cause allergy symptoms. Surveys have shown that as many as 70 percent of Americans believe they are allergic to at least one particular food. Yet, a food allergy may be one of the most under-diagnosed conditions in this country because scientific testing has been inaccurate, it is expensive, and it demands carefully informed patients and technicians. As I've already explained, allergic rhinitis with its persistent nasal congestion can easily cause sinus infections, and a significant percentage of the allergic symptoms are probably caused by food. If you suspect a food allergy, then I would suggest a food–elimination diet to confirm the diagnosis. Eliminate from your diet for at least three weeks the foods that are most likely to produce nasal allergy symptoms: cow's milk and all dairy products, wheat, rye, oats, chocolate, corn, oranges, eggs, and artificial food coloring. After that, begin to introduce each of these foods into your diet at the rate of one every three days. It should be obvious to you which foods cause your nose to react.

Allergy *skin tests* are medicine's most definitive method of diagnosing the cause of allergic rhinitis from airborne substances such as pollen, animal dander, etc. They involve injecting bits of suspected allergens in different places under the skin, or applying them to scratches on the arm or the back. If a particular area swells, reddens, and itches, the patient more often than not is allergic to that substance.

Most physicians agree that allergies result from aberrant functioning of the immune system, and that they tend to run in families. But there is no mention within the medical community of an emotional component causing allergies, nor is there any explanation for the tremendous increase in the number of allergy sufferers in the past twenty years. My "sandpaper" theory holds that as we breathe polluted and particulate-laden air 23,000 times a day, we are causing chronic irritation ("rubbing the surface raw") and inflammation of the nasal mucous membrane. This creates a hyperreactive membrane that, given the right genetic predisposition, emotional stress, and adequate exposure to an allergen, can precipitate a lifetime of allergies.

The nose and sinuses have become the "weak spot" in the bodies of people with chronic sinusitis and allergies. Although not life-threatening illnesses, they affect their victims daily as energy-draining conditions that can have a profound impact on their ability to enjoy life. Physicians now recognize them as systemic diseases, i.e., affecting the whole body. As the gateway and defender of the lungs, the nose and sinuses have a vital function to perform. As millions of sick sinuses and noses fail to protect the lungs by filtering out bacteria, viruses, pollutants, and pollen, and are unable to humidify and warm dry and cold air adequately, we are beginning to experience an epidemic of life-threatening lung disease.

Table 4.1

Diagnosing and Recognizing the Symptoms of Colds, Sinusitis, and Allergies

Primary symptoms—almost always present
Secondary symptoms—frequent but less often present

THE COMMON COLD

Primary:
- Preceded by high stress; too much going on at once
- Preceded by a sore throat
- Nasal congestion
- Runny nose
- Thin clear/white nasal mucus
- Fatigue
- Mild muscle aching
- Lasts for four to seven days

Secondary:
- Headache
- Sore throat
- Cough
- Low-grade fever

SINUS INFECTION (ACUTE SINUSITIS)

Primary:
- Preceded by the common cold
- Preceded by unexpressed anger or unshed tears
- Head congestion (facial or head fullness)
- Head or facial pain (headache, cheek, tooth, or eye pain)
- Thick green/yellow nasal or especially postnasal mucus drainage (down back of throat)
- Extreme fatigue
- Lasts for two or more weeks

Secondary:
- Preceded by allergies or by prolonged exposure to air pollution, smoke, or toxic fumes
- Fever

- Sore throat
- Cough
- Hoarseness
- Nasal congestion
- Lasts for several months

ALLERGIES, HAY FEVER, OR ALLERGIC RHINITIS

Primary:
- Preceded by personal or family history of allergies, eczema, or asthma
- Intermittent symptoms: either seasonal (pollen), food-related, environmentally or emotionally triggered
- Positive allergy skin tests
- Thin, clear/white nasal mucus
- Nasal congestion
- Sneezing
- Itching of nose, eyes, or throat
- Symptoms relieved with antihistamines, food elimination, environmental clearing, or stress reduction

Secondary:
- Persistent or perennial symptoms
- Postnasal drip with intermittent sore throat, cough, or hoarseness
- Wheezing, difficulty breathing
- Skin rash
- Allergic "shiners" (dark circles under eyes)

Chapter 5

THE CONVENTIONAL MEDICAL TREATMENT FOR SINUSITIS, ALLERGIES, AND OTITIS MEDIA (MIDDLE EAR INFECTION)

I n allopathic (conventional) medical schools, doctors are taught to diagnose and treat disease. They learn that body and mind are separate and distinct compartments of a human being, with little interaction between the two. They are trained to focus their attention almost exclusively on the body, and they do so in militaristic terms. They think of the immune system as a defense force on constant alert to protect the body against invasion by bacteria, viruses, allergens, and cancer cells; but they are in a quandary as to how the immune system can be weakened enough to allow infection, allergy, and cancer to occur. Consequently, conventional medicine plays only a reactive role in treating the body: a specific symptom appears and the doctor prescribes drugs or surgery to vanquish or treat it.

What does it mean to treat an ailment? This usually depends on what the condition is. In some instances, treatment implies a cure, with the expectation that the problem will not recur. These treatments are most often surgical. For example, appendicitis is treated with an appendectomy.

At other times, to treat means to relieve symptoms of a chronic condition that has no known cure. These conditions range from cancer and AIDS to the common cold and sore throat. They also include chronic sinusitis and allergic rhinitis. Relief of symptoms constitutes the bulk of a physician's work; almost 75 percent of all ailments fall into this treatment realm.

ACUTE AND CHRONIC SINUSITIS

The treatment of acute sinusitis is in yet another category. Acute sinusitis is most often a viral infection in one or more of the sinus cavities. However, most primary care physicians do not differentiate between a virus and bacteria, and therefore treat most cases of acute sinusitis as if it were a bacterial infection. The goal of treatment is to kill the bacteria, open the blocked sinus duct, and restore the mucus-and-cilia cleansing system, while relieving symptoms. Acute sinusitis does have a cure, but the chances of it recurring at some point, either months or years later, are very high.

Acute sinusitis is not a simple infection to treat. Doctors seldom identify the bacteria that cause the infection (or determine if it is a bacteria or virus), so they select an antibiotic to combat the bacteria most likely to have caused the infection. The antibiotic is taken by mouth and absorbed into the bloodstream. Because of the relatively poor blood supply in the sinuses, it usually takes several days before the effect of the drug is felt, especially in adults. Strong antibiotics in relatively high dosages taken for long periods of time are often required.

The next objective is to open the blocked sinus duct and the ostium so that the infected mucus can drain from the sinus. A decongestant opens the duct by shrinking the swollen mucous membrane. However, most decongestants have a drying effect, which thickens the mucus and *prevents it* from draining. Many commercial decongestants also contain an antihistamine, which is also quite drying.

Acute sinusitis is an infection without an accepted standard treatment program. Since it is most often treated as a bacterial infection, antibiotics have been, and continue to be, the primary component of the conventional medical treatment. However, if there was one drug that always worked for everyone, this would be a very brief discussion, and I would not have to devote most of the chapter to the subject. The reality is that the efficacy of treatment varies with each patient and with the physician who is administering the treatment. During the past decade, physicians have had to employ greater creativity, using a vastly expanded arsenal of antibiotics, decongestants, expectorants, and nasal corticosteroid sprays to succeed in treating sinus infections.

Antibiotics

The bacteria most often responsible for causing sinus infections in both adults and children are *Streptococcus pneumoniae, Hemophilus influenzae,* and *Moraxella catarrhalis.* During the 1990s, doctors have found a marked increase in the incidence of *Staphylococcus aureus* and *Pseudomonas aeruginosa* in cases of chronic sinusitis, perhaps because of improved diagnostic techniques.

Nasal endoscopy is a procedure usually performed by allergists and ENT physicians using a rod lens telescope that is inserted into the nasal cavity. It permits superior visualization of the interior of the nose, including the opening of ostia, currently being referred to by physicians as the ostio-meatal complex. Intranasal endoscopy can be performed in an office setting using only topical anesthesia, and is easily tolerated by the unsedated patient. It can identify pathologic changes, assist in making the diagnosis of sinusitis, and help to obtain samples of pus for culture. This is a much more accurate method for identifying the bacteria (or determining if it is a bacteria or a virus) causing the sinus infection than the random nasal swabs that were used in the past. The procedure is also useful for monitoring patient response to medical therapy and for assessing the need for subsequent therapy. Most ENT doctors consider the widespread use of diagnostic nasal endoscopy the greatest single recent advance in sinusitis management.

The physicians who treat the vast majority of patients with acute sinusitis are primary care doctors—family practitioners, internists, and pediatricians, most of whom do not perform nasal endoscopy.

Unfortunately, the antibiotics that effectively treat all the bacteria that cause sinusitis are quite expensive. As sinus infections become more difficult to treat, especially those caused by *Staphylococcus aureus,* researchers have come to the rescue with ever more powerful antibiotics.

For the past twenty-five years the drug of choice has been amoxicillin, unless there is an allergy to penicillin. The usual dosage is either 250 or 500 mg (125 or 250 mg in children) three times a day. Both are taken for ten days. This is a routine first step, but it is a hefty dose of antibiotic! Adult patients are told that they should notice definite improvement, with the yellow mucus beginning to clear, in about four to five days. In children the response is usually faster, with fever, nasal drainage, and cough markedly reduced after about forty-eight hours. Patients are instructed to take the medicine for the entire ten days. If this instruction is not followed, the infection often remains. Many physicians routinely prescribe amoxicillin for fourteen days, instead of ten, to reduce the number of treatment failures. For the majority of patients with acute sinusitis, a ten-day course of amoxicillin is all they will need.

In spite of their compliance with instructions, more than 10 percent of patients will call or return to the office shortly after the tenth day, still complaining of most of their symptoms. Some will report that they felt much better while on the antibiotic, but that as soon as they stopped taking it the symptoms recurred. Others will say they experienced no improvement whatsoever. For this reason many physicians are now using Augmentin (amoxicillin/clavulanate) or TMP/SMX, Bactrim, or Septra (trimethoprim/sulfamethoxazole) as their first choice for an antibiotic instead of amoxicillin.

If amoxicillin is unsuccessful, with the second attempt at treatment, a different antibiotic is selected. The second-choice antibiotics have a bit broader spectrum of efficacy than amoxicillin; all are much more expensive. Table 5.1 lists the second-

Table 5.1

Second-Step Antibiotics for Sinus Infections—after Amoxicillin

Best drugs for killing both Streptococcus pneumoniae *and* Hemophilus influenzae *(listed in order of efficacy; those on the same line are roughly equivalent):*
Augmentin
Ceclor, Cefzil, Ceftin, Lorabid
Biaxin, Zithromax
Bactrim, Septra, Cotrim
Vantin

Best for killing Staphylococci *and* Pseudomonas:
Augmentin
Ceclor, Cefzil, Ceftin, Lorabid
Duricef, Ultracef, Keflex, Cefanex, Anspor, Velosef
Bactrim, Septra

step drugs that are commonly used for the treatment of sinus infections—both acute and chronic sinusitis.

A small but growing percentage of patients are still not cured following a ten-day course of a second-step antibiotic, or their infection returns again shortly after they finish. It sometimes helps to take a two- or even three-week course of the antibiotic and gradually taper it off over the last five to seven days. This seems to allow the body's immune system a better chance to take over for the antibiotic. Whatever the reason, this strategy does appear to be more effective than abruptly stopping the drug a patient has been taking for two to three weeks.

Patients who do not respond to antibiotics are good candidates for further diagnostic evaluation with a CT scan or nasal endoscopy to see if there is a physical obstruction of the sinus.

During the past twelve years, I have worked with several hundred patients suffering from chronic sinusitis both locally and from more than thirty different states. I have spoken to a multitude of people through Sinus Survival workshops and seminars, and received many letters and questions from others, both through the mail and more recently the Sinus Survival Web site (www.sinussurvival.com). Most of them who have severe sinusitis. Their stories are striking in their similarity. Almost every one of them had taken multiple antibiotics for their infections, some continuously for a year or more, and yet, they were still sick. Many had already undergone sinus surgery, while others had it recommended to them by their physicians.

Antibiotics have been and continue to be the foundation of conventional medical treatment for a sinus infection. But at this point I rarely prescribe these drugs. I'll do so only for patients who have strictly adhered to the Sinus Survival Program for 10 days and have seen no improvement with their infection. It is also OK for someone with a sinus infection who has one or two sinus infections per year and has not been taking antibiotics for other reasons. As you will soon learn, antibiotics are not usually necessary in treating sinus infections. I'm convinced that *the overuse of antibiotics in treating acute sinusitis has become one of the three primary causes of the epidemic of chronic sinusitis.* (The other two are air pollution and emotional stress.)

To be more accurate, I should say the abuse of antibiotics and our dependence upon them in treating a myriad of problems, not just sinus infections, lies at the root of the problem. In recent years new strains of antibiotic-resistant bacteria, called supergerms, have appeared with a vengeance. According to the Centers for Disease Control and Prevention, 19,000 hospital patients die annually from antibiotic-resistant infections, and another 58,000 people die because of complications attributable to bacterial infections. Many of the people suffering from chronic sinusitis are still sick because their sinuses are infected with antibiotic-resistant bacteria.

Stuart B. Levy, M.D., professor of Medicine, Molecular Biology, and Microbiology, and director of the Center for Adaptation Genetics and Drug Resistance at Tufts University School of Medicine, believes that "up to 50 percent of all antibiotic use in the U.S. today is actually misuse, and some experts estimate that half of all prescriptions written may not even be needed." Dr.

Levy is the author of *The Antibiotic Paradox*. The paradox is that the same antibiotics that prevent bacteria from killing people also breed antibiotic-resistant supergerms.

Just as our own species continues to evolve, so do bacteria. They are able to adapt to the attacking antibiotics, and the overuse of these medications provides countless opportunities for bacteria to get to know their enemy and change accordingly. And it's not just overprescribing by physicians that has created this problem. Most livestock are routinely given antibiotics to fight infections, often in low doses, and milk is allowed to contain eighty different antibiotics. As we ingest antibiotic-laden meat and dairy products, we are contributing to breeding resistant bacteria. Our habit of stopping antibiotic use as soon as symptoms improve also allows resistant strains to survive and flourish.

There is growing evidence that antibiotics interfere with the body's own immune system, hence weakening our ability to fight off the offending bacteria. Another extremely damaging aspect of taking antibiotics is that they destroy the friendly bacteria in our digestive tract, which allows for the overgrowth of candida organisms. The subsequent infection of the sinuses by candida has become a primary focus of the Sinus Survival Program in treating chronic sinusitis. This subject will be discussed in depth in Chapter 6.

If you believe you must have antibiotics in order to overcome your infection, then take them for the duration (usually ten days) in order to wipe out all of the pathogenic bacteria. Follow that course of antibiotic with acidophilus powder or capsules to replenish the good bacteria in the intestine. There are a number of recommendations in chapters 6, 7, and 8 that will allow you to strengthen your immune system while you're taking an antibiotic, and when you are not.

James Hughes, director of the National Center for Infectious Diseases at the federal Centers for Disease Control and Prevention says, "We're facing a serious global problem with antimicrobial resistance now. It affects nearly all of the pathogens we previously considered easily treatable." *Beyond Antibiotics,* by Drs.

Michael A. Schmidt, Lendon H. Smith, and Keith W. Sehnert, is an excellent reference book on this subject.

Decongestants and Expectorants

The decongestants are specifically used to open the ostia and sinus ducts while relieving the symptoms of head, nasal, and ear congestion, headache, facial pain, and, to some extent, sore throat and cough. Expectorants, which are mucus thinners, can help to relieve the same symptoms.

The challenge of using a decongestant is to find one whose benefits outweigh its side effects. Decongestants are readily available in many familiar over-the-counter (OTC) products, such as Dristan, Contac, Allerest, Drixoral, Actifed, Dimetapp, Triaminicin, and a host of other cold remedies. However, every one of these contains an antihistamine in combination with the decongestant. Given the drying effect of antihistamines and the subsequent thickening of the mucus, I am convinced they do more harm than good. They are fine if all you are trying to treat is a cold, but I believe that in many instances they have actually helped a cold progress into a sinus infection. If you have a history of sinus problems, I would advise you to avoid antihistamines. If you are not sure about the ingredients of an OTC product, ask a pharmacist.

The most common ingredients in both prescription and OTC decongestants are pseudoephedrine, phenylpropanolamine, and phenylephrine. Each works in much the same way to shrink swollen mucous membranes and reduce nasal and sinus congestion. Many products contain these decongestants in combination. Some, available only by prescription, include two of these ingredients; others only one, along with a pain reliever or an expectorant or cough suppressant.

There is a wide range of choices at the pharmacy. The following is a guide to lead you through the confusing maze of cold and sinus preparations. Before you begin the process, it would be helpful to ask yourself what it is you are treating. What are the symptoms that most trouble you? Are you stuffed up? Or is it the headache, the cough, the sore throat, or the thick mucus that you would most like to eliminate? Since you probably have more than one symptom, you will be looking for a decongestant in combination with something else. However, unless allergies triggered your sinus infection, choose anything but an antihistamine. I recommend the preparations in tables 5.2 through 5.6. If all you need is a plain decongestant, then Sudafed in a tablet, caplet, chewable, or liquid form is an excellent choice. Sudafed also offers the option of a 4-, 12-, or 24-hour tablet. If you have a lot of thick mucus draining, don't want a decongestant, and would like a simple expectorant, Robitussin is a good OTC choice, while Fenesin, Humibid, and Organidin are all good prescription drugs.

Tables 5.2, 5.3, and 5.6 all list OTC products. Please follow the dosage instructions on the bottle or package. The drugs in Table 5.4, which your doctor may prescribe, contain the same decongestants and expectorants as those found in the OTC products. The primary difference is that these drugs contain higher doses and are long-acting, continuing to work for up to twelve hours. The exceptions are Entex and Dura-Gest capsules; the latter is both a brand-name drug and used by most pharmacists as the generic form of Entex. These short-acting products can be taken every four to six hours and contain two deconges-

Table 5.2

Decongestants with Analgesics (OTC)

Advil Cold and Sinus Tablets and Caplets
Alka-Seltzer Plus Cold & Sinus Medicine
Motrin IB Pain Reliever Tablets, Caplets, and Gelcaps
Sine-Aid Sinus Medication Caplets, Gelcaps, and Tablets
Sine-Off No Drowsiness Formula Caplets
Sinutab Sinus Medication
Sudafed Cold and Sinus
Sudafed Sinus Tablets and Caplets
Tylenol Sinus Tablets, Caplets, and Gelcaps

Table 5.3

Decongestants with Expectorants (OTC)

Robitussin-PE Syrup
Triaminic Expectorant
Sudafed Non-Drying Sinus Liquid Caps

tants, phenylephrine and phenylpropanolamine, in combination with the expectorant guaifenesin. I find them more effective in the treatment of acute sinusitis than the long-acting preparations. Avoid them if you have high blood pressure. They can also cause insomnia in adults, but some young children experience the opposite side effect and become drowsy. Omitting the bedtime dose usually eliminates the insomnia.

I usually don't encourage patients to take the decongestant on the same rigid schedule as the antibiotic, or for the entire ten-day course. I tell them to take it regularly for the first four to five days, then gradually taper off. If they still experience head and sinus congestion, they should continue the ten-day course. Patients with active sinus infections should avoid air travel because of the pressure changes and poor air quality found on airplanes.

Table 5.4

Decongestants with Expectorants (Rx)

Deconasal II Tablets
Dura-Gest Capsules
Dura-Vent Tablets
Entex Capsules
Entex LA Tablets
Entex Liquid
Guaifed Capsules
Guaifed-PD Capsules
Respaire-60 Capsules
Respaire-120 Capsules

If they can't, I recommend taking a decongestant approximately two hours prior to the scheduled landing, along with using a decongestant nasal spray shortly before takeoff.

Decongestant Sprays

An OTC alternative for those with extreme head and nasal congestion or sinus pain is nasal decongestant spray. There are several twelve-hour varieties from which to choose, including Afrin, Dristan, Sinex, Neosynephrine, and Vicks. These should be used with great caution and only for two or three days at most. They can easily become addictive! They produce what is called a rebound effect, which means that as their decongestant effect wears off and the head and nasal congestion return, the feeling of stuffiness is worse than it was before using the spray. This elicits a strong desire to spray again, and a vicious cycle begins. Be careful!

If you have been using a spray regularly and are unable to stop, you probably need some help. Consult with your physician and tell him honestly what has been happening. I have had a high success rate helping patients to break this habit with the following regimen:

- Throw away the nasal spray.
- Take a tapered dose of cortisone over a one-week period, either Medrol (the generic name is methylprednisolone) in the 4-mg dosepak or 5 mg of prednisone. These are prescription drugs that relieve inflammation.
- Take forty capsules of Entex or Dura-Gest in a tapered schedule: one capsule three times a day over seven days; then one capsule two times a day over seven days; followed by one capsule daily over seven days.
- Use moisture—including saline nasal spray, a humidifier, and steaming in the bathroom (refer to the Moisture and Irrigation section in Chapter 7)—and one or more of the natural decongestants listed under "Stuffy Nose" in Table 1.6, "Natural Quick-Fix Symptom Treatment" (p. 19).

Remember that it is extremely difficult to keep your sinuses healthy with *continued* use of a decongestant nasal spray. However, one instance in which it can be quite helpful is during air travel. If you have a stuffy nose before embarking on your trip, plan to use the spray shortly before take-off. If allergies are believed to be contributing to the sinus infection, **nasal corticosteroid sprays** are often prescribed. These will be described in the "Allergies" section on page 92.

Antitussives (Cough Suppressants)

If a patient's chief complaint is a cough that interrupts sleep, I will withhold the bedtime dose of decongestant and substitute a strong prescription cough suppressant containing either codeine or hydrocodone in combination with a decongestant, an expectorant, or both. Such antitussives can cause drowsiness, which is why I rarely recommend them for daytime use. Besides, these people are already tired from having a sinus infection. They don't need any additional sedation. The most commonly prescribed antitussives for sinus patients are listed in Table 5.5. If a cough suppressant is indicated for use during the day, especially in children, there are several similar OTC combination drugs from which to

Table 5.5

Antitussives with Decongestants (D) and/or Expectorants (E) (Rx)

Duratuss HD (D, E)
Hycomine Pediatric Syrup (D)
Hycomine Syrup (D)
Hycotuss (E)
Robitussin A–C (E)
Robitussin-DAC (D, E)
Tussi Organidin NR (E)
Tussi Organidin DM NR (E)
Vicodin Tuss (E)

Table 5.6

Antitussives with Decongestants (D) and/or Expectorants (E) (OTC)

Benylin Multisymptom (D, E)
Benylin Cough Suppressant Expectorant Liquid (E)
Children's Sudafed Cold & Cough Liquid (D)
Comtrex Deep Chest Cold
Robitussin-CF Liquid (D, E)
Robitussin Cold & Cough Liqui-Gels (D, E)
Robitussin Maximum Strength Cough & Cold (D)
Robitussin Pediatric Cough & Cold Formula (D)
Sudafed Severe Cold Formula Caplets & Tablets (D)
Sudafed Cold and Cough Liquid Caps (D, E)
Theraflu Maximum Strength Non-Drowsy Formula Caplets (D)
Triaminic AM Cough and Decongestant Formula (D)
Triaminic DM Syrup (D)
Tylenol Cold Medication No Drowsiness Formula Caplets & Gelcaps (D)
Tylenol Cough Multisymptom Severe Congestion (D, E)
Tylenol Cough Medication with Decongestant, Multisymptom (D)
Vicks 44D Cough & Head Congestion Relief (D)
Vicks 44E (E)
Vicks DayQuil Liquid and Liquicaps (D)
Pediatric Vicks 44e (E)

choose. They can be taken by both adults and children. The most commonly used and easily found are listed in Table 5.6.

Analgesics (Pain Relievers)

To relieve the frequent symptoms of headache, facial pain, and sore throat, I recommend the OTC pain relievers Advil, Motrin, and Nuprin. Both contain ibuprofen, which not only relieves pain but reduces inflammation. (To some extent, ibuprofen also can lower a fever.) Both pain relievers are dispensed in 200-mg tablets, and they are safe for *adults* in dosages of three or even four at a time if the pain is especially severe. Some of the worst sinus headaches often accompany a drop in barometric pressure, and will require the higher dosage. This dosage, however, should be taken with food, especially if there is a history of stomach ulcers. Since the headache is usually accompanied by some degree of nasal and/or head congestion, the Advil Cold and Sinus Caplets or Motrin IB Pain Reliever Tablets are effective options available to sinus sufferers.

Aspirin has the same effects as ibuprofen but doesn't seem to be as strong. Tylenol and other acetaminophen-containing products are simply analgesics, with no anti-inflammatory effect on the mucous membranes of the sinuses. However, if lowering a fever is the primary objective or you prefer taking acetaminophen to ibuprofen, or you are treating a child for acute sinusitis, then Sudafed Cold & Sinus is the drug of choice.

Sinus Surgery

If you have completed several courses of antibiotics, have strictly adhered to all of your primary care physician's recommendations, and you are still infected, your next step is often a referral to an ear, nose, and throat specialist. Otolaryngologists are the professionals usually assigned the task of treating the most challenging chronic sinus sufferers—Type 1—described in Chapter 4. The sinus patients in this group suffer the most discomfort. Before arriving at the specialist's office, they might have been fighting a sinus infection for several months to a year, and in many cases, two or three years. Most of them have already been through multiple courses of antibiotics without success. Their physicians have given up; these patients are considered treatment failures.

The initial evaluation by the ENT doctor usually includes the application of a topical decongestant in the nose and a nasal bacterial culture, followed by a physical examination of the nose, throat, and sinuses. The specimen for the culture is usually obtained using nasal endoscopy and needs to be obtained right from the opening of the sinus ducts (ostia) or else it will be of little value. The ENT specialist is attempting to identify the specific bacteria that are infecting the sinuses. The bacteria found in the nose are not usually the same as those infecting the sinuses. The culture should be performed by someone who has had a lot of experience with endoscopy and in locating the ostia so that the results will be a true reflection of the bacteria that are actually causing the infection. This test is critical to the selection of the most effective antibiotic. As a result of the more accurate performance of this test, many specialists have seen a dramatic increase in *Staphylococcus aureus* and *Pseudomonas aeruginosa* in the sinuses. These have been among the most difficult bacteria to treat.

Subsequent diagnostic procedures may include a sinus CT scan to determine if, after a course of an antibiotic, there are any lingering pockets of infection; nasal endoscopy, to see if there is any obstruction around the ostia; a nasal cytogram, a microscopic inspection of cells from the nasal mucous membrane; and a complete battery of skin and/or blood tests to identify possible allergies.

The initial treatment usually includes a ten-day to two-week course of one of the second-step antibiotics (see Table 5.1). If this fails—meaning either that there is no improvement or that the infection is still present on the CT scan or recurs shortly after the antibiotic is stopped—further evaluation using one or more of the diagnostic procedures previously mentioned will be necessary. Depending on the results, either a different antibiotic or surgery will be offered.

Sinus surgery has improved dramatically over the past fifteen years. If there is an obstruction of the ostio-meatal complex (the opening of the sinus duct into the nasal passage), surgery is usually recommended. The endoscope has taken sinus surgery to an even higher level of success. The most common endoscopic sinus surgery is a bilateral middle antrostomy, in which the maxillary sinus ostia are enlarged from 2 mm to about 10 or 12 mm (approximately the width of a dime). This procedure is a marked improvement over the surgery that created naso-antral windows—the most common procedure prior to endoscopic surgery. The opening of a naso-antral window was about the same size as the opening created by an antrostomy, but it went entirely through the bony medial wall (nasal side) of the maxillary sinus. The new procedure is not only less destructive but preserves the normal direction of mucus flow in the sinus. Mucus naturally flows out through the sinus duct and into the nose. The fact that the naso-antral window was not in the best position to enhance drainage greatly diminished its rate of success, despite the large opening it produced. Many patients who have had this surgery, or the Caldwell-Luc operation or ethmoidectomy (other surgical procedures not performed as often anymore), continue to have sinus problems and not infrequently require additional surgery.

Endoscopic surgery has been widely performed since 1988 and it is clearly an improvement over the previous procedures. About one half of the approximately 6,000 otolaryngologists in the U.S. have received training in endoscopic surgery, and in 1998 performed over 200,000 of these procedures. They are performed on an outpatient basis under local anesthesia, and patients can expect to miss only about one week of work. It is certainly not inexpensive, with surgeons charging anywhere from $3,000 to $10,000 for the procedure. However, it is still a long way from a guaranteed cure for chronic sinusitis. What I am observing with increasing frequency is that many people experience short-term improvement, six months to one year, and then begin the cycle of sinus infections and antibiotics over again. One difference seems to be that they are not as uncomfortable with their infections as they were prior to surgery. This is probably because their sinuses are able to drain more easily. Other people I've treated have seen no change in their condition following this surgery.

I've recently learned about an otolaryngologist, Reuben Setliff, M.D., from Sioux Falls, South Dakota, who has pioneered a minimally invasive type of endoscopic surgery. He is reporting better long-term results than with the standard procedure.

In spite of technological and therapeutic advances, sinus surgery has been and will continue to be most successful in those instances in which it eliminates one or more of the obstructive causes of sinusitis, such as polyps, cysts, mucoceles, an enlarged or distorted nasal turbinate (turbinate hypertrophy), and a deviated septum. But even in these cases, the surgery is still treating the symptom, not the cause. What is responsible for stimulating the growth of the polyps, cysts, and swollen turbinates in nasal mucous membranes to such an extent that a congenital deviated septum is now all of a sudden obstructing the sinus from draining? Most ENT surgeons claim that there is no known cause for these phenomena. They just happen. Many patients who have had polyps surgically removed have seen them recur. And what about the other surgical cases of chronic sinusitis that do not involve one of these obstructive causes? Has the diagnosis of fungus or candida been considered? Have all therapeutic options been tried prior to the decision to have surgery? In most cases they have not, because all of the physical, environmental, emotional, mental, social, and spiritual factors that contribute to sinus disease have not been addressed. Until they are incorporated into the therapeutic approach, the conventional medical treatment for chronic sinusitis will continue as a symptom-focused regimen, and chronic sinusitis will remain a largely incurable problem with the prognosis "You're going to have to learn to live with it."

For the most part, the conventional medical treatment for the other respiratory diseases is also based on relieving symptoms with medication. Unlike sinusitis, there is no "last resort" surgical procedure available "if all else fails."

ALLERGIES

The treatment for allergic rhinitis, or hay fever, besides removing the offending allergen, consists of medication and allergy desensitization injections.

Eliminating the allergen is usually a bit of a challenge. Avoiding allergenic foods can be relatively simple, but getting rid of the family pet if you're allergic to cats, or escaping from pollen, is much more difficult. One option for allergic cat owners is to wash the cat once a month, and within three to eight months it will stop making the offending allergen in its saliva. You will have created a nonallergenic cat.

You can minimize pollen exposure by taking refuge in sealed, air-conditioned office buildings and houses, where filters cleanse most of the offending pollen from incoming air. For those allergy sufferers unconcerned with domestic decor, the NIH recommends the following steps to achieve a dust-free and dust mite–free bedroom: Remove carpeting, upholstered furniture, heavy curtains, venetian blinds, fuzzy wool blankets, and comforters stuffed with wool or feathers. Empty the room, scrub it and everything that is to be returned to it, and thereafter thoroughly clean the room every week. If replacing curtains, hang some that are lightweight and can be laundered weekly. Replace the comfortable chairs with wooden or metal ones that can be scrubbed, and keep clothing in plastic zippered bags and shoes in closed boxes off the floor.

For temporary relief of mild allergies, doctors usually prescribe antihistamines. For years these drugs almost always caused drowsiness, but now there are a few that do not have this inconvenient side effect. Claritin, Zyrtec, and Allegra are all nonsedating prescription options. There are a number of OTC antihistamines, either alone or in combination with decongestants (see tables 5.7 and 5.8). Since nasal congestion is a primary symptom of allergies, it is usually recommended that you take a decongestant/antihistamine combination. The stimulant effect of the decongestant sometimes counteracts the sedation of the antihistamine. However, if you don't need a decongestant, most of the drugs listed in Table 5.7 are also available as an antihistamine only. I would recommend trying some of the OTCs before opting for a prescription. The latter are considerably more expensive. A one-month prescription of Claritin, Zyrtec, and Allegra can range from $50 to $75. Claritin is usually the most expensive of the three. As a reflection of the prevalance and severity of allergies, as well as of our quick-fix conditioning, it is interesting to note that Claritin is by far the most heavily advertised drug in America. In 1999, $94 million was spent in promoting Claritin, with Zyrtec ranked #4 at $39 million. (To give these statistics more perspective, Viagra ranked third at $44 million.)

Table 5.7

Decongestant and Antihistamine Combinations (OTC)

Actifed Cold & Allergy Tablets
Benadryl Allergy/Congestion Tablets and Liquid
Chlor-Trimenton 4 Hour Allergy/Decongestant Tablets
Chlor-Trimenton 12 Hour Allergy/Decongestant Tablets
Contac Continuous Action Nasal Decongestant/Antihistamine 12
　　Hour Capsules & Caplets
Coricidin D Decongestant Tablets
Dimetapp Tablets, Liq-Gels, Extentabs & Elixir
Drixoral Allergy/Sinus Extended-Release Tablets
Nasalcrom CA Caplets
Singlet Caplets
Sinutab Sinus Allergy Tablets and Caplets
Sudafed Cold & Allergy Tablets
Tavist-D Caplets
Triaminic Syrup
Triaminicin Tablets
Tylenol Allergy Sinus Caplets, Gelcaps, & Geltabs
Children's Tylenol Allergy-D Chewable Tablets & Liquid

　　Many allergy sufferers also derive significant benefit from the antiallergic and anti-inflammatory effects of the prescription corticosteroid nasal sprays such as Beconase, Vancenase, Nasalide, Nasonex, and Nasacort. Cromolyn sodium has a similar action and is available as a nasal spray (Nasalcrom) and as an eyedrop (Opticrom). The effect of the spray seems to be enhanced if used after nasal irrigation. Irrigation removes the mucus secretions so the prescription spray does not sit on the mucus but hits the lining of the nose directly. The irrigation also removes allergens such as pollen and dust. A seasonal pollen allergy sufferer, especially one who is also prone to sinus infections, should use the spray on a maintenance schedule throughout most of the allergy season, about one to two months. Long-term use of these cortisone sprays, beyond three months, seems to cause chronic irritation, inflammation, and increased mucus secretion. This is less of a problem with the aqueous-based than the Freon-based sprays. The potentially serious side effects that can accompany the oral administration of corticosteroids, such as Prednisone, are not a risk with the sprays since they are very minimally absorbed into the bloodstream.

A recent and effective addition to the pharmaceutical treatment of allergies is the intranasal antihistamine, Astelin Nasal Spray. If your primary symptom is a runny nose, without congestion or itching, your doctor may prescribe Atrovent Nasal Spray, an anticholinergic. This group of drugs work well as drying agents for excessive mucus secretions.

If you are not satisfied with the symptomatic relief you have received from antihistamines and steroid nasal sprays, your next step will often be a visit to an allergist. Depending upon the results of a battery of allergy skin tests, you may then be considered a candidate for allergy desensitization injections. These shots, containing very small amounts of the offending allergen(s), will often be given a few days apart early on, and progress to monthly injections that can last for several years. People with severe pollen allergy seem to benefit most from this course of treatment, while those with mold, dust mite, and animal dander allergies do not fare as well. Why the shots do and sometimes don't work remains a mystery. Whether or not they do, however, they are consistently an expensive treatment option.

Conventional medicine has recognized the importance of heredity in causing allergies, and continues to develop better diagnostic tools and more effective medications to both identify the allergen and nullify its effects. But a guaranteed or permanent cure for the sneezing and stuffy and drippy nose of allergic rhinitis is still a long way off.

OTITIS MEDIA

The ear is not typically thought of as being a part of the respiratory tract. But the fact that the middle ear space is lined by the same ciliated mucous membrane as the nose and sinuses, and is connected through the eustachian tube (also lined by the same respiratory epithelium) to the back of the nose and throat, technically establishes the middle ear as an integral component of the respiratory tract. It is also impacted by the same factors that adversely affect the nose, sinuses, and lungs, although not as directly. One Canadian study found that children exposed to secondhand cigarette smoke at home before age three are twice as likely to get serious, persistent or recurrent middle ear infections.

Middle ear infection, medically known as acute otitis media, is the most common diagnosis in children treated by physicians and accounts for nearly one third of all doctor's visits for children up to age five. Due to the position and anatomy of the eustachian tube, ear infections are very often seen in conjunction with acute sinusitis. The bacteria that most often cause this infection are the same as those responsible for sinus infections. I once heard an ENT physician say that anytime he sees an adult with otitis media, he or she always has an underlying sinus infection.

When otitis media is present, sinusitis may be ignored or even remain unrecognized. Young children will usually have a fever above 101°F. These patients are extremely uncomfortable, and their ear pain becomes the focus of attention for both doctor and patient. But unlike a blocked and infected sinus, the infected middle ear space has the opportunity to drain through the rupture of the eardrum. This common occurrence relieves the pain and often resolves the infection. The conventional medical treatment of otitis media is usually the same as that of acute sinusitis; therefore, if the diagnosis of sinusitis is missed, the sinus infection will usually get better anyway. In adults with otitis media, however, I would recommend more regular use of a decongestant than I would for children, and for a longer period of time (three times a day for at least ten days) than I would with sinusitis. This is because adults with middle ear infections routinely complain of "stuffiness" in their ears long after the pain has gone, even after two or three weeks.

Even though the evidence has been mounting that antibiotics are not effective against most middle ear infections (many are caused by a virus), particularly in children, and may even contribute to recurring infections because they interfere with the body's own immune system, the Centers for Disease Control and Prevention reports that they are prescribed for acute otitis media 99 percent of the time.

In a report released in 1994, the Project on Government Oversight, an independent watchdog group in Washington, said that a researcher at the National Academy of Sciences' Institute of Medicine concluded that antibiotics were no more effective than placebos in treating middle ear infections. Yet, the Department of Health and Human Services still recommends antibiotics for ear infections. The use of antibiotics can reduce the risk of the potentially serious complications of otitis media, such as mastoiditis (an infection of the bone behind the ear) and meningitis, which occurs in one out of four thousand ear infections. Analgesics and decongestants are also usually prescribed. Most effective for this acute problem are the decongestant nose drops.

Many young children have repeated episodes of acute otitis media, as often as four or five times a year. They usually begin with a cold. After multiple courses of antibiotics, many of these children are referred by their pediatrician or family doctor to an ENT physician, who will very often perform surgery. The procedure is one in which a tube (called a tympanostomy tube) is placed through the eardrum to facilitate drainage from the middle ear space. This is the most common operation for children that requires general anesthesia, numbering about one million procedures in the United States annually. Some studies have shown that this surgery results in a greater incidence of hearing loss than nonsurgical treatment.

This is not only unfortunate, in many cases it is also unnecessary. One study has found that about a quarter of middle-ear surgeries to insert tympanostomy tubes in children are "inappropriate." This study, published in the April 1994 issue of the *Journal of the American Medical Association,* also concluded that another one-third of these surgeries may be questionable. This means that several hundred thousand children in the United States may be having tubes surgically inserted in their ears that offer no demonstrated advantage over less invasive therapies, while also placing them at greater risk for undesirable outcomes.

As you can easily see, there is a clear and consistent pattern with the conventional medical treatment of the most common chronic respiratory diseases. The orientation is entirely on the body and, more specifically, treating the physical symptoms of one particular dysfunctional part. In searching for the causes of disease on only a microscopic, cellular, and tissue level, medical science narrows the focus even further, and usually fails to determine the source of illness. Why does one individual get sick, and another does not? What are the factors that weaken immunity, or maintain health? As a result of the physically limited and narrow disease-oriented scope of medical research, pharmaceutical drugs and surgery have become the primary, and almost only, weapons wielded by physicians in their battle against the enemy—disease. If it's infected or inflamed, then blast it with powerful antibiotics and corticosteroids. If too much histamine is being released, then counterattack with antihistamines. And if there is an obstruction preventing drainage, then cut it out or create a new opening.

This approach has been extremely successful at saving lives and in effectively treating acute illness. But for the most part, conventional medicine has failed to cure chronic disease. As you've just learned, the overuse of some of these medications has actually contributed to the epidemic of respiratory disease. The narrow perspective of the conventional approach has not allowed for the exploration of alternatives to surgery, resulting in many millions of unnecessary surgical procedures costing billions of dollars. While conventional medicine has brought us miraculous technological advances in treating disease, it has also taken us to the brink of financial ruin. The cost of health care in America currently exceeds $1 trillion. The "business of caring" has become much more of a business, with a lot less caring. Perhaps the time has come to heed the words of former Surgeon General C. Everett Koop, M.D., who continues to warn us: "Beware the medical-pharmaceutical complex!"

Chapter 6

HEALING YOUR BODY: PHYSICAL AND ENVIRONMENTAL HEALTH

I f you would rather not learn to live with your chronic sinusitis or allergies and a diminished quality of life, I would like to take you on a journey into an exciting new (yet ancient) frontier of medicine. For the past twelve years I have been practicing *holistic medicine* while treating respiratory disease and a variety of other so-called incurable conditions. The Sinus Survival Program, as outlined in chapters 6, 7, and 8 of this book, is the foundation of that practice. *Commitment* to this approach has resulted in at least a significant improvement or in most cases a cure of chronic sinusitis. This success stems primarily from the basic *health* orientation of the holistic approach. Rather than focusing on the disease and treating its symptoms—they are certainly not ignored, just perceived differently—holistic medicine addresses *causes* while restoring balance and harmony to the whole person. It goes far beyond the "quick fix" (outlined in Chapter 1) or the repair of a "broken part," and through *attentive listening* to your body, leads you to an understanding of what can be learned from your physical pain and to use that knowledge to change and heal your life. My own miserable sinuses have led me to a condition of health I never knew existed. I was guided on this healing path by the words of Hippocrates, "Physician, heal thyself." In the remainder of this book, I'd like to guide you on a similar path leading not only to the healing of your nose, sinuses, or anything else causing you dis-ease, but to a state of holistic health. By taking the Wellness Self-Test in Chapter 2, you can measure your present state of well-being. I'd recommend repeating this test every two or three months to gauge your progress.

In addressing causes, the holistic approach does not often lend itself to the "quick fix" to which our society has become so accustomed. Whether our need is for food, energy, information, entertainment, transportation, communication, or health care, we look to satisfy it in the fastest, simplest, and most effortless way. Science and technology have attempted to keep pace with our desire for speed and ease, and indeed they have performed incredible, at times almost miraculous, feats that have allowed an ease of living never before experienced in human history. However, there is a price to be paid for all of this comfort. Technology is helping us to destroy our environment—to pollute our air, poison our food and water, deplete our soil, thin our protective ozone layer, decimate our forests at the rate of one acre every second, and cause the extinction of nearly 100 species of plants and animals *daily!* Our own species, *Homo sapiens,* may not be far behind.

Sinus disease may be the proverbial canary in the coal mine. (Miners often take canaries with them into mines to use as an early-warning sign of oxygen depletion or of the presence of toxic gases. If the canaries die, the miners know it is time to get out of the mine.) There is already overwhelming evidence that the health of the entire human respiratory tract is rapidly deteriorating. More than one third of all Americans suffer from some form of respiratory disease, and more people are dying from asthma, chronic bronchitis, emphysema, and lung cancer than ever before. By destroying the quality of our air and our environment, we appear to be in the process of destroying ourselves. Many of us are becoming "human canaries," and it is time to get out of the "coal mine" and change the way we live as individuals and as a society.

CAUSES

Holistic medicine emphasizes harmony and integration within individuals, between them and their community, and with the planet itself. To address the burgeoning state of disharmony and imbalance that exists today both within our bodies and on the earth, we must begin by confronting the causes of our dis-ease and restoring our own health. I strongly believe that *air pollution* is the primary cause of the epidemic of respiratory disease. The mucous membrane lining the entire respiratory tract from the nose to the lungs is subjected to a relentless assault of toxic pollutants with almost every one of our 23,000 daily breaths.

If we were able to maintain a strong immune system, we might be able to withstand the onslaught of the pollutants without getting infected, allergic, asthmatic, or bronchitic. However, the combination of environmental and emotional toxins has significantly *weakened the human immune system*. In recent years we have developed a number of disorders related to an impaired immune system. These diseases, which were unknown or quite rare as recently as twenty years ago, are now turning into epidemics. The Epstein-Barr virus, the cause of mononucleosis, is now in part responsible for chronic fatigue syndrome. Besides the four respiratory diseases (asthma, chronic bronchitis, emphysema, and lung cancer), herpes simplex infections, candidiasis, "ecologic illness," lupus (systemic lupus erythematosus), multiple sclerosis, and AIDS (acquired immunodeficiency syndrome) are all examples of this phenomenon. As you will soon learn in the section about psychoneuroimmunology (Chapter 7), emotional stress can also have a profound impact on immune function. This is not a new development, but it is a relatively recent scientific discovery. The heightened stress levels pervading the planet, together with the environmental pollution, seem to have created a potentially devastating situation for normal immune function.

As more people contract these illnesses, the job of the primary care physician is becoming even more challenging than it already was. Managed care (HMOs, PPOs) has become the dominant force in America's health care system. The foundation of these medical insurance companies is built upon primary care physicians and the concepts of cost-effective and preventive medicine. Although they profess to want better health for their subscribers (HMO = Health Maintenance Organization), like any other business, their chief objective is to make money. One of the essential ways of attaining that goal is by insisting that all patients be seen first by a primary care physician. These family doctors, internists, and pediatricians are often overwhelmed with too many patients and can be financially penalized if they refer too many people to specialists. They have neither the time nor, in most cases, the training to teach their patients how to maintain good health. (Medical school is almost entirely focused on the diagnosis and treatment of disease.) The result is that not infrequently many physicians attempt to reduce medical costs by prescribing medication over the phone, thereby avoiding an office visit. They also save money for the insurance company by minimizing referrals to specialists and caring for more seriously ill patients than they did previously. (A 1997 survey of over 12,000 primary care doctors think the scope of care they are now expected to provide is too big.) The result of both of these common practices is that *antibiotics and corticosteroids are often over-prescribed,* which can lead to antibiotic-resistant supergerms, candidiasis, and immune suppression. This disturbing development is, sadly, another major contributor to the epidemic of respiratory disease, and has also resulted in significantly diminishing the quality of health care in this country.

Think of the Sinus Survival Program as a course in self-healing and optimal health. In this and the following two chapters, that follow, you will be provided with a prescription for improving six components of health, while treating each of the primary causes of sinusitis and allergies. I have referred to several books for those who would like to explore these areas in greater depth. I have tried to simplify each component and have suggested "exercises" to help you find your own path to a greater level of physical, environmental, mental, emotional, spiritual, and social fitness. These exercises must be practiced regularly in order to be effective. (However, if a particular exercise feels too uncomfortable to you, then stop.) If you are willing to be patient and practice—remember, it took years for you to develop your current state of health—I promise that you will feel better. Keep in mind that although this is a course with a lot of homework, there are no exams or grades, so enjoy yourself!

You will first learn how to heal the sensitive and "wounded" mucous membranes by nurturing them with optimal air and moisture and removing irritants from your environment. There are numerous methods to strengthen a weakened immune system and many treatment options in lieu of antibiotics and other powerful drugs with potentially harmful side effects. Although I infrequently prescribe most of these medications or recommend surgery, there are instances in which they are the preferable choice. Holistic medicine is *not* an alternative to conventional medicine but a complement. It is also the most therapeutically sound and cost-effective approach to the treatment of chronic disease that I've found in nearly thirty years of practicing medicine. By taking responsibility for your own health, you become not only your own healer but a highly skilled practitioner of preventive medicine as well. I believe that the holistic model for self-care presented on the following pages will become an essential part of the foundation of primary care medicine in the twenty-first century.

ENVIRONMENTAL HEALTH

Harmony with your environment (neither harming nor being harmed)
Awareness of your connectedness with nature
Feeling grounded
Respect and appreciation for your home, the Earth, and all of her inhabitants

Contact with the Earth; breathing healthy air; drinking pure
water; eating uncontaminated food; exposure to the sun, fire,
or candlelight; immersion in warm water (all on a daily basis)

Over the past decade I have met with air filtration, humidifica-
tion, negative ionization, and indoor air pollution experts; allergists; specialists in environmental medicine; and ecological
architects. With their guidance and their state-of-the-art technology, I have learned a great deal about environmental health.
The information that follows is a result of that education.

There is nothing more important to human health and survival than the quality of the air we breathe. The sinuses and the
nose, our first line of defense against unhealthy air, are a sensitive gauge of air quality. Ideal quality is rated by clarity (freedom
from pollutants), humidity (between 35 and 55 percent), temperature (between 65° and 85°F), oxygen content (21 percent of
total volume and 100 percent saturation), and negative ion content (3,000 to 6,000 .001-micron ions per cubic centimeter).
Air that is clean, moist, warm, oxygen rich, and high in negative
ions is the healthiest air a human being can breathe.

Not only are we dependent on oxygen for survival, but every
part of the human body thrives with a maximum supply of oxygen. If your respiratory tract is defective because of a nasal, sinus, or lung ailment, or if the amount of oxygen available in the
air is relatively low (for example, air high in carbon monoxide,
air at higher altitudes, or stale indoor air), your body is receiving
less than its optimal requirement of oxygen.

Negative ions are air molecules that have excess electrons.
Negative ions vitalize or freshen the air we breathe. The earth itself is a natural negative-ion generator. Health spas have always
been located in areas high in negative ions (3,000 to 20,000 per
cubic centimeter of air), such as along seacoasts, near rushing
streams and waterfalls, in mountainous areas, and in pine forests
(pine needles cause negative ions to be generated in the surrounding air). Although unproven, there is speculation that negative ions increase the sweeping motion of the cilia on the

respiratory mucosa, and subsequently enhance the movement of mucus and the clearing or filtering of inhaled pollutants. They also help to reduce pain, heal burns, suppress mold and bacterial growth, and stimulate plant growth, and they contribute greatly to our sense of well-being and comfort.

Positive ions, on the other hand, are air molecules lacking electrons. Pollen can carry fifty or more positive charges per grain of pollen. This positive charge slows the cilia and the clearing of mucus, and in so doing can cause some degree of nasal congestion. Most man-made pollutants result from combustion processes (auto/truck exhaust, smokestacks, cigarette smoke, etc.), which leave the pollutants with a positive charge. Heating and ventilation systems tend to produce air containing an excess of positive ions. Aircraft cabins have been tested and found to contain an excessively high amount of positive ions. This obviously contributes to the "stuffy" feeling of airplane air, and also helps to explain why so many of my patients have developed sinus infections following air travel.

The negative ion content of indoor air can be as low as 10 to 200 negative ions per cubic centimeter. This is considered to be "ion-depleted" air and is a significant component of "sick-building syndrome." Ion-depleted air is also created by heating/cooling systems; window air conditioners; air cleaners (including HEPA filters), which "scrub" negative ions from the air; and the screens of television sets and computers, which have a high positive charge that draws negative ions out of the air and neutralizes them. Most of the factors in our environment responsible for depleting the beneficial negative ions also produce an excess of unhealthy positive ions.

The majority of Americans spend 90 percent of their time indoors, where, the EPA says, the air can be as much as 100 times more polluted than outdoor air. Few of us live in clean, moist environments that are warm year-round; even fewer live in the mountains, on a beach, or in the woods. For the 92 million people whose sinuses, noses, and lungs are already feeling the pain that comes from breathing unhealthy air, and for anyone else who wants to enjoy optimum health, here are some ways to minimize the risks of breathing poor-quality air and to prevent respiratory disease.

Location

Where we live, work, play, or otherwise spend our time is critical to our health. If you are considering a move and need help in evaluating a potential location, use this list from Richard L. Crowther's book *Indoor Air: Risks and Remedies:*

- Locate in houses and buildings that minimize the impact of outdoor air pollution.
- Locate in a city, town, or county that has minimal air pollution.
- Locate on a hill rather than in a valley, where pollution is more apt to concentrate.
- Do not locate near a major highway or traffic intersection.
- Do not locate next to a parking lot.
- Do not locate downwind from a power plant, chemical plant, or processing plant.
- Do not locate near industrial operations.
- Do not locate near businesses that emit pollutants.
- Do not locate near a railroad line that carries hazardous materials.
- Do not locate near airfields.
- Do not locate on land farmed with pesticides and chemical fertilizers.
- Locate away from agricultural fields that are sprayed.
- Do not live under or near high-voltage power lines.
- Locate away from stagnant waterways.
- Locate out of the air pollution or "seepage" range of oil or gas wells.
- Locate a safe distance from any mining operations.
- Locate close to a park, near a forest, or within a natural setting.

- Locate in a small, healthful rural or seacoast community.
- Consider the effect of altitude on air quality.
- Consider prevailing daily and seasonal wind patterns.
- Before moving to a city, review an air quality record of the past several years.
- In urban or rural locations, consider sites for passive solar orientation and exposure.
- South-sloping sites are preferable for drainage and solar advantage.
- Avoid being in a "shadow path" during winter months in a cold climate.
- Avoid sites with high levels of radon or radioactivity.
- Before buying a property, get soil, radon, and water tests (if a well is planned).
- Check municipal water quality.

In addition, if allergies are a problem for you, it would be helpful to check with the local allergy society on the predominant allergens in that area. I would also suggest living there for at least one month before making the commitment to move.

It is unlikely that all of these locational criteria can be met, but they can provide a basis for a thorough evaluation. If you are going to relocate and have the freedom to choose, avoid the following regions: southern California, the Northeast, and the Texas Gulf Coast. The healthiest air can be found along the West Coast (with the distinct exception of the Los Angeles metropolitan area and southward), rural areas along the Gulf Coast (other than Texas), and the west coast of Florida. I used to think that Hawaii was the optimum healthy environment until I heard from a *Sinus Survival* reader living on the big island of Hawaii. He told me that both he and his wife had recently developed terrible sinus problems, as had many of their friends. For nearly fourteen years the active volcanoes on that island have been spewing lava (600,000 cubic yards per day) and volcanic ash. When the lava hits the ocean water, it produces hydrochloric acid. This in combination with the ash has created a serious problem of toxic visible pollution that is threatening to ruin "paradise," or at least the respiratory tracts of many of its residents, and some of the aesthetic value of Hawaii as well. Apparently this volcanic pollution is, to some degree, affecting most of the Hawaiian islands and has resulted in many people moving back to the mainland.

Ecological Architecture

If you are contemplating the construction of a new home, the concept of ecological architecture could help considerably in creating a healthy environment. *Ecology* is defined in Webster's *New World Dictionary* as "the branch of biology that deals with the relationship between living organisms and their environment." Used as a modifier for the word *architecture,* it simply means the design of a dwelling that is sensitive to human health and gentle to the earth. Once we have considered the microclimate and the site, our biological needs, behavior patterns, and, most important, our budgetary limitations, nature will then dictate the design. Self-sufficiency through use of sun, air, earth, and water for heating, cooling, ventilation, and even electrical power is a realistic goal of an ecological design.

Common objectives regarding construction methods and materials include:

- Avoiding the use of plastic or other materials made of toxic ingredients that harmfully outgas (give off toxins and/or fumes) in the indoor environment
- Using nontoxic natural materials in preference to synthetic materials
- Designing with concern for sensitivities, allergies, or chronic health problems
- Being aware that nature's ecologic sustainability and well-being should not be diminished by what is built
- Taking the responsibility to conceive, design, build, and furnish a home or building to a "healthy home" ecological ethic

This is a holistic approach emphasizing the ecological bond between site and architecture. Preservation and wise use of our planet's resources in construction and throughout the lifetime of a home is fundamental to ecological design. For the sinus sufferer, a home must be clean, moist, warm, and oxygen and negative ion rich. The fact that it is designed in harmony with the atmosphere and the earth makes this an environmentally healthy concept.

I fully appreciate that most readers of this book will neither move nor design their own home as a result of what they read here. However, I want to present as many environmental treatment options as possible. Each can have a profound impact on your state of health and ultimately your quality of life.

Healthy Homes

You can create an oasis of healthy indoor air in your own home. In the desert an oasis provides water. In the sea of hazardous air in which we live, a healthy home or business can provide an oasis in which to breathe life-enhancing air.

Solving the problem of indoor air pollution entails both treatment and prevention. There is a company in Denver, called Healthy Habitats, that has been on the leading edge of this field for about twelve years. The owner of the company, Carl Grimes, has worked with me and a number of my patients to transform our unhealthy homes and offices into healthy ones. The procedures and techniques he employs adhere to the following guidelines:

- Prevention—avoid bringing pollutants into the home and workplace.
- Identify the source and develop a plan for isolating or removing the pollutant from the "breathing zone," or the surrounding area from which you obtain your breathing air, e.g., an infant's breathing zone includes the floor and carpeting.
- Reduce ambient pollution with ventilation, filtration, and ionization.

Grimes considers the three primary sources of pollution to be:

- Particulates—dust, pollen, dander, construction debris, and smoke
- Microorganisms—bacteria, viruses, molds, and dust mites
- Chemicals— personal care products, cleaning products, office equipment, and building/construction materials (see Table 3.1)

The type of treatment depends upon the type of pollution. For example, HEPA filtration might be used for particulates, charcoal for chemicals, and the drying of a wet crawl space could be the best option for eliminating microbes. Ozone has also been effective for persistent microorganisms; however, when a home is cleaned with ozone, the residents are advised to vacate the premises for two to three days.

Molds are rapidly becoming one of America's chief health hazards and one of the leading causes of chronic sinusitis. The 300 percent increase in asthma over the past twenty years has also been linked to molds. In addition to the overuse of antibiotics, many of us are being exposed daily to high levels of mold. The problem has resulted primarily from modern home design—more airtight, with air-conditioning and heating systems recirculating contaminated air; materials used; and most importantly *water leaks.* Molds can grow wherever it's damp, so it's important to quickly fix any leaks, regularly clean air ducts and furnace filters, be on the lookout for discoloration of walls or ceilings and any unusual odors, and empty (daily) and clean (weekly) humidifiers on a regular basis.

Several excellent books are available on the subject of healthy homes. Those that I recommend are: *Starting Points for a Healthy Habitat,* by Carl Grimes (GMC Media); *The Nontoxic Home and Office* by Debra Lynn Dadd (Jeremy P. Tarcher, Inc.); *The Healthy House* by John Bower (Lyle Stuart, Inc.); and *Your Home, Your Health and Well-Being* by David Rousseau (Ten Speed Press).

Air Cleaners and Negative-Ion Generators

As many as one million hospital admissions a year are attributed to poor indoor air quality. In recent years, as the EPA and private health organizations have publicized the problem of indoor air pollution, we have seen a proliferation of several hundred types of air cleaners, almost as many as there are indoor air pollutants. According to Michael Berry, Ph.D., former manager of the EPA's Indoor Air Project, the most potentially harmful pollutants are radon and the "biologicals," including pollen, mold, plant spores, dust mites, bacteria, and viruses. The pollutants most harmful to the respiratory tract are less than one micron in size. Regardless of their origin, size, or health-damaging effects, air pollutants can be described as free-floating particles in the air. Figure 6.1 shows the specific size ranges of the most common pollutants. The unit of measurement used for tiny air particles is the micron. An average hair strand is 100 microns thick, and about 400 one-micron particles would fit into the dot over the *i* in the word *micron*. The primary job of air cleaners is to remove as many of these particles as possible, the biologicals as well as the combustion products, particulates, chemicals, fumes, and odors (see Table 3.1). Radon, if present, requires the sealing of basement cracks and improvement of basement ventilation. Most air cleaners do not remove radon from the air. However, some air cleaners with high particle removal efficiency (HEPA, etc.) can remove some of the radon "daughters" (attached radon) that are in particulate form. A study at the Harvard School of Public Health determined that a negative-ion generator is a highly effective means of removing the attached fraction of radon (the radon daughters), although it does not reduce the unattached (gaseous) fraction of radon.

The strategy for solving the problem of indoor air pollution involves air cleaning and improved ventilation. Air cleaning devices can include furnace filters, portable stand-alone units, and negative ion generators. The efficiency of air cleaners is evaluated by their ability to filter a certain percentage of a certain size

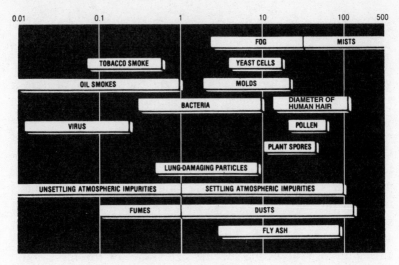

FIGURE 6.1. *Relative size of common air contaminants.*

of pollutant. The HEPA filter (an acronym for high-efficiency particulate arrestor) removes 97 percent of all 0.3-micron particulates and larger. This includes pollen, plant spores, most animal dander, dust, wood, and tobacco smoke, fumes, bacteria, and some viruses. This type of filter is standard equipment for most hospital operating suites, and is found in many of the more expensive freestanding air cleaners. It requires a strong fan or a booster fan to move air through it due to its increased efficiency.

The ULPA (Ultra Low Penetrating Air) filters were originally created to purify the air in semiconductor clean rooms. The Bionaire company has now made this new technology available to clean the air in homes. ULPA air purifiers are equipped with a superfine filter that removes a remarkable 99.999 percent of all airborne particles as small as 0.1 micron. The filter traps such allergens as tobacco smoke, pollen, dust, dust mites, mold, and bacteria. For best performance, it is recommended that ULPA filters be changed every six months to one year.

Negative-ion generators were originally designed to restore a more natural and beneficial level of negative ions to indoor air.

In the course of their use for biological benefit, it was discovered that free-floating ions quickly attach to airborne particles and cause them to agglomerate and precipitate from the air, or be drawn to grounded surfaces such as walls, metal surfaces, etc. Ionizers are highly effective air cleaners, removing particles as small as .001 micron, which would include viruses, dust, pollen, cigarette smoke, and all other airborne particulate pollutants. Compared to air cleaners with fans or blowers, ionizers are more likely to be operated full-time since they are totally silent (no fan) and consume only pennies of electricity per month.

However, in order to increase the speed with which an ionizer cleans the air, many manufacturers produce ionizers with excessive ion output. This has two undesirable effects: (1) The ion density established by these ionizers exceeds many times the natural range found outdoors, resulting in much the same adverse effects as breathing air with too few negative ions. A well-designed negative-ion generator will generate enough ions to be effective but will not exceed an upper limit that would make it biologically undesirable. (2) An excessively high ion density also causes a significant amount of pollutants to be driven to the walls and other grounded surfaces, resulting in the buildup of a dirty residue. Again, a well-designed ion generator will minimize such "plating," and this effect can be further reduced by placing the ionizer at least two feet from the nearest wall.

It has been my good fortune, and that of my patients, to have worked with a "pioneer" in negative-ion technology. For nearly thirty years Rex Coppom, owner of Air Tech International in Longmont, Colorado, has been developing state-of-the-art negative-ion generators. For almost eight years many of my patients have been using his Sinus Survival Air Vitalizer, a small unit that will clean the air of a 150- to 200-square-foot room and maintain an ideal level of negative ions. It costs $150, which is about one half to one third the price of a HEPA room air cleaner, which is somewhat less efficient in its cleaning capacity and has no negative ions. I have received many testimonials about its beneficial effects—dramatic headache relief, diminished nasal congestion, cessation of snoring, better sleep, more energy, fewer allergy and asthma attacks, general feelings of well-being, and diminished odor and symptoms resulting from secondhand cigarette smoke. I was amazed at how quickly it cleared the smoke from my kitchen during an oven-cleaning session that went somewhat awry. Ionization equipment is currently available for automobiles and aircraft cabins—both of which have far less than optimum air.

Electronic air cleaners (both central and freestanding) produce positive ions as they filter the air. On their first day of operation they are 85 percent efficient on all 1-micron particles and larger, but in order to maintain that efficiency they require cleaning every two weeks. For most of us, this makes them impractical and inconvenient. They also produce ozone, which, as discussed in Chapter 3, can be a potential health hazard.

To obtain a furnace filter, go to a hardware or building-supply store. Many of them carry the 3M pleated filter, under the brand names Filtret and Electret. These are excellent furnace filters and cost about $15. They should be replaced every one to two months during the winter and while central air conditioners are being run regularly. They are far more efficient than the $2 to $4 varieties found in supermarkets. There are several other brands of pleated furnace filters which are similar in efficiency to 3M.

The Dupont Wizard dust cloth is an interesting product that does a better job of dusting than can be obtained from liquid or spray dust cleaners. They are used dry, can be washed, and cost $2.

Air Duct Cleaning

When the air duct system of my thirteen-year-old home was cleaned for the first time, I was amazed at what emanated from the ducts after two hours of high-intensity vacuuming. I thought to myself, "It's no wonder I suffered with sinus problems for so long!" If the air ducts are filthy, it is nearly impossible for your furnace filter to clean the air in your home. After the air is filtered, it still has to travel through the ducts before you breathe it. I recommend air duct cleaning as part of the environmental treatment program. Depending on the size of your home, an air duct cleaning service, using good equipment, could cost between $200 and $250. To find this type of company in your city, look in the Yellow Pages under "Furnaces, Cleaning and Repairing."

Carpet Cleaning

Carpets are one of the most common sources of indoor air pollutants. They are excellent traps and hold on to dust, pollen, and microorganisms. While this helps to keep those particles out of the breathing zone, their gradual accumulation can become great enough to create a sustainable culture of bacteria, yeast, dust mites, and mold. In fact, many allergists recommend that their patients dispose of all their carpets.

While it is true that carpets harbor pollutants, it is possible to keep them clean. This poses a challenge to the homemaker. Conventional vacuum cleaners are designed to remove and retain the visible dirt, which means particles greater than 10 microns. Most of the particles and microorganisms that are too small to be seen are also smaller than the pores in the vacuum cleaner bag. This allows most of them to blow through the bag and into the room, settling back onto the carpets and furniture. If a forced-air heating system is running, the airborne particles can be drawn into the air ducts, contributing to their contamination as well. Also, as the bag fills, airflow decreases, causing uneven cleaning.

To prevent these problems I suggest a vacuum cleaner that uses either a HEPA-type filter or water-capture. Either one removes even subvisible dust and bacteria from the air. The water-capture types also have a continuously maximum airflow because they won't clog like a bag or filter. Both of these vacuums are expensive, costing between $500 and $1,000.

However, there is a much less expensive alternative. Dupont Hysurf vacuum cleaner bags have 1-micron pores and cost only $5. They appear to have the equivalent cleaning efficiency of the $500-plus "allergy" vacuum cleaners. Their major problem is that they are difficult to find. Some janitorial supply houses and medical supply stores have them. They can also be obtained from Sinus Survival Products.

Many people have their carpets professionally cleaned. However, due to their chemical composition, the most common cleaning agents are often worse than having dirty carpets. Alcohols, petroleum distillates, ammonia, dry-cleaning substances, and scents often cause headaches, mental "fuzziness," lethargy, and a general feeling of discomfort. Cleaning-agent residues may often cause respiratory irritation.

Before contracting with a carpet cleaner, check his references and insist on a non-scented cleaning agent that uses no petroleum distillates, alcohol, ammonia, dry-cleaning-type chemicals or enzymes, and has no suds that can be left in the carpet. Check his work to be sure he leaves no damp areas. This ensures maximum removal of all agents and enhances drying time. If the carpet stays wet for several days, bacteria and molds can grow rapidly.

Ventilation, Oxygen, and Plants

All indoor spaces, whether residential, commercial, industrial, or recreational, require some type of ventilation to provide breathable air for occupants, to furnish combustion air for cooking and heating, and to remove stale air filled with toxins and particulates. Commercial buildings are required by code to have even more efficient ventilation systems than residences. The American Society of Heating, Refrigerating and Air-Conditioning Engineers (ASHRAE) says that air should be replaced at the rate of 15 cubic feet per minute per person, but most systems fall below this minimum standard.

Improving ventilation will help relieve indoor air pollution as long as the outdoor air isn't dirtier than the air it is replacing. Local pollution sources, such as fumes from toxic waste leakage, wood burning, a neighboring industrial plant, a heavily trafficked highway, or crop spraying can render outdoor air unacceptable for indoor ventilation. Several days a year Los Angeles residents are advised to keep all windows and doors closed and ventilation ducts shut to prevent the heavily polluted outdoor air from entering homes and businesses. In areas like this it becomes a challenge to balance the health benefit of highly oxygenated outdoor air and the liability of the pollutants that come with it. Outdoor aerobic exercise presents a similar dilemma. If you live in a heavily polluted environment, I recommend exercising outside and ventilating your home and office well when outdoor air is good, but exercise indoors and keep windows and doors closed during periods of heavy pollution.

Air-conditioning systems are a helpful means of ventilation for people with respiratory and allergy problems. These systems remove excess moisture from the air, lowering its temperature. In less humid conditions there is a reduction of molds and spores, and with the windows closed there is also a marked decrease in pollen from the outdoors. Air conditioning, however, does deplete negative ions from the air.

Natural cross-ventilation is effective in reducing indoor air pollution if the placement of the intake vents is low and the outlets for the flow-through air are high. Operable windows on commercial buildings and a good location for the outdoor air intake—away from garage entrances or loading docks—are also important factors in improving indoor air quality. Mechanical ventilation with exhaust fans can certainly help in removing indoor pollutants, but such fans are most efficient when used in a confined space. Private offices or single-occupant rooms where smoking, cooking, and other fume-producing activities take place are ideal environments for mechanical ventilation.

Rooms producing commercial toxic or odoriferous fumes; spaces subject to bacterial and viral contamination, such as rest rooms; and indoor areas that present specific respiratory hazards all need optimized ventilation. Mold is a special problem in moist conditions. Adequate ventilation along with sunshine can help to reduce moisture and subsequently suppress mold.

The technology of ventilation can be complex, but the basic principle of displacing interior air with outdoor air and increasing the rate of fresh airflow is critical to treating the problem of indoor air pollution. Besides natural cross-ventilation and exhaust fans, other devices used to enhance ventilation and indoor air quality are air-to-air heat exchangers, makeup air units, attic fans, vortex fans, and ceiling fans. Remember that even if the "fresh" air is filthy, an effective air cleaner combined with good ventilation is still a winning combination.

Adequate ventilation not only helps reduce indoor air pollution but is the primary source of indoor oxygen. Plants can offer an aesthetically pleasant secondary source. Although the oxygen output from indoor plants is not great, plants with large leaf surfaces that grow rapidly are capable of enhancing air quality. Attached greenhouses and atria filled with plants that effectively absorb carbon dioxide and oxygenate the air (spider plants do this very well) can improve the indoor environment while humidifying the air.

In the early 1990s, studies conducted at the John Stennis Space Center in Mississippi showed that plants can also act as effective filters. Former NASA scientist Bill C. Wolverton, Ph.D., has spent the past thirty years studying the ability of plants to clear volatile organic chemicals from indoor air. Wolverton predicts that within twenty years plants will be governmentally mandated in new buildings as a matter of public health.

According to the EPA, the most plentiful of the organic chemicals in the average indoor environment is formaldehyde. It is released from a host of household furnishings, including synthetic carpeting, particleboard (used to make bookcases, desks, and tables), foam insulation, upholstery, curtains, and even so-called air fresheners. Common house plants such as chrysanthemums, striped dracaena, dwarf date palms, and especially Boston ferns are excellent filters for removing formaldehyde. Spider plants are also effective in removing carbon monoxide; areca palms are best at filtering xylene, the second most prevalent indoor organic chemical; and English ivy is good for filtering benzene, ranked third on the EPA's list. Aloe vera, philodendron, pothos, and ficus were also found to reduce levels of organic chemicals.

The Foliage for Clean Air Council, a communications clear-inghouse for information on the use of foliage to improve indoor air quality, recommends a minimum of two plants per 100 square feet of floor space in an average home with eight- to ten-foot ceilings.

Plants can help improve indoor air as oxygenators, filters, and humidifiers.

Prevention

Prevention of indoor air pollution involves eliminating pollutants at the source. Doctors who specialize in environmental medicine and some allergists can do skin and blood tests to help you identify pollutants to which you are particularly sensitive or allergic. These doctors are not always easy to find, nor are the tests always definitive, but they can help. With the use of environmentally sensitive architectural principles, a healthier home can be created. A major preventive strategy is the use of interior materials that emit no pollutants. Natural products such as wood, cotton, and metals are preferable to the lower-cost synthetic materials such as particleboard, fiberboard, polyester, and plastics.

Choosing to forgo a fireplace or wood-burning stove would be helpful, as would using a high-efficiency furnace with a sealed combustion unit to vent exhaust gases to the outside. Switch to nontoxic cleaning substances, including ordinary soap, vinegar, zephiran, and Air Therapy. (You can find a listing of such cleaners in *Nontoxic, Natural, & Earthwise,* by Debra Lynn Dadd.) Smoking should be relegated to the outdoors or to a well-ventilated enclosed space. If radon levels exceed the acceptable EPA standard of 4 picoCuries per liter of air, radon control measures should be implemented. Formaldehyde from insulation can be eliminated by using the substitutes of cellulose and white fiberglass insulation.

Humidification

According to Dr. Marshall Plaut, chief of the asthma and allergy branch at the National Institute of Allergy and Infectious Diseases (part of NIH), "Dry air triggers asthma and nasal congestion." I, too, have been convinced for quite some time that dry air, and especially cold and dry air, is a major contributor to sinusitis and chronic bronchitis. As a chronic irritant to the sensitive nasal mucous membrane, dry air can also contribute to a greater susceptibility to allergies. Studies on patients with allergic rhinitis have shown that warm, moist air can improve nasal congestion and other allergy symptoms.

Optimum indoor air quality requires air containing between 35 and 55 percent relative humidity. Moisture provided by room humidifiers can greatly benefit anyone with a respiratory condition. These humidifiers are most helpful in the winter (heavy "sinus season" runs from November through March), even in humid, cold-weather climates, because most heating systems dry the indoor air considerably.

Room humidifiers, also called tabletop models, have sufficient capacity to humidify a medium- to large-size room. Each type has some drawbacks. Ultrasonic models can emit an irritating white dust. So can cool mist models, which require the use of distilled water or an expensive demineralization cartridge, unless you have very soft water. Steam-mist models, also called vaporizers, can scald if you get too close to the mist they produce or if you tip them over by accident. Evaporative models, the most prevalent type, can become a breeding ground for bacteria. The warm-mist units are my first choice. They produce a mist just slightly warmer than room air, use tap water, require no filter, and are able to kill bacteria. Their only drawback may be that they use more electricity than the other types. I've been quite pleased with the performance of the Bionaire Clear Mist 5 (CMP-5), a warm-mist unit that I have used for the past six winter seasons. The tabletop humidifiers can cost from $30 to $120.

The larger humidifiers, called consoles, can humidify an average-size house, cost from $100 to $200, and are all the evaporative type. Although I've had no personal experience with these, I know that *Consumer Reports* has given a high rating to the Bionaire W-6S, as well as to the Toastmaster 3435 and Emerson HD850.

Central or in-duct humidifiers, those that attach to the furnace, are more convenient but often do not humidify an individual room as well as a portable humidifier can when the door to the room is closed. In the past the major problem with central humidifiers has been that most of them were the reservoir type, with a tray of standing water that breeds mold and bacteria. I recommend the flow-through type of central humidifier, e.g., Aprilaire or General, which eliminates the stagnant water problem and is easy to maintain. Depending on the model, size of your home, and installation, this humidifier would probably cost about $250 to $650.

Humidifiers are not the only option for moisturizing your home. The installation of waterfalls, indoor spas, and swimming pools will all add a lot of moisture to the house, but of course they are expensive to install and maintain. It may surprise you to learn that even the moisture from human breath and sweat, along with that from cooking, baths, showers, and plants, adds significantly to a home's humidity. If your bedroom is dry, hang a wet towel on a hanger in the room.

If you rarely suffer jolts of static electricity when you touch metal objects such as doorknobs, then the air in your home is probably humid enough. For a more precise test, you'll need a hygrometer. You can find these humidity measuring devices at most hardware stores. The one I've been using is the Bionaire Climate Check, a digital device that measures both temperature and humidity.

PHYSICAL HEALTH

High energy and vitality
Freedom from, or high adaptability to, pain, dysfunction, and
   disability

A strong immune system
A body that feels light, balanced, strong, flexible, and has good
  aerobic capacity
Ability to meet physical challenges
Full capacity of all five senses and a healthy libido

After almost thirty years as a family physician, it has become
quite clear to me that for anyone experiencing physical discomfort, life is not much fun. I am assuming that the majority of you
have either chronic sinusitis or allergies. There is probably a
small percentage of readers suffering from something other than
a respiratory ailment and an even smaller group who feel fine
physically but are interested in experiencing a greater degree of
health. I am making an educated guess that most of you would
not have gone to the trouble of buying and reading this book if
you do not have at least one very uncomfortable physical symptom that has not been relieved with the treatment you've been
using. The focus of holistic medicine is on restoring health to
the whole person—body, mind, and spirit—and on addressing
the causes of dis-ease. But I have found that it's extremely difficult for individuals to improve their mental or spiritual health if
their bodies are not functioning properly and they're in constant
pain, having trouble breathing, or have no energy.

The holistic approach to physical fitness will allow you to develop far greater awareness and appreciation for your body. You
will learn how to listen to the messages your body is communicating on a daily basis and allow your body to heal itself.
Through this heightened sensitivity you will develop more vitality and energy, a more powerful immune system, and the ability to perform personally challenging physical feats. But your
first order of physical "business" is "to get rid of this damn
_____!"

Symptom Treatment

I would recommend beginning the Sinus Survival Program with
an aggressive approach to treating the symptoms of your sinusi-

tis or allergies, or any other chronic condition. This includes consulting with your physician and making sure that you have treated your ailment with the best methods that conventional medicine has to offer, even if they provide only symptomatic relief. However, it is essential that you try to determine if the benefits of that treatment, such as drugs and surgery, outweigh the liabilities. As I've previously mentioned, in the case of chronic sinusitis, the continued use of antibiotics (more than three courses within a six-month period) is potentially more of a detriment than an asset. If you have been taking multiple antibiotics for months or years, follow the recommendations in this chapter, especially those for treating candida. They will provide you with a natural, safe, and effective alternative to the chronic use of antibiotics, while you undo the damage done by the antibiotics. I realize that it may sound like too great a risk, but stopping antibiotics is invariably the first step most of my patients must take before they can cure chronic sinusitis. But suppose you've started on the Sinus Survival Program and then develop a sinus infection, which is certainly not an uncommon occurrence. (Remember this is a healing *process,* not an instant cure, and you have yet to address all of the possible factors that trigger your infections.) In this instance, if you then follow all of the recommendations in the "treating sinusitis" column in the table on pages 13–15 for ten days to two weeks and see *no* improvement, then you might consider taking an antibiotic. Although this situation rarely occurs, it can happen.

As you begin the Sinus Survival Program, it is often helpful to rate each of your symptoms on a scale of 1 to 10, with 1 being an almost incapacitating symptom and 10 being perfectly normal (no symptom). You can use the Symptom Chart (pp. 125–126) and rate yourself at the end of each week. It provides you with both an objective (most of the symptoms can be measured objectively—you can either see, hear, or feel them) and subjective (especially energy level) means of monitoring your progress. You don't need anyone else or an X ray or lab test to tell you how well you're doing.

The foundation of the physical aspect of holistic medical treatment is to love and nurture your body with safe and gentle therapies. You should have a much better idea of how to do that, especially for your respiratory tract, after reading this chapter. Remember that the essentials of the Physical and Environmental Health Components of the Sinus Survival Program are condensed in tables 1.1, 1.2, and 1.3 on pages 13–16 and again in this chapter on pages 183–186.

GOALS

The primary goals of the Physical and Environmental Health Components of the Sinus Survival Program are:

(1) To heal the mucous membranes lining the nose, sinuses, and lungs
(2) To strengthen the immune system
(3) To significantly reduce the overgrowth of *Candida albicans* (yeast)

As you begin this physical and environmental approach to treating your symptoms, remember the images that I've mentioned earlier in the book—the fine sandpaper abrading the sensitive mucous membranes, or the onslaught of pollutants assaulting the lining of the entire respiratory tract with every breath, 23,000 times a day. *It is the healing of this chronically irritated and inflamed mucous membrane that should now become the object of your treatment plan.* This dysfunctional and weakened membrane is a primary cause of most of your symptoms. Suppose you now replace that earlier image of assaulting with one of gently caressing and bathing that delicate mucosa with perfectly fresh, clean, warm, and moist air with every breath you take. You're loving and nurturing your nose and sinuses. This healing vision can be expanded in any way you'd like. But it is important to keep it in mind, since it will help to keep you on the right track as you choose different treatment options. For instance, if your nose is really stuffed up, you may opt for soothing steam rather

Symptom Chart

Began Sinus Survival Program on _____
Rate Symptoms from 1 (worst) to 10 (best = normal)

SYMPTOM	BEGIN ____ (date)	END WEEK 1	END WEEK 2	END WEEK 3	END WEEK 4	END WEEK 5	END WEEK 6	END WEEK 7	END WEEK 8	END WEEK 9	END WEEK 10	END WEEK 11	END WEEK 12
Head congestion (fullness)													
Nasal congestion (stuffy nose)													
Postnasal drip													
Headache													
Yellow/green mucus (from nose)													
Yellow/green mucus (back of throat)													
Sneezing													
Itching: nose, throat													
Ear congestion (ears plugged up)													
Sore throat													
Swollen glands (in neck)													
Cough—dry													

SYMPTOM	BEGIN ____ (date)	END WEEK 1	END WEEK 2	END WEEK 3	END WEEK 4	END WEEK 5	END WEEK 6	END WEEK 7	END WEEK 8	END WEEK 9	END WEEK 10	END WEEK 11	END WEEK 12
Cough—wet/mucusy													
Shortness of breath													
Wheezing													
Fatigue (rate energy level)													
Avg no. of hrs. sleep													
Other symptoms:													
Medications: (pharmaceutical drugs) (use a "√" if still taking drug)													
Vitamins/herbs supplements (use a "√" if still taking)													

than blast your already inflamed membranes with a decongestant nasal spray. It works almost as quickly; it's just not quite as
convenient. But most important, it heals rather than harms as it
treats your symptoms.

AIR AND BREATHING

The first step is to change the quality of the indoor air you're
breathing—in essence, to create healing rather than harmful or
irritating air. All of the recommendations mentioned in the
"Environmental Health" section are helpful. But at the very
least I would start with a negative-ion generator in your bedroom and, if you can afford it, in your workplace as well. Within
three to four weeks I would add a warm-mist humidifier in the
bedroom, along with plants in the house, an effective furnace
filter, followed by air duct and carpet cleaning. If the expense
does not deter you, then a central humidifier installed on the
furnace will complete your indoor air enhancement program.
You may not create optimal indoor air, but you'll be close. Try
to keep your thermostat between 65° and 70° F, and relative
humidity between 35 and 55 percent. It is also helpful to have an
instrument that measures both humidity and temperature. I use
the Bionaire Climate Check.

There may be nothing more important to our health than the
quality of the air we breathe, but the way in which we breathe
is also essential. We can live for weeks without food and days
without water, but if we stop breathing for more than two or
three minutes, we die. Breathing is the single most important
physical function we perform, yet almost all of us breathe inefficiently. For the most part we aren't even conscious of our
breath, and spend hour after hour breathing shallowly into the
chest, depriving ourselves of the tremendous energy and revi-
talizing power that proper breathing can provide.

The primary purpose of breathing is to deliver **oxygen** to
every cell in every tissue and organ in the body while removing
carbon dioxide. Oxygen's primary role in the body is to produce

the energy required for every basic bodily function via its inter-action with ATP. Since the cellular content of ATP is responsi-ble for the body's total energy levels and its ability to perform all of its functions, adequate oxygen levels are essential for our overall health. When our oxygen intake is reduced, ATP is di-minished as well.

A variety of environmental factors can also contribute to oxygen deficiency, including high carbon monoxide and smoke pollution, smog, and high altitude. (Oxygen content decreases by over 3 percent every thousand feet above sea level.) The pri-mary cause of chronic reduced oxygen levels in the body, how-ever, is due to shallow and inefficient breathing patterns. Typically, most of us habitually breathe in through the chest, failing to breathe deeply and fully. This unconscious and ineffi-cient method of breathing significantly reduces our oxygen sup-ply. By simply learning how to improve the way you breathe, you can considerably improve your health and ensure that your cells remain in an oxygen–rich state.

Breathing through the abdomen instead of through the chest is a simple yet powerful way to improve energy and flow of oxy-gen, enhance digestion, relieve stomach pain and flatulence, and diminish stress. Since most of us rarely breathe through our bel-lies, learning to do so at first may seem odd. Yet, *abdominal* breathing is easy to do. Just direct your breath in and out through your belly. If you do so correctly, your chest will not move. You can easily check this by placing one hand on your belly and the other on your chest. As you breathe, the lower hand should move, while the hand on your chest should remain motionless.

Don't get discouraged if you are unable to accomplish this on your first try. Make it a practice to spend a few minutes each day breathing abdominally (working up to 20 to 30 minutes a day is recommended), along with regular brief sessions whenever you notice yourself feeling tense or irritable. Abdominal breathing can also be performed in conjunction with meditation (see Chapter 8).

WATER, MOISTURE, AND NASAL HYGIENE

Next to oxygen, **water** is our most essential nutrient, and drinking enough water to satisfy your body's needs may be the simplest, least expensive self-help measure you can adopt to maintain your overall good health, in addition to the health of your mucous membranes.

Our adult bodies are 60 to 70 percent water (an infant's body is about 80 percent), and water is the medium through which every bodily function occurs. It is the basis of all body fluids, including blood, digestive juices, urine, lymph, and perspiration, which explains why we would die within a few days without water.

Water is vital to metabolism and digestion and helps prevent both constipation and diarrhea. It is also critical to healthy nerve impulse conduction and brain function. Some of water's other vital functions in the body are:

- Enhancing oxygen uptake into the bloodstream (the surface of the lungs must be moistened with water to facilitate oxygen intake and the excretion of carbon dioxide)
- Maintaining a high urine volume, helping to prevent kidney stones and urinary tract infections
- Regulating body temperature through perspiration
- Maintaining and increasing the health of the skin
- Maintaining adequate fluid for the lubrication of the joints and enhancing muscular function, particularly during and after exercise or other strenuous activity
- Moistening the mucous membranes of the respiratory tract, which in turn increases resistance to infection and allows the sinuses to drain more easily

Because water is so important to our health, all of us need to make a conscious effort to stay well hydrated, since most of us lose water faster than we replace it. For example, we lose one pint of water each day simply through exhalation. We also lose the same amount through perspiration, as well as three additional pints per day through urination and defecation. Exercise and heat exposure, especially in a dry climate, also increase water loss in the body. The percentage of body water content also decreases with age. All told, on average, each of us loses two and a half quarts of water (80 ounces) per day under normal conditions. Therefore, it is essential that the same amount or more be replenished daily.

Unfortunately, most Americans don't come close to consuming that much water per day. As a result, many of us are chronically dehydrated. When we think of dehydration, we may envision a lost soul in the desert, dying of thirst. However, most conditions of dehydration are not that dramatic, so that dehydration all too often is unsuspected and therefore undiagnosed. Meanwhile, its insidious effects can wreak havoc on our health by chronically impacting every one of our bodily functions. The results are:

- Reduced blood volume, with less oxygen and nutrients provided to all muscles and organs
- Reduced brain size and impaired neuromuscular coordination, concentration, and thinking
- Excess body fat
- Poor muscle tone and size
- Impaired digestive function and constipation
- Increased toxicity in the body
- Joint and muscle pain
- Water retention (edema), which can result in a state of being overweight and also impede weight loss
- Hyperconcentration of blood with increased viscosity, leading to higher risk of heart attack

Even though you may not be feeling thirsty, you may nonetheless be one of the millions of Americans who are chronically dehydrated. Observation of your urine is one simple way to determine if you are. If your urine is heavy, cloudy, and deep yellow, orange, or brown in tint, it's more than likely that you are dehydrated. The urine of a properly hydrated body tends to be light and nearly clear in color, similar in appearance to unsweetened lemonade. As your water intake approaches your daily need for it, you will notice the appearance of your urine changing accordingly. (Remember that B vitamins will also turn urine a dark yellow.)

Because dehydration is so deceptive—it can occur without symptoms of thirst—in general, we need to drink more water than our thirst calls for. This does not mean coffee, soft drinks, or alcohol, all of which contribute further to dehydration. Even processed fruit juices and milk are not healthy substitutes for water because of the sugar and possible pesticides in the former and the hormones and antibiotics in the latter.

The exact amount of water a person needs depends on a number of individual factors, such as body weight, diet, metabolic rate, climate, level of physical activity, and stress factors. Some health professionals recommend that we all drink 8 eight-ounce glasses of water a day. A more accurate rule of thumb is to drink half an ounce of water per pound of body weight if you are a healthy but sedentary adult, and to increase that amount to two thirds of an ounce per pound if you are an active exerciser. This means that a healthy, sedentary adult weighing 160 pounds should drink about 10 eight-ounce glasses of water per day, while an active exerciser should drink 13 to 14 eight-ounce glasses. If your diet is particularly high in fresh fruits and vegetables, your daily water intake needs may be less, since these foods are 85 to 90 percent water in content and can help restore lost fluids. Herbal teas, natural fruit juices (without sugar added and diluted 50 percent with water), and soups that are sugarless and low in salt (the thinner the better) are also acceptable substitutes for drinking water.

Nearly as important as the amount of water you drink is the *quality* of your water. Simply put, if you aren't drinking filtered water, then your body is forced to become the filter. Still, it's impossible to generalize about whether you should drink tap, bottled, or filtered water. (Distilled water is not recommended for drinking because it lacks necessary minerals and can also leach them from your body.) In some communities, water purity is so high that it requires no treatment, while other water sources are contaminated with high concentrations of lead and radon, the two worst contaminants.

Another issue related to our drinking water is chlorination. Since chlorine was first introduced into America's drinking water supply in 1908, it has eliminated epidemics of cholera, dysentery, and typhoid. Multiple studies, however, now suggest an association between chlorine and increased free radical production, which can lead to a higher incidence of cancer. On the positive side, chlorine is effective in eliminating most microorganisms from drinking water. (One notable exception is the parasite *Cryptosporidium,* which is resistant to chlorine.)

Unless you live in one of the communities that supplies pure water, drinking tap water is not recommended, especially since the majority of health-related risks present in drinking water occur from contamination that is added *after* the water leaves the treatment and distribution plant. This includes pipes that run from municipal systems into your home, lead-soldered copper pipes, and fixtures that contain lead and may leach lead or other toxic metals (such as cadmium, mercury, and cobalt) into your tap water. Therefore, if you drink tap water, it would be a good idea to have the water from your tap tested, regardless of the claims from your local water utility. You can get started by calling your local health department for a referral for testing.

Because of the growing concerns regarding tap water, increasing numbers of Americans now choose bottled water for drinking and cooking purposes. This can not only prove to be expensive, but also may not be as safe as you think. Regulations mandated for the bottled-water industry are similar to those followed by the public water treatment industry and currently do not include required testing for *Cryptosporidium* and many other contaminants. Moreover, 25 percent of bottled water sold in this country comes from filtered municipal water that is then treated. For this reason, perhaps the healthiest choice regarding your drinking water is to invest in a water filter. Reverse-osmosis filters appear to be the most effective home water-filtering systems presently available. But there are also some distillation and carbon filters that are able to reduce lead in water significantly. There are carafe-style filters for the kitchen faucet that cost about $25, under-the-sink models for $400, and point-of-entry units that purify the water as it enters the house. These can cost as much as $1,250.

Since it is impossible to always know for certain whether what we drink or eat is completely safe, do the best you can. To get in the habit of drinking enough water spread your intake throughout the day (drinking very little after dinner), and don't drink more than four eight-ounce glasses in any one-hour period. It's also best to drink between meals so as not to interfere with your body's digestive process. Make your water drinking convenient; keep a container of water at hand, in your car, or at your desk, and don't wait until you feel thirsty to start drinking. Most important, be sure that there's always a bathroom nearby.

Moisture helps empty the sinus of its thick, infected mucus, and in doing so helps restore normal cilial function and relieves nasal and head congestion, headache, sinus pain, and sore throat. Warm, moist air is best, and the easiest place to get it is in the bathroom. Steamers can now be installed in showers, or simply close any doors and windows and turn the shower on hot to create steam. You then have the choice of either getting in the shower—after adjusting the temperature, of course—or just sitting and relaxing in the steam until you run out of hot water. Make a conscious effort to breathe through your nose. Hot towels applied over the face can also be helpful.

As most of us do not have an endless supply of hot water or steamers, making a steam room of the bathroom can be done only two or three times a day. What about the rest of the time? If you are staying home from work, your best source of moist air is a humidifier placed by your bed, with the bedroom door and windows closed. Most humidifiers are quiet and very effective in producing a moist environment in an enclosed space. They are available in pharmacies, department stores, and hardware stores under a variety of brand names. The one I know best and with which I have enjoyed excellent results is the Bionaire-Clear Mist 5 (CMP-5). It quietly yet powerfully puts out warm moisture, can cover an area of up to 1,600 square feet, and is relatively easy to clean. The Kenmore Warm Mist is the identical unit, and it is available at most Sears stores. These units cost about $125. Although the ideal humidifier has probably not yet been designed, while writing this new edition of *Sinus Survival* I began using the Slant/Fin GF-200. This warm mist humidifier uses ultraviolet germicidal technology to produce 99.999 percent germ-free mist. It costs under $100.

The cool-mist ultrasonics put out a fine mineral dust unless distilled water is used to fill them, and the warm ultrasonics have a tendency to break down. Steam humidifiers or vaporizers can become quite hot, which could be a concern if you have small children. The ultrasonic humidifiers with a demineralizing component seem to have eliminated most problems. Whatever your choice, be sure the reservoir tank opening is large enough to allow for cleaning. Wipe and cleanse the tank at least weekly with vinegar water; otherwise it becomes a breeding ground for molds, which are becoming a more common cause of chronic sinusitis. During treatment for a sinus infection, the humidifier should be used every night while you sleep. It's also a good idea to fill it and turn it on as soon as you come home from work so your bedroom will be warm and moist by the time you're ready for bed. The moisture is very helpful in relieving the infection's cough and sore throat during the night. To minimize mold, I would empty the humidifier every morning and allow it to dry out.

Another device I've been using preventively on myself and recommending to patients as part of their treatment program is the *Steam inhaler* (see Fig. 6.2). It's extremely effective for thinning and loosening the thick infected mucus stuck in the sinuses, and can also be quite soothing to dry and irritated mucous membranes. A drop of eucalyptus oil added to the unit while you are steaming enhances its beneficial effect. (If you are treating a sinus infection you can also add a drop or two of tea tree oil.) It works extremely well as a nasal decongestant and for

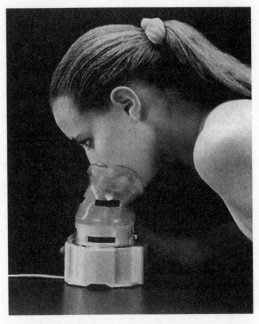

FIGURE 6.2.   *Steam inhaler.*

relieving sinus headaches. If used just prior to nasal irrigation, a procedure that I'm about to explain, it will greatly increase the benefit of the irrigation. The Steam inhaler I use is made by Kaz, costs about $50 and unfortunately is no longer readily available. Complete information on where to obtain any of the products I mention is listed in the Product Index at the end of the book.

Assuming your environment is relatively dry, as indoor air tends to be during the winter months in most parts of the United States, you can provide moisture with a saltwater (also called *saline*) *nasal spray.* There are several commercial products available in pharmacies. However, you can make your own saline spray by mixing one third of a teaspoon of non-iodized table salt and a pinch of baking soda in an eight-ounce cup of lukewarm bottled water (without chlorine) and dispensing it from a spray bottle. You can use sea salt without iodine. Spray into each nostril while closing off the other nostril and simultaneously inhaling. This is nonaddictive and can be done as often as you like throughout the day. It has no negative side effects, except for the curious looks you will get from those wanting to know what in the world you are doing.

The *Sinus Survival Spray,* a botanical saline nasal mist, has been a highly effective addition to the Sinus Survival Program. Formulated by Dr. Steve Morris, a naturopathic physician from Mukilteo, Washington, and myself, we have been using it on ourselves and recommending it to our patients for more than six years, with excellent results. In addition to saline, which makes up the bulk of the spray, the ingredients include:

- Berberis: acts as an antibacterial, antifungal, and anti-inflammatory
- Selenium: a powerful antioxidant with antiallergic and anti-inflammatory capability
- Aloe vera: has antifungal properties and relieves irritation
- Grapefruit-seed extract: an excellent antifungal

The first three ingredients are all soothing and healing to the nasal mucous membranes. The selenium has allowed the product to be used as part of the allergy treatment program as well as for sinusitis. I've even used this spray as an eyedrop and found it quite soothing for dry and irritated eyes caused by air pollution and arid conditions. (Berberine has been described in a medical journal as being effective for treating inflammations of the cornea.) When the spray bottle is turned upside down, it can function as an eyedropper. The Sinus Survival Spray is available in many health food stores and can also be obtained through Sinus Survival Products.

An even more effective way of moisturizing is *saline irrigation.* This procedure can result in dramatic relief from pain by reducing swelling in the nasal passages, causing a reduction of pressure in the sinus, as well as helping to empty the sinus of its infected mucus. Saltwater sprays also irrigate, i.e., wash out some mucus, bacteria, and dust particles, while reducing swelling. However, they don't do it as well as the following irrigation methods. Throughout the past decade I've heard many people comment that nasal irrigation, using any of the first three techniques described below, has been the *single most helpful component* of the entire Sinus Survival Program. Irrigation should be done three to four times a day for acute sinusitis and once or twice for a milder chronic condition. Many former sinus sufferers continue to irrigate daily on a preventive basis, even after curing their chronic sinusitis.

Mix the saline solution for irrigation fresh each day in one cup of lukewarm bottled water. Add one third of a teaspoon of non-iodized table salt or sea salt and a tiny pinch of baking soda, thus making the solution close to normal body fluid salinity and pH. Irrigating with plain water is usually somewhat uncomfortable. Use the full cup of saline solution for each irrigation (one-half cup for each nostril). Lean over the sink, with the head rotated so that the nostril to be irrigated is directly above the other nostril, while using one of the following methods. Always blow your nose *very* gently after irrigating.

Method 1   For the past six years I have been recommending the use of the Neti Pot, and more recently SinuCleanse, for nasal irrigation (see Fig. 6.3). It is a small porcelain pot with a narrow spout (SinuCleanse is plastic with a very similar shape and size and is ideal for traveling). This is probably the most gentle and convenient method for irrigation. Because of this, people with chronic sinusitis are much more apt to use this method on a regular basis, both therapeutically in treating an infection and preventively. SinuCleanse is sold with packets of hy-

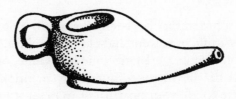

FIGURE 6.3.   *Neti Pot.*

pertonic saline to mix with water, making this method even more convenient. The Neti Pot is made by the Himalayan Institute in Honesdale, Pennsylvania, and is available in many health food stores. SinuCleanse is available through Sinus Survival Products.

Method 2 Use an angled nasal irrigator attachment (the Grossan nasal irrigator is available at some pharmacies) on a Water Pik appliance. Set the Water Pik at the lowest possible pressure and insert the irrigator tip just inside one nostril, pinching your nostril to form a seal. Irrigate with your mouth open, allowing the fluid to drain out either your mouth or nose. Repeat the procedure in the other nostril.

Method 3 Completely fill a large, all-rubber ear syringe (available at most pharmacies) with saline solution. Lean over the sink and insert the syringe tip just inside one nostril, so that it forms a comfortable seal. *Gently* squeeze and release the bulb several times to swish the solution around the inside of your nose. The solution will run out both nostrils and may also run out of your mouth. Repeat this for each nostril until one cup of saline solution is used, or until the solution is clear.

Method 4 For very small children, irrigate with ten to twenty drops of saline solution per nostril from an eyedropper.

If you are using a decongestant nasal spray or a corticosteroid nasal spray, use them only *after* the saltwater nasal irrigations.

These methods obviously require more effort than the saline nasal sprays, but many patients comment on how much more helpful it is.

Another solution that has been effective in irrigation is called Alkalol. It is a mucus solvent and cleaner, and can be used with the saline solution in a 1:1 ratio (one half saline, one half Alkalol) with all of the methods previously mentioned. You will probably have to ask your pharmacist to order it for you, as it is not usually available, but Alkalol is very inexpensive.

Water, moisture, and nasal hygiene, i.e., saline spray, steam, and irrigation, can also help to relieve the symptoms of dry, crusted nasal membranes that are common with chronic sinusitis and often prone to nosebleeds. You can apply Neosporin ointment or even better Ponaris nasal emollient (ask your pharmacist to order it) to the nasal membranes twice daily with a Q-tip or your little finger.

The beneficial effects of nasal irrigation for chronic sinusitis are obvious to anyone with this condition who has irrigated regularly. However, it was not until a group of Spanish physicians performed a recent study in Madrid on allergy sufferers that the benefits of irrigation for allergies was documented. They found that irrigating the nose with saline three times a day during the grass pollen season (May to July) significantly reduced the allergic response to grass. This finding also supports the critical role of the nasal mucous membrane in the allergic response. And it reinforces the primary objective of the Sinus Survival Program: *to heal the mucous membranes!*

HYDROTHERAPY

Other than drinking, irrigating, moistening, bathing, or soaking in it, I've found that water can be therapeutic by virtue of its temperature. While taking a shower, increase the temperature as much as you are able to tolerate and allow this hot water to strike your face, especially the area around your nose and sinuses. To prolong your tolerance, you can move your face from side to side or in a circular motion. If you are congested or have a sinus infection, this technique will help relieve the congestion and allow the sinuses to drain.

Both as a therapeutic and preventive measure that can strengthen the immune system, I also recommend turning off the hot water completely and allowing the cold water to strike your mid-chest for about a minute. I learned this technique from Dr. Steve Morris in 1989. He explained that it is a commonly prescribed hydrotherapeutic technique in naturopathic medicine for stimulating the thymus gland—an important component of the immune system located in your chest cavity directly under the sternum (breastbone). I've been practicing this technique routinely ever since, just before I finish showering. I can't be certain what it's doing for my thymus, but it definitely stimulates the rest of my body!

DIET

"We are what we eat." I have heard that saying many times, but it never made much of an impact until I began changing my diet in the process of treating my own chronic sinusitis. I am now convinced that most chronic medical conditions can be helped significantly by a healthful diet. With specific regard to the respiratory tract, the change I recommend most is to *avoid milk and dairy products.* The protein in milk tends to increase and thicken mucus secretions. If you would like to compensate for the loss of calcium in your own or your child's diet, the following foods are especially rich in calcium: broccoli, kale, sesame seeds and sesame seed butter, tofu, sea vegetables, and soy cheese. You can also buy a liquid calcium and magnesium combination at most health food stores. An adequate daily dose for an adult female is 1,200 mg of calcium and 500 to 600 mg of magnesium.

Sugar should also be avoided, especially if you suspect that candida is contributing to your sinusitis. A nutritionist once asked me, "Would you fill the gas tank of your car with sand?" She felt that filling your body with sugar is equally destructive. Yet, the average American eats or drinks about 150 pounds each year, which is about the equivalent of 41 teaspoons of sugar every day! It seems to be in almost everything, from nearly all breakfast cereals to spaghetti sauce. Sugar not only has no nutritional value, it is also harmful.

The following are only a few of sugar's health-depleting effects:

- Sugar weakens the immune system, increasing susceptibility to infection and allergy and further exacerbating all other diseases caused by diminished immune function.
- Sugar has been shown to be a risk factor for heart disease *and may be more harmful than fat.*
- Sugar stimulates excessive insulin production, thereby causing more fat to be stored in the body; lowers levels of HDL cholesterol (the healthy cholesterol); increases the production of harmful triglycerides; and increases the risk of arteriosclerosis (hardening of the arteries).
- Sugar contributes to diminished mental capacity and can cause feelings of anxiety, depression, and rage. It has also been implicated in certain cases of attention deficit disorder (ADD).
- High sugar intake is associated with certain cancers, including cancer of the gallbladder and colon. Recently sugar has also been implicated as a causative factor in cases of breast cancer.
- Excessive sugar in the diet is a primary contributor to candidiasis (intestinal yeast overgrowth), which can lead to a host of health problems, including gastrointestinal disorders, asthma, bronchitis, sinusitis, allergies, and chronic fatigue.

If you still feel a need to satisfy your sweet tooth, substitute modest amounts of pure honey or maple syrup to decrease the risk of these adverse effects.

Caffeine is a drug to which more than half of all Americans are addicted. Chronic sinusitis sufferers are especially prone to this addiction since fatigue is often such a prominent symptom. Caffeine is a diuretic that can contribute to dehydration and increased mucus production. The average person drinks two and a half cups of coffee a day, or 425 mg of caffeine. Coffee has roughly three times the caffeine of tea. Caffeine is a stimulant that we consume to have more energy. But the quick fix it provides lasts for only a few hours, only to leave us with a greater sense of fatigue and irritability when the effect wears off. Our

Table 6.1

Caffeine Amounts (mg)

COFFEE (5-OUNCE CUP)
Decaffeinated instant: 2
Decaffeinated brewed: 2–5
Instant: 65–100
Percolated: 65–125
Drip: 115–175

TEA (5-OUNCE CUP)
Bag, brewed for five minutes: 20–60
Bag, brewed for one minute: 10–40
Loose, black, five-minute brew: 20–85
Loose, green, five-minute brew: 15–80
Iced: 25 to 70

SOFT DRINKS (12-OUNCE GLASS)
Cola: 45
Mountain Dew: 55

CHOCOLATE
Cocoa, 5-ounce cup: 4–6
Milk chocolate, 1 ounce: 3–6
Bittersweet chocolate, 1 ounce: 25–35

solution for this state of low energy is usually to drink another cup of coffee or tea or another bottle of caffeine-rich soda pop. Your entire body suffers as a result of being on a perpetual "roller coaster" of ups and downs. Since one of your primary goals in treating sinusitis is to strengthen your body, it is best to avoid anything that may weaken it.

The evidence seems to indicate that limiting ourselves to one or possibly two cups (of a weaker strength) of coffee per day would be relatively safe (200 mg or less per day). However, the majority of us drink more than that and are therefore at higher risk for a variety of health problems including high blood pressure; increased risk of cancer, heart disease, and osteoporosis; poor sleep patterns; anxiety and irritability; dizziness; impaired circulation; urinary frequency; and gastrointestinal disorders. Caffeine also causes loss of calcium from muscle cells and can interfere with the blood clotting process by decreasing platelet stickiness.

Taken in moderation, however, caffeine has been shown to enhance mental functioning, improve both alertness and mood, and reduce risk for gallstones. It appears that 200 mg or less of caffeine per day may be safely tolerated by most individuals. Prominent cancer researcher John Weisburger, director emeritus of the American Health Foundation, believes that tea is an effective antioxidant (see p. 149), and that the chemicals in tea may help counteract carcinogens in food, especially in grilled, fried, and broiled meat. Researchers at the National Institute of Nutrition, in Rome, found that black and green tea raise antioxidant activity in the blood by 40 to 50 percent. Other studies have found that black and green tea can reduce the risk of fatal heart disease and some cancers. These teas can be found in most health food stores and some supermarkets.

Reactions to caffeine vary widely from person to person and stem in part from genetic differences in the way the body metabolizes it. Smoking reduces the effect of caffeine, while pregnancy and birth control pills can enhance it.

The best way to break caffeine addiction is to do it very *gradually,* over a period of a few weeks or even months. Start by substituting noncaffeinated beverages such as herbal tea or a roasted-grain beverage for one of your normal cups of coffee each day. Over time, cut back further while increasing the number of substitute beverages and beware of the possible withdrawal symptoms of headache, nervousness, and irritability. Typically these will pass within a day or two. Also avoid other caffeinated drinks, such as soft drinks (particularly colas), cocoa, chocolate, and nonherbal teas.

The regular intake of good fats is essential to our health. Unfortunately, most of us are getting too much *unhealthy fat* in our diets. Primary sources of these harmful fats include red meats, milk and other dairy products, and the hydrogenated trans fats found in margarine, cooking fats, and many brands of peanut butter. These fats are also found in many packaged foods, including most commercial cereals, which also tend to be loaded with sugar.

In addition to milk and dairy increasing mucus production. unhealthy fats lead to arteriosclerosis and the buildup of plaque on the inner lining of the arteries, where over time they obstruct the flow of blood and the transport of oxygen and nutrients to the body's internal organs. This obstruction, in turn, can lead to heart attacks, angina, stroke, kidney failure, and pregangrene in the legs.

The excessive intake of unhealthy fats is also associated with certain cancers, including cancer of the breast, colon, rectum, prostate, ovaries, and uterus. This is particularly true of the saturated fats derived from meat products.

Obesity, which is increasing to epidemic proportions in this country, is also directly related to excessive fat (and sugar) intake. Obesity is a serious disease condition by itself, but if prolonged, it can contribute to many other forms of illness, including adult-onset diabetes.

Becoming aware of your fat intake and minimizing the amount of harmful fats you consume is an important step toward optimal health.

Salt is another ingredient that is far too prevalent in many diets, and it poses particular dangers for certain people who suffer from high blood pressure. Many of us have been conditioned since childhood to crave salt, but its overuse draws water into the bloodstream. This, in turn, increases blood volume, causing higher blood pressure levels. Too much salt also upsets the body's sodium-potassium balance, thereby interfering with the lymphatic system's ability to draw wastes away from the cells.

Although some salt can be used in cooking, a good rule of thumb is to avoid adding salt to your food once it is served.

Refined, or simple, carbohydrates, such as those found in white breads and in pastas made from white flour, are another group of health-threatening agents. When eaten in excess, these types of foods overstimulate insulin production and produce the same excessive fat storage in the body that results from eating too much sugar. This can lead to the onset of diabetes and obesity. The rise in obesity among American children is due in part to a diet heavy in sugars and refined carbohydrates and lacking in nutritious alternatives, notably fruits and vegetables.

Several recent studies have shown that certain carbohydrates previously promoted as being "whole" sources of starch are very rapidly digested and absorbed. As a result, they elevate blood sugar fully as much as sugar itself, contributing to all the problems cited earlier for sugar. Most carbohydrates have been carefully analyzed and assigned a *glycemic index* rating. A high glycemic index indicates that a food acts much as sugar does in the body; food sources with a low glycemic index are assimilated much more slowly and therefore offer much better nutritional value. High glycemic index foods include corn flakes, puffed rice, instant and mashed potatoes, white bread, maltose, and, of course, sugar itself. Foods with a low glycemic index include whole grain cereals (oats, brown rice, amaranth, kamut, millet), legumes (beans, peas, peanuts, soybeans), pumpernickel breads, whole wheat pastas, pearled barley, bulgur wheat, sweet potatoes, apples, oranges, yogurt, and fructose.

Alcohol is another example of a substance that when taken in moderation may enhance health but when consumed in excess can cause a variety of serious problems. A growing body of research now indicates that one or two beers or a glass of wine per day can be beneficial to health as a way to relieve stress and to improve digestion. In fact, studies have shown that complete abstainers from alcohol have a slightly shorter life expectancy than those who drink in moderate amounts. Unfortunately, for many men especially, alcohol and moderation usually "don't mix."

Although most people drink in order to feel better, evidence indicates that alcohol can significantly contribute to feelings of depression, loneliness, restlessness, and boredom, according to studies conducted by the National Center for Health Statistics. In addition, very moody people are also three times more likely to be heavy drinkers (three or more drinks per day).

If candidiasis is aggravating your chronic sinusitis, don't drink any alcohol for at least three months during treatment. Aside from the social stigma surrounding excessive alcohol consumption, too much alcohol can also contribute to obesity; increased blood pressure; diabetes; colon, stomach, breast, mouth, esophagus, laryngeal, and pancreatic cancers; gastrointesrinal disorders; impaired liver function; impaired mental functioning; and behavioral and emotional dysfunctions. If you are having difficulty in bringing your alcohol consumption under control, seek the help of a professional counselor.

Try to decrease your consumption of *food additives.* These include chemical preservatives (such as BHA, BHT, sodium nitrite, and sulfites), artificial colors, and artificial sweeteners (including saccharin, aspartame [NutraSweet], and cyclamates). Almost every one of these additives has been shown to have a potential health risk.

Perhaps our biggest problem with food is our enormous American appetite. We eat about 40 percent more *calories* than we need, and obesity (weighing 20 percent above ideal body weight) has become epidemic. A massive nine-year U.S. study on caloric intake involving two dozen laboratories, sixty government and university researchers, and 24,000 rats and mice is currently in its eighth year. The results of restricting caloric intake by 40 percent have had a dramatic impact on increasing longevity. The most prominent advocate of human caloric restriction is Roy L. Walford, M.D., an immunologist at the University of California at Los Angeles, who has raised some of the world's oldest mice using caloric restriction. His findings are described in his books *Maximum Life Span* and *The 120-Year Diet.*

Our society has chosen food as its greatest treat, and unfortunately the most highly prized foods not only have no nutritional value but ultimately can make us sick. Now that I have eliminated many of your life's greatest pleasures—ice cream, soda pop, sugar, coffee, and alcohol—as well as 40 percent of your calories, I hope you are still with me. I'm sorry. I can tell you, though, that when I stopped eating my evening bowl of ice cream nearly eight years ago, I thought it would be a lot more difficult than it turned out to be. What happens is that shortly after making these dietary changes, you will begin to appreciate new rewards: more energy, less mucus, fewer pounds, and a great feeling of accomplishment that comes from applying self-discipline toward doing something beneficial for yourself. Remember, too, that these are just recommendations, not commandments. My own guideline on this subject is "Everything in moderation, including moderation." I do believe, however, that if you are miserable with sick sinuses, you should try to adhere as closely as possible to these suggestions. Try to make at least a three-month commitment to this diet.

A *healthy diet* is generally rich in organic fruits and vegetables, whole grains (e.g., brown rice, bulgur, wheat, oats, amaranth, millet, quinoa, barley, and couscous), legumes, and fiber—abundant in bran cereals, beans, apricots, and prunes. Raw foods are usually better than cooked. Good sources of protein are nuts, seeds, fish, turkey and chicken (free-range), and the soybean products tofu and tempeh. The foods that most strengthen the immune system are also highly beneficial to those whose sinus condition is caused by nasal allergies; these are garlic, onions, citrus fruits, and horseradish.

In January 1992 the U.S. Department of Agriculture unveiled a new shape for the ideal American diet: a pyramid built on a base of grains (see Fig. 6.4).

This is a very brief discussion of nutrition. Classes on the subject or consultation with a nutritionist would help you tailor a healthy diet to your personal tastes. Two books often recommended by nutritionists are *Food Is Your Best Medicine* by Henry G. Bieler, M.D., and *Vibrant Health from Your Kitchen* by Bernard Jensen, N.D.

If you have followed the preceding recommendations without a noticeable improvement in your condition, I suggest eliminating from your diet for at least three weeks the foods that most commonly produce the *allergic reactions* that may cause chronic sinusitis, allergies, and asthma: cow's milk and all dairy products,

Food Guide Pyramid

A Guide to Daily Food Choices

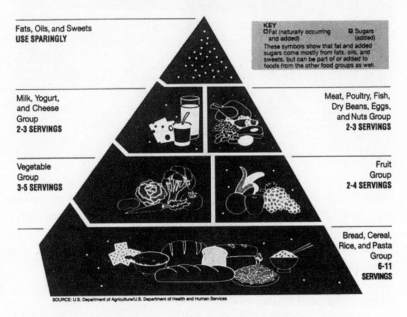

Fats, Oils, and Sweets
USE SPARINGLY

KEY
☐ Fat (naturally occurring and added)   ● Sugars (added)
These symbols show that fat and added sugars come mostly from fats, oils, and sweets, but can be part of or added to foods from the other food groups as well

Milk, Yogurt, and Cheese Group
2-3 SERVINGS

Meat, Poultry, Fish, Dry Beans, Eggs, and Nuts Group
2-3 SERVINGS

Vegetable Group
3-5 SERVINGS

Fruit Group
2-4 SERVINGS

Bread, Cereal, Rice, and Pasta Group
6-11 SERVINGS

SOURCE: U.S. Department of Agriculture/U.S. Department of Health and Human Services

FIGURE 6.4.   *Food guide pyramid.*

wheat, chocolate, corn, white sugar, soy, yeast (brewer's and baker's), oranges, tomatoes, bell peppers, white potatoes, eggs, fish, shellfish, cocoa, onions, nuts, garlic, peanuts, black pepper, red meat, aspirin, artificial food coloring, coffee, black tea, beer, wine, and champagne. I realize how difficult this can be, but it only need be for three weeks. After that, begin to reintroduce each of these foods into your diet at the rate of one every three days. Pay attention to your body and note any new symptoms such as headache, nausea, diarrhea, gas, or mental "fog." It then should be obvious to you which food, if any, causes your body to react.

I wish there were some way to make dietary change both simple and easy. If there were, I am sure it wouldn't have taken so many years for my family's diet to have reached the healthy point it has—and even that was with the added impetus of my daughter Carin's wish to be a vegetarian. If there is a good health food store not too far from your home, try to shop there and try using one of their cookbooks. The salespeople are usually very helpful. Many supermarkets now have health food sections. Take a few extra minutes on your next trip to see what looks good. Be a little adventurous, but do try to implement change gradually. This transition should not be made in two weeks. Those who take their time have a much greater chance of maintaining their healthy diet. Although there are many powerful therapeutic measures to help your nose, sinuses, and lungs, few are more valuable than eating only food that is nourishing and non-allergenic to your body.

VITAMINS, HERBS, SUPPLEMENTS, AND ANTIOXIDANTS

In case you hadn't noticed, life in urban America can be extremely stressful. Almost daily we are exposed to chemical stress, emotional stress, and infection. Each type of stress has numerous sources. Chemical stress, for example, may come from polluted air, polluted water, food pesticides, insecticides, heavy metals, or, worst of all, radioactive wastes. More than ever, we are exposed to a myriad of foreign chemicals, both commercially synthesized and naturally occurring in our environment. The 1989 Kellogg Report stated that 1,000 newly synthesized compounds are introduced each year, which amounts to three new chemicals a day. The current number of foreign chemicals (called xenobiotics) now totals around 100,000 and includes drugs, pesticides, industrial chemicals, food additives and preservatives, and environmental pollutants. Toxic chemicals easily find their way into our bodies through the air we breathe, the food we eat, and the water we drink. We also ingest foreign chemicals when taking medicinal or illicit drugs, or when using alcohol or tobacco.

Compounding this problem is the fact that the soil in which our foods are grown is greatly depleted of the trace minerals needed to create and maintain health. Many of our foods are shipped, frozen, stored, and warehoused, reaching us weeks or months after being harvested. Degeneration of their nutrient value occurs at each stop. Cooking methods, such as boiling and frying, also contribute to nutrient loss once the food reaches our kitchens and restaurants. Moreover, the standard American diet has become increasingly devoid of nutrients and overburdened with empty calories and nonfood additives. Therefore, even though the body is designed to eliminate toxins, it cannot always handle the overload present in today's environment. Unfortunately we still know very little about the magnitude of the harmful effects caused by our continual exposure to these chemicals. In this book you're learning about some of these toxic effects on the respiratory tract. There are several studies that reveal a strong correlation between high exposure to air pollutants and pesticides and contracting cancer. David Abbey, Ph.D., a professor of biostatistics at Loma Linda University, found that women living in the Los Angeles area have a 37 percent greater risk of developing *all forms of cancer* as a result of high exposure to particulates than women who live in cleaner air environments. His studies also revealed a 125 percent higher risk for both men and women of getting lung cancer from high levels of ozone pollution.

We are learning that all stressors—chemical, emotional, and infectious—harm us by weakening our immune systems with highly toxic molecules called free radicals. According to Deepak Chopra, M.D., author of *Quantum Healing: Exploring the Frontiers of Mind/Body Medicine* and *Ageless Body, Timeless Mind,* free radicals are the "metabolic end-products in the body of environmental pollution, food toxins, carcinogens, and emotional toxins."

Free radicals, or oxidants, are very unstable and highly reactive molecules that contain one or more unpaired electrons. They try to capture electrons off other molecules to gain stability, a process known as oxidation. Antioxidants are substances that significantly delay or inhibit oxidation. They neutralize free radicals by supplying electrons.

Medical research has already implicated free radicals as causative factors in many diseases (e.g., arthritis, cancer, mental disorders, cataracts, and heart disease) as well as in susceptibility to infection and in accelerating the process of aging. In fact, over the past thirty years, research has revealed a common factor in every degenerative disease of our time: cell damage as a result of free radicals. Denham Harman, M.D., of the University of Nebraska says, "Today it seems very likely that the assumption that there is a basic cause of aging is correct and that the sum of deleterious free radical reactions going on continuously throughout the cells and tissues is the aging process or a major contribution to it."

Free radicals are responsible for most cellular damage. Fortunately our bodies manufacture antioxidant enzymes within the cells for protection against free radicals, and also employ antioxidant nutrients (e.g., vitamin A, carotene, vitamin E, vitamin C, selenium, and zinc) supplied by our diet. As long as there is an adequate supply of oxygen, water, antioxidant nutrients, and enzymes in the body, cell damage is minimized. When any one of these is deficient, cell damage is accelerated, as in the process of aging and in disease. Through their critical role in helping to prevent disease, *vitamins, acting as antioxidants, can offer considerable help to our body's immune system.*

When disease, including any of the chronic respiratory diseases, is present, the cells are overrun with an excess of free radicals and the immune system cannot maintain its protective shield. This occurs when stress lowers our body's production of antioxidant enzymes to a level less than our needs. Unfortunately, city living makes it difficult to avoid most of our stressors. It is a wonder that the majority of us are free of a chronic disease. For those who have not been as fortunate, and for anyone interested in strengthening their body's natural defenses, practicing preventive medicine, or experiencing a greater degree of physical health, the following recommendations for vitamins, herbs, and nutritional supplements will help.

Vitamin C

In 1970 the distinguished chemist and Nobel prizewinner Linus Pauling turned his attention to the benefits of megadoses of vitamin C in the prevention and treatment of colds. The verification of his findings by other researchers has been complicated primarily by the great variability in the dosages and types of vitamin C that have been used. In my experience, vitamin C has been extremely effective in the treatment and prevention of colds, allergies, and sinus infections. In that colds are the most common cause of acute sinusitis, their prevention is good preventive medicine for sinusitis. In addition to its antioxidant properties, vitamin C is essential to the manufacture of collagen, the main supportive protein of skin, tendon, bone, cartilage, and connective tissue; has an anti-inflammatory effect, especially in some autoimmune diseases such as lupus and rheumatoid arthritis; can block allergic reactions and rebuild healthy mucous membranes, making it a natural antihistamine; facilitates the absorption of dietary iron; enhances the immune response and white blood cell activity; and, in conjunction with vitamin E, strengthens arterial walls. In a recent study conducted by researchers from the USDA and National Institute on Aging, vitamin C was shown to provide greater protection against cholesterol buildup (by raising HDL—the "good" cholesterol) and reduce the risk of heart disease.

The average daily dose for cold prevention is 3,000 mg. If you already have a cold or sinus infection, I recommend as much as 15,000 mg a day. Take this amount in divided dosages, either 5,000 mg three times a day with meals (to avoid stomach upset, it is best to take most vitamins with food) or 2,000 to 3,000 mg every two to three hours, preferably in a powdered form as ascorbate or Ester C. These are much more easily absorbed and more potent than ascorbic acid—the more common form of vitamin C found in fruits, vegetables, and most commercial brands of vitamin C. You can also take time-released vitamin C capsules or tablets that are assimilated over twelve hours. Most other vitamin C tablets last for only six to eight hours. This high dosage for colds and sinus infections should be maintained for several days, or until your symptoms begin to improve. Taper off very gradually over the next two weeks to get back down to the usual daily dose of 3,000 mg. Dr. Pauling's prescription: At the first sign of a cold, take 1,000 mg or more of vitamin C every hour during the waking hours. Possible side effects of dosages above 3,000 mg are diarrhea, bowel gas, and cramps. But these symptoms are more likely to occur with the pure ascorbic acid form of vitamin C. If you experience these symptoms, cut back on your next dose by 1,000 mg. A less common side effect is the development of kidney stones. This can usually be prevented by drinking the recommended daily amount of water or by taking 75 mg of vitamin B_6 a day.

Another method for taking vitamin C, called titrating to bowel tolerance, was developed by Robert Cathcart, M.D. Cathcart has treated over 9,000 patients with large doses of ascorbic acid, some as great as 100,000 mg a day. He believes the maximum relief of symptoms is obtained at a point just short of the amount that produces diarrhea. According to Dr. Cathcart, the amount of vitamin C that can be taken orally without causing diarrhea when a person is ill may be as much as ten times the amount he or she would tolerate if well. Using this method, he claims success treating a host of viral infections, including colds, influenza, mononucleosis, and viral pneumonia; environmental and food allergies; cancer; rheumatoid arthritis; hepatitis; and yeast infections.

There is quite a variation in the strength of different brands of vitamin C. For instance, 1,000 mg of ascorbate is better absorbed than 1,000 mg of ascorbic acid. Once ascorbic acid is absorbed into our bloodstreams, it reacts with many minerals, such as sodium, calcium, magnesium, and zinc to form ascorbates. It is in this form, as ascorbates, that vitamin C enters the trillions of cells in our bodies. Taking vitamin C in ascorbate powder is the most effective way to enhance absorption.

Vitamin C, as an antioxidant, is a free-radical scavenger. Studies have shown that our bodies can use a lot more of it when we are under stress. Use your own discretion in varying your dosage, depending on the degree of stress you think you have experienced that day. If it was a high air pollution day or if you had a rough time at work, take more than the 3,000 mg. The same recommendation holds true for all of the other vitamins and herbs I will mention in the following sections. Vitamin C and all of the other vitamins and herbs are more effective if eaten in the natural form of food rather than taken in pill or powder forms. The foods highest in vitamin C, in roughly descending order, are guavas, oranges, cantaloupe, strawberries, red chili peppers, red sweet peppers, green sweet peppers, kale, parsley, collard greens, turnip greens, mustard greens, broccoli, brussels sprouts, and cauliflower. Their vitamin C content is higher when eaten raw. It is also more nutritious (less calories and more fiber) to eat raw fruit than to drink fruit juice.

Linus Pauling died in 1994 at age 93 of prostate cancer. He reportedly took 10,000 mg of vitamin C every day.

Vitamin A and Beta-Carotene

Most vitamin A comes from its precursor, beta-carotene, which is converted to the vitamin form in the gastrointestinal tract. Beta-carotene is a substance in carotenoids, which are usually found in yellow, orange, or red foods. Listed in roughly descending order of vitamin A content, these include carrots, sweet potatoes, yams, kale, spinach, mangoes, winter squash, cantaloupe, apricots, broccoli, romaine lettuce, asparagus, tomatoes, nectarines, peaches, and papayas. Vitamin A itself can be obtained directly from consumption of cod liver oil, liver, kidney, eggs, and dairy products.

Vitamin A helps to maintain the integrity of mucous membranes, is required for growth and repair of cells, is necessary for protein metabolism, protects night vision, and protects against cancer. Beta-carotene has been shown to have an effect as an anticancer nutrient—a discovery made by Japanese researchers more than twenty-five years ago. It is also a powerful antioxidant and a potent immunostimulator. In research conducted by Charles Hennekens, M.D., of Harvard Medical School, beta-carotene was found to reduce dramatically (by 50 percent) strokes and heart attacks in people who already have cardiovascular disease. Adequate beta-carotene in the diet should supply the vitamin A you need, but vitamin A deficiency in the United States is not uncommon. According to a survey by the U.S. Department of Health, Education, and Welfare, about 60 percent of women and 50 percent of men have intakes below the standard set for good nutrition. Pure vitamin A can be toxic to the liver in prolonged dosages greater than 50,000 IU (international units) a day, but beta-carotene is not. The only side effect of high doses of beta-carotene is yellowing skin, which is not dangerous and disappears when levels are reduced. For sinus infections it is recommended that you take beta-carotene at 25,000 IU three times a day. After the acute infection has been resolved, this dosage can be reduced to once or twice a day and continued indefinitely for prevention of both sinusitis and allergies.

Vitamin E

The specific functions of vitamin E are unclear, although it is recognized as a powerful antioxidant and can help protect against heart attack and stroke. Some studies have shown vitamin E to raise levels of the desirable cholesterol, HDL. According to Nabil Elsayed, Ph.D., a professor of public health at UCLA, "You will definitely improve your chances of resisting smog if you increase your vitamin E intake." He believes that vitamin E can significantly reduce lung damage from ozone. Another study indicates that E helps to prevent asthma. For people with sinusitis, allergies, and asthma, 400 IU of vitamin E daily are recommended and should be taken as mixed tocopherols. When it is combined with selenium, vitamin E becomes twice as potent. This dosage need not be reduced as the symptoms of infection subside. Foods highest in vitamin E are crude and unrefined soybean oil and wheat germ oil, fresh wheat germ, whole grains, raw nuts (most varieties), and all green, leafy vegetables.

Multivitamins

There are many comparable multivitamins from which to choose. Make sure your choice has all of the B vitamins and is yeast-free. Take one daily whether you have any of the respiratory conditions or not, and in addition to the vitamin supplements A, C, and E.

Minerals

The two minerals that seem most effective in aiding the body's immune system are *selenium* and *zinc*. An article in the *Journal of the National Cancer Institute* said that men with lower levels of selenium in their blood were most likely to develop cancers of the lung, stomach, and pancreas. Low selenium levels might also be linked to bladder cancer and asthma. Selenium is an antioxidant that breaks down leukotrienes, an allergy-related compound. To treat symptomatic sinus infections and allergies, I recommend either selenium citrate, aspartate, or picolinate in a dosage of 200 micrograms (mcg) daily, or selenium in a combination pill with vitamin E. Foods high in selenium are whole-wheat products, fish, whole grains, mushrooms, beans, garlic, and liver. Selenium can be toxic to the body, so don't maintain a daily dosage much greater than 200 mcg for a prolonged period of time.

Zinc appears to be critical to the release of vitamin A from the liver, helps to convert beta-carotene to vitamin A, and is vital to the process by which new cells are produced and protein metabolized for repair of body tissues. People with sinusitis and allergies should take between 40 and 60 mg of zinc picolinate or oratate daily when symptomatic, and 20 to 40 mg daily for preventive maintenance. The foods highest in zinc are beef liver and the dark meat of turkey. For men, zinc is the most essential nutrient for maintaining a healthy prostate.

Magnesium is a mineral that, during an allergic reaction, supports lung function by relaxing the smooth bronchial muscles. It's also an antihistamine and is used intravenously to stop asthma attacks. The recommended dose for treating and preventing both sinusitis and allergies is 500 mg daily.

Herbs, Botanicals, and Other Remedies

It has been estimated that nearly 25 percent of all pharmaceutical drugs are made from plants, herbs, leaves, bark, or roots. In September 1990, cancer researchers asked the Department of the Interior for federal protection for the Pacific yew, a tree found in the ancient forests of the Pacific Northwest whose bark provides a scarce new cancer-fighting drug. The fact that we are destroying global forests so rapidly, especially the rain forests, means that we are eliminating potentially lifesaving drugs without even knowing it. Many species of plants are becoming extinct before botanists can determine their value. There are still a few human cultures remaining that depend almost entirely on naturally occurring vegetation for their medicines.

Onions; the herbs garlic, echinacea, and berberis; and bee propolis all seem to strengthen the immune system to such an extent that they may be called natural antibiotics. I recommend all of them to patients fighting a sinus infection. They can be taken in addition to a pharmaceutical antibiotic in the form of a capsule, liquid, or tea. Good reference books for medicinal herbs are *A Textbook of Natural Medicine* by Joseph Pizzorno, N.D., and *The Complete Botanical Prescriber* by John Sherman, N.D.

Garlic, a member of the lily family, is a perennial plant, cultivated around the world, that has been prescribed throughout history to treat a variety of ailments. Egyptians have been using it for almost 5,000 years, and the Chinese for at least 3,000 years.

Hippocrates and Aristotle cited many therapeutic uses for garlic, including the relief of coughs, toothaches, earaches, dandruff, hypertension, atherosclerosis, diarrhea and dysentery, and vaginitis. It can be effective as an antibacterial, antiviral, antifungal, antihypertensive, and anti-inflammatory agent. At the National Cancer Institute, garlic has recently shown promise in fighting stomach and colon cancer. Garlic is for the most part nontoxic, although it does cause bad breath. Many brands of processed garlic are available at health-food stores in pill, capsule, and liquid forms. Raw garlic is best, up to one clove per day.

Echinacea is at the top of the list of immunity-enhancing herbs. A perennial herb native to the American Midwest, it serves as an immunostimulator, wound healer, and anti-inflammatory, antiviral, antibacterial, and antineoplastic (cancer). For treating sinus infections and colds, it can be taken as a liquid (tincture), in a dosage of 20 to 30 drops four to five times a day; or in capsules, 200 mg three times a day. Think of echinacea as you would an antibiotic. It must be taken regularly in order to have a therapeutic effect, but if taken beyond three weeks it is possible to build up a tolerance to its therapeutic effect. Naturopathic physician Dr. Steve Morris has grown some of the highest-grade echinacea in America, on his farm near Seattle. He recommends to his patients that they take the herb daily until their symptoms are completely gone, and continue for another three to four days beyond that point. Two possible, but very infrequent, problems with echinacea: (1) allergic reactions in people with ragweed allergy; and (2) as an immune stimulant, it may increase any overactivity of the immune system, such as allergies. Echinacea can also act to prevent allergies, particularly when taken just prior to exposure to allergies or before your pollen season begins. Its anti-inflammatory properties can also help to relieve allergy symptoms.

Berberine is an active ingredient of *goldenseal,* a perennial herb native to eastern North America and cultivated in Oregon and Washington State. Due to its popularity, goldenseal has become an endangered herb. Because of this, I am recommending the use of berberis aquafolium instead of goldenseal. Berberis does not cause the allergic reactions sometimes seen with goldenseal, and most importantly research has shown that berberine has antibacterial, antifungal, and antiparasitic activity. For treating a sinus infection, you can take twenty to thirty drops three times a day.

Bee propolis is an extract from the bee's body (it is *not* bee pollen), and it comes in both liquid and capsules. The dosage is 500 mg three times a day. If you use the liquid form, follow the instructions on the bottle. Bee propolis appears to enhance immune function.

There are a growing number of products available containing the herb *ephedra,* a natural decongestant and bronchodilator, from which many of the pharmaceutical decongestants have been derived. Ephedra combined with herbal expectorants is an effective natural method of treating sinusitis, asthma, and allergy symptoms. There are a number of products available in health food stores containing ephedra in combination with other beneficial herbs. The Chinese herb Ma huang is also ephedra. Those on heart or blood pressure medications should only take ephedra under medical supervision.

Recently, several vitamin companies have introduced products that combine many of the antioxidants with other medicinal herbs. If any are available at your health food store, you may be able to fulfill the foregoing recommendations with just one type of tablet or capsule.

Proanthocyanidin, a type of bioflavonoid, is a relatively new antioxidant, discovered more than thirty years ago by French professor Jack Masquelier, Ph.D., at the University of Bordeaux. After extensive testing—it is considered to be one of the most investigated nutritional supplements on earth—it is being sold in the United States under the brand name *Pycnogenol,* or as *grape-seed extract.* The latter is less expensive, and research has shown it to be even stronger than Pycnogenol. While both are natural plant products in the bioflavonoid "family," Pycnogenol is made from the bark of the European coastal pine tree and its more potent counterpart comes from the seeds of grapes.

Proanthocyanidin is fifty times more powerful an antioxidant than vitamin E and twenty times more than vitamin C. The earliest clinical tests verified its use for improving conditions of the arteries and capillaries, in prevention of infections, as an anti-inflammatory (especially for arthritis), and for anti-aging. Most European physicians consider it to be their first choice for hay fever, and it is also widely used for asthma. Like many other bioflavonoids, this substance is helpful in treating allergies because it prevents the release of histamine. One 100-mg capsule daily would be a good addition to a daily preventive antioxidant regimen. For treating allergies, the dosage of grape seed is 100 to 200 mg three times a day. It is best taken on an empty stomach. Sinus Survival Grape-Seed Extract, containing Masquelier's original OPC (proanthocyanidin), can be obtained through Sinus Survival Products (see the Product Index).

For readers whose primary complaint is a persistent postnasal drip, or just a lot of clear nasal mucus drainage without a sinus infection, an effective remedy may be *Omega-3 essential fatty acids* contained in fish oil. Fish oil can be found in the health food stores in a variety of products such as EFA (essential fatty acids) or as EPA/DHA combinations. Good food sources of omega-3 EPAs include cold water fish (salmon, sardines, tuna), wild game, flax seeds and flaxseed oil, canola oil, walnuts, pumpkin seeds, soybeans, and leafy greens. If you choose to treat your excessive mucus problem by taking EFA capsules, then begin with a dosage of two or three capsules a day, then add one a day up to eight or ten capsules or until your symptoms have improved. Then maintain this dosage for at least a month before gradually tapering back down to one capsule a day. If you are a good candidate for the fish oil treatment, you may have several of the following symptoms: dry eyes; dry mouth or excessive thirst; sensitivity to cold and heat; dry skin everywhere except face and scalp, which are too oily; cracking on the sides of your heels and fingertips; breaking of fingernails (in layers); rough skin on your thighs, buttocks, and the backs of your arms. The most common side effect of this treatment is belching. This can be minimized by refrigerating the capsules and taking them cold. Diarrhea and a flulike syndrome are also possibilities. Fish oil has also been found to be effective for the treatment of arthritis and chronic urticaria (hives).

Flaxseed oil is an omega-3 option that is readily available in both liquid or capsule. You cannot cook with it; it must be refrigerated; and the recommended dosage is one tablespoon twice a day.

Other natural remedies for chronic sinusitis and the other respiratory conditions are *peppermint oil* and/or *eucalyptus oil*. I put a very small amount (one drop) of peppermint oil on my fingertip, then wipe it around the *outside* of both nostrils. The oil, which acts as a stimulant and decongestant, seems to improve circulation to the nasal and sinus mucous membranes. This enhances the effect of breathing clean and moist air. I like to spray my nose with the saline spray or stand in front of the humidifier and then apply the peppermint oil. It feels wonderful!

Eucalyptus oil has a similar effect. It can be inhaled either with or without steam, although the former method is more effective. I recommend spraying V-VAX, a highly medicinal eucalyptus oil, into the Steam Inhaler several times over the course of 15 to 20 minutes of steaming. Without steam, the eucalyptus can simply be applied to a tissue, which you can then hold in front of your nose while breathing through your nose (if it isn't too congested) for a few minutes. After an initial cough, this usually feels very soothing to the entire respiratory tract, while very effectively relieving nasal congestion and sinus headaches. There are approximately 730 different varieties of eucalyptus trees, but only eleven are rated medicinal by the U.S. and British pharmacopeia (drug directory). V-VAX, imported from Australia, is rated number one. I have tried others that are not as effective in treating the symptoms of sinusitis. V-VAX can also be used as a nontoxic germicide for cuts, burns, and cold sores, and as an effective topical pain reliever for arthritis and muscle soreness. It is available in some health food stores and through Sinus Survival Products.

EXERCISE, PHYSICAL ACTIVITY, AND REST

No discussion of physical health would be complete without including the subject of exercise and physical activity. Regular exercise has the potential to contribute more to the condition of optimal health than any other health practice. Yet, in spite of exercise's many proven benefits, we are becoming an increasingly sedentary nation. This is especially true of our children, who are becoming fatter (25 percent are overweight), weaker, and slower than ever before.

Numerous studies show that sedentary people, on average, don't live as long or enjoy as good health as those who get regular aerobic exercise in the form of brisk walking, running, swimming, cycling, rebounding, or similar workouts. In fact, some researchers now believe that lack of exercise may be a more significant risk factor for decreased life expectancy than the *combined* risks of cigarette smoking, high cholesterol, being overweight, and high blood pressure. Simply put, *being unfit means being unhealthy.*

The benefits of regular exercise and physical activity include lessening of tension and *decreased* "fight or flight" response, depression, anxiety, smoking, drug use, and incidence of heart disease and cancer; *increased* self-esteem, positive attitudes, joy, spontaneity, mental acuity, mental function, aerobic capacity, and enhanced energy; *increased* muscular strength and flexibility; and *improved* quality of sleep. Regular exercise also results in an increased muscle-to-fat ratio and increased longevity (people who are least fit have a mortality rate three and a half times that of those who are most fit).

Some of the more pronounced benefits of regular exercise occur with older women. A seven-year study conducted by the University of Minnesota School of Public Health tracked the physical activity levels of over 40,000 women, all of whom were postmenopausal and ranged in age from 55 to 69. The results showed that women who exercised at least four times a week at high intensity had up to a 30-percent lowered risk of early death compared to women in the same age group who were sedentary. But even infrequent exercisers among participants in the study (once per week) experienced reduced mortality rates.

In selecting an exercise program, choose a blend of activities that will increase *aerobic capacity, strength,* and *flexibility.* A regimen focused solely on strength conditioning, such as weight lifting, while providing strength, does little to increase aerobic capacity and can even diminish flexibility. Adding a stretching routine and an aerobic workout on alternate days will provide a much more effective exercise practice.

Aerobic Exercise

The word *aerobic* means "with oxygen." Aerobic exercise refers to prolonged exercise that requires extra oxygen to supply energy to the muscles. In general, aerobic activities cause moderate shortness of breath, perspiring, and doubling of the resting pulse rate. A few words of conversation should be possible at the height of activity; otherwise the workout may in fact be too strenuous.

Aerobic exercise is based on maintaining your *target heart rate,* producing greater benefits to the cardiovascular system and providing more oxygen to the body than any other form of exercise. To determine what your target heart rate should be, use the following formula: 220 minus your age, multiplied by 60 to 85 percent. Keep in mind that 60 percent is considered low-intensity aerobic exercise, with 70 percent being moderate and 85 percent being high intensity. For example, a 40-year-old's target heart rate is between 108 and 153 beats per minute. To accurately determine your pulse, use your index and middle finger to feel the pulse on the thumb side of your wrist or at your neck, just below the jaw. Using a watch with a second hand, count the number of beats in 60 seconds, which will give you your heart rate in beats per minute (or count for 15 seconds and multiply by 4).

When you have attained your target heart rate (after about five to ten minutes of exercising), try to maintain it for at least twenty minutes. It is also beneficial to coal down by working out at a slower heart rate and with less intensity for an additional five to ten minutes before you end your session.

The most convenient forms of aerobic exercise involving the least amount of wear and tear on the body are brisk walking, hiking, swimming, rebounding (jumping on a mini-trampoline), and cycling. Cross-country skiing, if convenient, can also provide a very good aerobic workout. Jogging can also be effective, but to avoid injury, it is recommended that you stretch thoroughly before and after each run, use good running shoes and orthotics—if indicated—and supplement with vitamin C, calcium, and collagen to strengthen your bones, cartilage, muscles, and tendons. Treadmills, rowing machines, stair climbers, stationary bikes, and cross-country ski machines also offer an opportunity for excellent indoor aerobics, as do low-impact aerobics classes. Racquetball, handball, badminton, singles tennis, and basketball provide good aerobic workouts as well.

The keys to a successful aerobic routine are consistency and comfort. Aerobic conditioning does not have to entail a great deal of time, nor does it have to be painful. Find an activity that you can enjoy and keep it fun. Remember, too, that low to moderate aerobic exercise for 45 minutes is just as beneficial as high intensity for 20 minutes. *Do not begin any aerobic activity in the heat of an emotional crisis, especially intense anger.* Wait at least 15 to 20 minutes to avoid the risk of heart attack or arrhythmias that can be triggered under such circumstances. In addition, make sure your aerobic exercise precedes meals by at least half an hour, or follows them by at least two and a half hours, in order to avoid indigestion.

Exercise outdoors if you live or work where it is convenient and safe to do so (specifically with regard to automobile traffic and outdoor air quality and temperature). When you exercise, you may increase your intake of air by as much as ten times your level at rest. The combination of fresh air and sunshine provides greater health benefits than indoor exercise. For chronic respiratory disease sufferers, and for those practicing respiratory preventive medicine, air quality is a critical factor in determining where and when to exercise. Ozone, a very harmful air pollutant, is created by the combination of nitrogen oxides, hydrocarbons, and sunlight. A bright sunny day in the downtown area of most large cities will produce high concentrations of ozone. The EPA considers air unhealthy when ozone levels top 0.125 parts per million. However, in a study conducted by New York University's Morton Lippman, M.D., thirty healthy adults showed decreases in lung capacity during a half-hour of exercise at ozone levels below the federal limit.

I suggest scheduling exercise around the rise and fall of pollution levels. In the summer, ozone builds up during the morning, reaches its maximum late in the afternoon, and then ebbs in the evening. In the winter, ozone isn't such a problem, but cold night air can trap a layer of carbon monoxide, nitrogen dioxide, sulfur dioxide, and particulates that can linger into the early morning. A good general practice is to do outdoor exercise in the morning during the summer and in the evening during the winter.

If you are used to walking, biking, or jogging along main roads, lung specialists recommend that you stay away from these high-traffic areas during rush hour. Avoid waiting beside stop signs or stoplights, where carbon monoxide builds up. Henry Going, M.D., a UCLA pulmonologist, says, "I've seen guys jogging in place next to cars at stoplights. You might as well smoke a cigarette." On windy days pollution disperses quickly as you move away from the road. On calm days it can extend about sixty feet from either side of the road.

If all of these concerns pose too great an obstacle, if you live in a highly polluted city, or if you experience a wheeze, cough, or tightness in your chest during your workout, it's time to head indoors for aerobic exercise. Remember that mouth breathing during exercise bypasses the nose and sinuses, your body's natural air filter. Air pollution can therefore more easily aggravate asthma and chronic bronchitis during exercise. Ozone levels in most homes, gyms, and pools are about half that of the outdoors—even less with a good air-conditioning system.

William S. Silvers, M.D., a Denver allergist, has found that many patients with respiratory difficulties who exercise regularly and follow this with a wet steam exposure experience improved breathing and increased mucus flow and expectoration, and have less nasal and throat congestion. He recommends that following your twenty to thirty minutes of aerobic exercise, and after your heart rate has dropped to its pre-exercise level, you have five to ten minutes of exposure to wet steam. This can be done in either a steam room at a health club, the bathroom of your home, with a Steam Inhaler, or by standing over a boiling pot of water with a towel over your head. You should do nasal/chest breathing, which is best performed by taking a deep, slow inhalation through your nose and then breathing out from your chest. Do this as many days as you can, whether you exercise indoors or outdoors.

Moderate exercise is less strenuous than aerobic but still beneficial. In a research project at the University of Minnesota School of Public Health, moderate exercise was defined as rapid walking, bowling, gardening, yard work, home repairs, dancing, and home exercise, conducted for about an hour daily. A treadmill test determined that those who got this much leisure-time exercise had healthier hearts than those who got less or none. There was no added benefit in doing more than an hour's worth of physical activity. Robert E. Thayer, Ph.D., a professor of psychology at California State University, Long Beach, has found that brisk walks only ten minutes long can increase people's feelings of energy (sometimes for several hours), reduce tension, and make personal problems appear less serious. Not only does it nourish mind and body, *walking is also by far the easiest, safest, and least expensive (you need only comfortable shoes) form of exercise.* Briskly walking two miles at 3.5 to 4 miles per hour (15-minute miles) burns nearly as many calories as running at a moderate pace, and confers similar fitness benefits. By swinging your arms, you'll burn 5 to 10 percent more calories and get an upper-body workout as well.

Strength Conditioning

Building and maintaining muscle strength is another essential component of your overall exercise program. Strength conditioning falls under the following three categories. *Strengthening without aids* includes calisthenics such as sit-ups, push-ups, jumping jacks, and swimming. *Strengthening with aids* includes chin-ups, dips, weight lifting, and training on weight machines. And *strengthening with aerobics* involves various forms of interval training that can be done running, bicycling, jumping rope, circuit training with weight machines, and working out on a heavy bag. The goal of interval training is to work intensively, reaching your maximum heart level for a short interval, then lowering the level of activity to recover. Repeating this process while maintaining your heart rate in its target zone reduces recovery time, strengthens various muscle groups, and conditions the cardiovascular system.

Weight training is perhaps the most popular form of strength conditioning exercise. To design a weight program to meet your specific needs, consult with a personal trainer, who will most likely advise you to work out two or three times a week. It isn't necessary to lift a lot of weight to build and tone muscle. If muscle tone and definition is your goal, best results will be achieved using less weight and more repetitions. To build mass, increase the amount of weight you use and do fewer repetitions. Remember to breathe out as you exert effort, and for free-weight exercises it is advisable to work with a spotter. Also, wear a weight belt to help keep your spine properly aligned. If you are unable to work with a personal trainer, refer to the list of recommended books for helpful guidelines in designing your strength conditioning program.

Increasing Flexibility

The final component of a good exercise program addresses flexibility. This includes stretching exercises, yoga, tai chi, and the Feldenkrais Method. Exercise that promotes flexibility also significantly contributes to strength and function by allowing the body's muscle groups to perform at maximum efficiency. Lack of flexibility can severely inhibit physical performance, increase the potential for injury, and compromise posture. Muscles exist in a state of static tension wherein contrasting sets of muscles exert similar force to create a state of balance. When muscles become weak or inflexible, this balance is disrupted, resulting in reduced function or postural misalignment. Additional benefits of muscle flexibility include improved circulation, enhanced suppleness of connective tissue (tendons and ligaments), decreased risk of injury, and greater body awareness.

Stretching exercises

Some form of stretching is recommended before and after both aerobic and strengthening workouts. Before you begin stretching, do five minutes of movement to warm up your muscles and body core. This will enhance your circulation and make stretching easier. Never stretch to the point of pain. Ideally, you should feel a tension in the affected muscle or muscle group that you are working. As you do, breathe into the stretch to elongate and relax the muscle group as you hold the posture for 20 to 30 seconds. Repeat each stretch at least twice. You should notice that your range increases on the second and third repetition. A few minutes of daily stretching will noticeably improve your well-being over time.

Yoga

Yoga, a Sanskrit word meaning to *yoke,* refers to a balanced practice of physical exercise, breathing, and meditation to unify body, mind, and spirit, making yoga one of the most effective and ancient forms of holistic self-care. The benefits of this five-thousand-year-old system of mind/body training to improve flexibility, strength, and concentration are well documented. There are a number of yogic systems; *hatha yoga* is most well-known in the West. Hatha yoga postures, or *asanas,* affect specific muscle groups and organs to impart physical strength and flexibility, as well as emotional and mental peace of mind.

There are a variety of hatha yoga forms available, and initially it is a good idea to receive instruction for at least a few months, due to the subtleties involved in yoga practice that are not apparent without firsthand experience of its practice under the guidance of a qualified yoga instructor.

Tai chi

Sometimes referred to as *meditation in motion,* tai chi or tai chi chuan, like yoga, is thousands of years old. It involves slow-motion movements integrated with focused breathing and visualization and is practiced daily by tens of millions of people in mainland China. The goal of tai chi is to move *qi* ("chee"), or *vital life force energy,* along the various meridians, or energetic pathways, of the body's various organ systems. According to traditional Chinese medicine, when the flow of *qi* is balanced and unobstructed, both blood and lymph flow are enhanced and the body's neurological impulses function at optimal capacity. The result is greater vitality, resistance to disease, better balance, stimulation of the "relaxation response," increased oxygenation of the blood, deeper sleep, and increased body/mind awareness. Although not as well known as yoga in this country, tai chi is rapidly gaining in popularity, and tai chi instructors can be found in most metropolitan areas. After being taught the basic movements of tai chi, you can practice them almost anywhere to instill a centeredness and sense of calm and to alleviate stress.

Aerobic exercise was an integral part of the program I used to cure my own chronic sinusitis, and it is still a big part of my daily routine. Initially it requires discipline. Start gradually and try not to push yourself too hard. Exercise does not have to hurt to be beneficial, in spite of the prevalent belief in "no pain, no gain." It won't take long before you start looking forward to it as one of the highlights of your day. The benefits that you will soon realize will help to increase your motivation to continue. You may eventually do it every day, although research has shown no increased cardiovascular benefits beyond five days a week (three times a week is minimum). However, exercise does much more than merely benefit your heart. As these aerobic workouts strengthen your heart and lungs directly, your ability to provide oxygen to every part of your body is enhanced—and this, after all, is the scientific basis of physical health. As a human animal, you can experience many of life's greatest pleasures only through your body. Regular exercise can add immeasurably to your enjoyment of life and heighten your sense of well-being.

Sleep and Relaxation

While diet, the use of supplements, and exercise can all benefit physical health and improve immune function, perhaps the most powerful and overlooked key to overall well-being is sleep. The average person requires between eight and nine hours of uninterrupted sleep, yet in the United States we average between six and eight hours, with an estimated 50 million Americans suffering from insomnia.

Lack of sleep and its resulting depression of the immune system can be a factor in many chronic health conditions and is a common cause of colds and sinus infections. Additional sleep is therefore an essential component in the holistic treatment of such conditions. Besides lowered immune function, sleep deprivation can also cause a decrease in productivity, creativity, and job performance and can affect mood and mental alertness. In cases of insomnia, most incidents of sleep deprivation are due to a specific stress-producing event. While stress-induced insomnia is usually temporary, it may persist well beyond the precipitating event to become a chronic problem. Overstimulation of the nervous system (especially from caffeine, salt, or sugar) or simply the fear that you can't fall asleep are other common causes.

Researchers have identified two types of sleep: *heavy* and *light*. During heavier, or nonrapid-eye-movement (NREM) sleep, your body's self-repair and heating mechanisms are revitalized, enabling your body to repair itself. During lighter, rapid-eye-movement (REM) sleep, you dream more, releasing stress and tension. (For more on dreams, see Chapter 7.)

Conventional medicine commonly prescribes sleeping pills for insomnia and other sleep disorders, but as with almost all medications, there are unpleasant side effects to contend with, as well as the risk of developing dependency. A more holistic approach to ensuring adequate sleep begins with establishing a regular bedtime every night so that you can begin to reattune yourself to nature's rhythms. By not awakening to an alarm clock, you allow your body to get the amount of sleep that it requires. Try going to sleep earlier if you find you still need an alarm clock. According to Ayurvedic medicine (the traditional medicine of India), the circadian rhythm, caused by the earth rotating on its axis every 24 hours, has a counterpart in the human body. Modern science has confirmed that many neurological and endocrine functions follow this circadian rhythm, including the sleep–wakefulness cycle. Ayurveda teaches that the ideal bedtime for the deepest sleep and for being in sync with this natural rhythm is 10 P.M. Unfortunately, most people with insomnia dread bedtime and go to bed later, when sleep tends to be somewhat lighter and more active. Ayurveda also states that eight hours of sleep beginning at 9:30 P.M. is twice as restful as eight hours beginning at 2 A.M. It is also important in resetting your biological clock to get up early and at the same time every day, regardless of when you go to bed. Establishing an early wake-up time (6 or 7 A.M.) is essential for overcoming insomnia. You'll eventually begin to feel sleepier earlier in the evening, and even if you aren't actually sleeping by 10 P.M., you'll benefit just by resting in bed at that hour.

Other natural remedies include:

- Vitamin B complex, 50 to 100 mg daily with meals; the best food sources of the B vitamins are liver, whole grains, wheat germ, tuna, walnuts, peanuts, bananas, sunflower seeds, and blackstrap molasses.

- Niacinamide (vitamin B_3) up to one gram (1,000 mg) at bedtime, for people who have trouble staying asleep, not falling asleep
- Calcium and magnesium, 500 to 1,000 mg of each within 45 minutes of bedtime
- Chamomile, passionflower, hops, skullcap, and especially valerian herbs; they are natural sedatives that do not alter the quality of sleep the way prescription and over-the-counter drugs do; they can all be taken as a tea, while valerian and passionflower are available in stronger dosages in a tincture form.
- Kava kava is another useful herb for both anxiety and insomnia; recommended dosage for sleep is two to three capsules (60 to 75 mg per capsule) an hour before bedtime.
- Tryptophan, three to five grams 45 minutes before retiring, and at least one and a half hours after eating protein; adding B_6 to the tryptophan along with fruit juice can improve results. Tryptophan is available by prescription only.
- 5-hydroxytrytophan (5-HTP), 100 to 250 mg before bed
- Melatonin, a hormone produced by the pineal gland in response to darkness, is most effective for difficulty falling asleep; recommended dosage ranges from 1 to 4 mg, one half hour to one hour before bed. Melatonin can also be used for sleep maintenance with a sustained-release 1-mg preparation.
- Hot bath or hot tub
- Breathing exercises and/or meditation to relax muscles and relieve tension

Most importantly, don't worry about lost sleep, since in most cases anxiety is what caused the problem in the first place. If you can learn to relax without drugs, you will have cured your sleeping problems while giving your immune system a powerful boost. Nearly all of the recommendations in chapters 7 and 8 will help you to achieve this goal.

Relaxation is another essential ability that promotes physical health. Derived from the Latin *relaxare,* meaning "to loosen," relaxation is a way to allow the mind to return to a natural state of equilibrium, creating a state of balance between the right and left brain. It is also a highly effective means of stress reduction.

Relaxation is a skill that can be improved upon with practice; therefore, it is recommended that you take time each day to relax. This can be achieved as easily as taking a few deep abdominal breaths or simply shifting your focus away from your problems and concerns, or through any activity that engages your creative and physical faculties. Such activities include reading and writing, gardening, taking a walk, painting, singing, playing music, doing crafts, or any other hobby that you enjoy for its own sake, without the need to be concerned about your performance. Committing two to three evening hours a week to the hobby or activity of your choice will help make relaxation a natural and regular part of your daily experience. The ability to relax and shift gears away from the competitive drive that compels most of us in our society holds the key to greater health.

ALLERGIES, HAY FEVER, AND ALLERGIC RHINITIS

Even more than chronic sinusitis, allergies have a strong **genetic** component. Often at least one parent or a sibling has had a history of hay fever, eczema, or asthma. The results of a number of studies have revealed that if one parent has allergies, there is up to a 25 percent chance that their children will develop allergies too. This number increases dramatically to 75 percent if both parents have allergies. There is a very small percentage of children who develop allergies even though neither parent has them. Along with the genetic predisposition, **airborne allergens** (pollen, mold, animal dander, dust mites, chemical exposures, etc.), together with **emotional factors,** are the primary *triggers* for precipitating the allergy symptoms. Polluted, dry, and cold air can act as an irritant that over the years can cause the nasal mucous membrane to become extremely sensitive and hyperreactive to pollen, mold, dander, dust, and smoke. The primary cause of allergies is a weakened immune system. Other physiologic factors that have been found to contribute to allergies are a diminished secretion of hydrochloric acid in the stomach and a magnesium deficiency, or a magnesium/calcium imbalance.

Foods can also cause nasal allergies. Food allergy ranks as one of the most common conditions in the United States, with as many as 12 million sufferers. Compounding this problem is the fact that millions of Americans are unaware that they are having negative reactions to the foods they eat. Ironically, the foods to which we react are the foods we crave the most. The foods that most commonly cause allergy are cow's milk and all dairy products, wheat, chocolate, corn, sugar, soy, yeast (both brewer's and baker's), oranges, tomatoes, bell peppers, white potatoes, eggs, fish, shellfish, cocoa, onions, nuts, garlic, peanuts, black pepper, red meat, coffee, black tea, and beer, wine, and champagne. Aspirin and artificial food colorings can also cause allergic reactions. But as holistic physicians know, any food can cause an unsuspected allergic reaction, even water. Milk is by far the most common food allergen contributing to hay fever. It is the protein in milk, not the fat, that is the offending allergen. Therefore, low-fat, skim, acidophilus-enriched milk, as well as ice cream, can all be a problem. In aged cheese, cottage cheese, and yogurt, the protein is partially broken down and the antigenic effect is not as great. In most cases it is the cumulative effect of the milk, pollen, mold, and pollution that causes the severe allergic reaction.

Doris Rapp, M.D., past president of the American Academy of Environmental Medicine and author of *Allergies and Your Family,* recommends the following method for detecting food allergies. Take your pulse in the morning, on an empty stomach. Count your heartbeat for a full minute. Then eat the food you wish to test. Wait 15 to 30 minutes, then retake your pulse. If your heart rate has increased by 15 to 20 beats per minute, chances are that you are sensitive to the food you ate. Another effective method for diagnosing food allergy is the "food elimination diet" described on page 147–148.

The symptoms of food allergy are many and usually occur within four days after eating the food in question, further contributing to the fact that food allergies are often overlooked as an underlying cause of poor health. In the case of joint effects, the symptoms can take seven to twelve days to manifest. Nearly every organ system of the body can be the target of food reactions, including the brain (foggy-headedness, headache), heart (rhythm disturbances), lungs (asthma), gastrointestinal tract (ulcers, colitis), veins (phlebitis), bladder (frequency, urgency, enuresis), and joints (arthritis). If you suspect you suffer from food allergies, consult a holistic physician or practitioner of environmental medicine, who offer a more comprehensive perspective on allergies and food sensitivities than more conventional allergy specialists do. To find such a physician in your area, contact The American Academy of Environmental Medicine, 10 E. Randolph, New Hope, PA 18938, (215) 862-4544. Modified cleansing diets are also helpful during your high-allergy seasons. These should be administered by a nutritionally oriented physician or a naturopath.

In Chapter 5, I outlined the conventional medical treatment for allergies. However, unlike the frequent ineffectiveness of antibiotics in treating chronic sinusitis, the non-sedating antihistamines and steroid nasal sprays usually serve as an effective quick fix for seasonal pollen allergy. If you are not satisfied with the conventional approach, would like to complement it or try a nonmedicated alternative, or you have perennial (year-round) allergies, it is possible to treat your allergy effectively, either airborne or food, without drugs and their potential toxic side effects.

Many of the recommendations in this chapter for treating chronic sinusitis are also effective for treating, preventing, and curing allergies, and can be found in tables 1.1, 1.2, 1.3, and 1.4 in both Chapter 1 and at the end of this chapter. The vitamins, herbs, minerals, and supplements that are particularly therapeutic for allergies are **grape seed; vitamins C, E, and A; zinc; selenium; magnesium;** and **echinacea.** Their use in treating allergies has already been discussed earlier in this chapter. In addition to these, I also recommend the following:

- Stinging nettles (*Urtica dioica*)—a natural antihistamine; dosage is 300 mg, one to three times a day.
- Ephedra or ma huang (*Ephedra sinica*)—this herb contains ephedrine, a highly effective natural decongestant and bronchodilator. Dosage is 12.5 to 25 mg two or three times a day. Should not be used if you have high blood pressure or are taking heart medication.
- Quercetin—a bioflavonoid usually found in blue-green algae that inhibits the release of allergic and inflammatory compounds and acts as an antioxidant and natural antihistamine. It works better if taken preventively before the allergy season begins and then continued throughout the season. It should be taken in combination with the digestive enzyme bromelain for better absorption. Total daily dosage is between 1,000 and 2,000 mg divided into three to six doses. Best taken on an empty stomach.
- Licorice (*Glycyrrhiza glabra*)—taken internally, licorice acts as an anti-inflammatory and antiallergenic. Externally it works similarly to topical hydrocortisone in treating itchy rashes. Dosage is 10 to 20 drops three times a day. Should not be used if you have high blood pressure or an enlarged prostate.
- Papaya (*Carica papaya*)—a natural decongestant and mucus thinner. Dosage is 1 or 2 tablets four times a day (dissolved in the mouth).
- Cayenne pepper—contains the potent flavonoid capsaicin, which reduces inflammation of mucous membranes and acts as a decongestant. It can be sprinkled on your food.
- Vitamin B_6—strengthens the immune system. Dosage is 200 mg twice a day.
- Hydrochloric acid—diminished secretion of hydrochloric acid in the stomach may be a contributing factor to allergies. Dosage is 1 or 2 tablets before meals.

- Pantothenic acid—strengthens the adrenal glands. Dosage is 500 mg three times a day.

If your predominant allergy symptoms are headache, then refer to the "Natural Quick-Fix Symptom Treatment" on pages 187–189. The eucalyptus oil, V-VAX, described on page 161 is particularly effective for headache. If you're suffering with itchy or swollen eyes, the following herbs are helpful:

- Pasqueflower (*Pulsatilla vulgaris*)—use this only in its homeopathic form, taken by mouth.
- Red eyebright (*Euphrasia officinalis*)—can be used as eyewash or compress, and eyebright tea can be used to relieve excessive mucus and nasal congestion.

An air cleaner or a negative-ion generator can also have a significant impact in treating allergies. Dr. ShihWen Huang, a professor at the Shands Teaching Hospital at the University of Florida in Gainesville, conducted an independent study on 90 children afflicted with perennial allergic rhinitis (43 of them also had asthma) and their families for at least three years. He placed an air cleaner, without ionization, in their homes for a full year. Their allergic symptoms were scored weekly by the parents, and the patients were evaluated every three months. The results of the symptom score showed: (1) improvement in quality of sleep (less snoring or mouth breathing) in 98 percent of the children; (2) improvement of allergic symptoms: sneezing 80 percent, scratchy throat 75 percent, nasal congestion 70 percent, cough 75 percent, wheezing 70 percent, better behavior or mood 65 percent, sinus infection 50 percent, postnasal drip 40 percent. The overall improvement was most apparent in 85 percent of the children during the first four months of the study. The parents also reported as a group: (3) 72 percent reduction in workdays lost; (4) 43 percent decrease in school days missed; (5) 49 percent reduction in emergency-room visits; (6) 63 percent decrease in clinic visits related to allergy problems; (7) 12 percent increase in clinic visits for non-allergy–related problems; (8) 76 percent reduction in over-the-counter drugs purchased; (9) 43 percent reduction in prescription drugs purchased. Dr. Huang's conclusions: (a) significant beneficial effects of adding an air-cleaner unit in the bedroom of allergic children with perennial rhinitis were observed with proper monitoring, and (b) more frequent changing of the filter (every four months) may maximize the effect of the air cleaner due to the difference in indoor pollution in each household.

Although I know of no similar study using negative-ion generators as air cleaners, I would strongly suspect that the benefits would be even more impressive.

In the following chapters you will learn how to use your mind and spirit together with the physical approach described in this chapter for treating your allergies. While the therapies you've just learned are quite effective, the holistic approach is needed for a greater degree of healing and possibly curing allergies.

COLDS

In medical terminology, the common cold is called nasopharyngitis or upper respiratory infection (URI); it is an inflammation of the respiratory tract. There are an estimated one billion colds every year in the U.S. The average adult develops two to four colds a year, usually between October and March. Children average six to ten colds, and people over age 60 have less than one cold per year. The common cold is the nation's leading cause of absenteeism, accounting for seven lost workdays per person annually.

We're now becoming more aware of the fact that the majority of these "colds" are actually sinus infections. Be suspicious if your cold has lasted longer than two weeks. We also know that the common cold is usually the trigger for causing acute sinusitis, and that the more of these infections we get, the greater the likelihood that we'll develop chronic sinusitis. That's why it's so important to either prevent colds or significantly reduce their adverse effects. Early recognition of the factors responsible for colds will allow you to make choices that can prevent the infection from ever getting a strong foothold in your body and making you sick. Recognizing the earliest symptoms of a cold and then treating it aggressively can also minimize its impact and prevent a subsequent sinus infection.

The first physical symptoms of a cold are usually a sore throat, fatigue, feeling weak or achy, clear, thin mucus drainage, nasal congestion, and possibly some sneezing. For a complete list of primary and secondary symptoms, refer to the chart on page 74.

Colds are caused by over 200 different viruses. In the late fall and winter, colds are usually caused by parainfluenza and respiratory syncytial viruses; while in spring, summer, and fall the predominant cold bug is one of the one hundred or more rhinoviruses. People become infected when exposed to the virus, either by inhaling it airborne or from contact with an infected surface, usually someone's hand. Rhinoviruses can survive for about three hours outside the nasal passages or on objects. The virus usually infects healthy cells by passing through the walls of the mucous membranes in the nose, eyes, or mouth.

Just as with any other illness, there are multiple factors impacting whether or not you get sick. Emotional stress, especially time pressure while attempting to accomplish too many things simultaneously, is perhaps the most prevalent risk factor in causing colds. This situation is often accompanied by a lack of, or not very restful, sleep. These factors combine to reduce immune responsiveness and weaken our resistance to the cold viruses to which we're frequently exposed during the winter months. Any of the previously mentioned environmental risks—cigarette smoke, heavy air pollution, or extremely dry or cold air—can irritate the mucous membrane of the nose or throat enough to allow the virus to enter the weakened cells.

There is very little that conventional medicine offers in the way of cold treatment for the simple reason that there is no remedy that has been scientifically proven. The conclusion of the medical community is that the therapeutic benefits of vitamin C, chicken soup (it's just the steam above the bowl that helps—

steaming water will have the same effect), rest and fluids, gargling, and most OTC cold tablets (especially those with a variety of ingredients) are overrated. Zinc gluconate lozenges did, however, test well in a study performed at the Cleveland Clinic. The zinc produced complete recovery in about four days, instead of a week in the untreated cold sufferers. The usual recommendations address the predominant symptoms:

- Decongestants—for a stuffy nose
- Antihistamines—for a runny nose
- Cough suppressants—to reduce cough
- Expectorants—to loosen mucus
- Aspirin or acetaminophen—to relieve muscle aches and/or fever

Your best line of defense against a cold is a strong immune system. Maintaining a healthy immune system is not only good prevention, but will also assist in a quicker and more complete recovery if you do get a cold. Some studies have shown that people who engage in moderate exercise are less likely to get colds, and they have fewer sick days.

If you respond quickly enough to the earliest signs of a cold, you can usually avoid the full force of the infection and not infrequently prevent the cold in its entirety. Chapter 7 will help you to heighten your emotional awareness to a point where you can recognize the emotional triggers of a cold early enough to defuse or release them. For nearly five years after curing my chronic sinusitis, I did not have one cold! This was a major contributor to my being able to maintain healthy sinuses. However, it takes time and practice to finely tune your emotional "antennae." If you're not quite there yet, at the first hint of a sore throat or nasal symptoms, do the following:

- Rest and get more sleep.
- Take vitamin C (in the form of Ester C or polyascorbate), between 15 and 20,000 mg in the first twenty-four hours; ei-

ther 5,000 mg three or four times a day, 2,000 mg every 2 hours, or 1,000 mg every waking hour. (If you get diarrhea, then reduce the dosage.) Very gradually taper this dose over the next three to five days.

- Take vitamin A (kills viruses), 150,000 IU daily for two to three days; you can take 50,000 IU three times on the first day, then gradually taper over the next two to three days.
- Take Yin Chiao, a Chinese herb, 5 tablets four or five times a day in the first 48 hours.
- Take garlic, eaten raw (one or two cloves a day) or in liquid or capsule form, 4000 mcg (of allicin) per day.
- Take echinacea or Echin Osha Blend®, (combination of echinacea with osha root and other herbs), 1 dropperful in water three to five times a day for three to five days; or 900 mg four times a day. Do not take echinacea if you're pregnant or have an autoimmune disease like lupus, MS, or HIV.
- Take zinc gluconate lozenges, containing at least 13 mg, every two hours.
- Gargle with salt water.
- Use a saline nasal spray hourly, preferably the Sinus Survival Spray containing antiviral herbs.
- Take lots of warm or hot liquids; take ginger root or peppermint tea; you can also include ginger, honey, lemon, cayenne, cinnamon, and a teaspoon of brandy.
- Take a hot bath and steam, adding a few drops of eucalyptus, peppermint, and/or tea tree oil.
- Take the "homeopathic vitamin Cs," *Aconitum* (monkshood) and ferrum phos (iron phosphate).
- Use acupuncture and acupressure, especially points 3, 4, and 8 (see diagram on p. 200).
- Eliminate dairy products and sugar and eat lighter foods; eat less protein; also include warm soups, steamed vegetables, and generous amounts of garlic, ginger, and onions.

The sooner you act, the more effectively this regimen will prevent the cold or lessen its severity and duration. The best treatment is obviously prevention, and that entails maintaining a strong immune system. A good preventive maintenance program is outlined in the tables on pages 183–185.

Keep in mind the basic objective of the physical aspect of holistic medical treatment: *Love your body.* By creating the uncomfortable symptoms of a cold, your body is sending you a very strong message: There is a need for nurturing that isn't being met. You've been "doing" too much and not caring enough for yourself. Your actions and behavior, in conjunction with your genetic and emotional makeup, have combined to create an imbalance that manifests as physical discomfort. If balance is not restored and the body's warnings are not heeded, the problem can progress into a dis-ease of greater magnitude, such as chronic sinusitis—a persistent state of imbalance and physical disharmony.

Many of the products included in these tables that are not readily available at most health food stores can be obtained by referring to the Product Index at the end of the book.

Other Quick-Fix Remedies

During the twelve years since the first edition of *Sinus Survival* was published, I have learned of many effective treatments for the symptoms of sinusitis and allergies. I was informed of the majority of them from readers of the book who were so excited by their results that they wrote to me. Most of these remedies were used in conjunction with the Sinus Survival Program and many have been incorporated into the Program or have been included in the list of "natural quick fixes" on pages 187–189. There are several others that I have not had the opportunity to personally experience or to use with patients. Some of those are described in the following paragraphs.

The first one came from a reader who used a remedy that combined a tablespoon of apple cider vinegar with a tablespoon or more of honey in a cup of hot water. She drank this "sinus cocktail" two to three times a day. It apparently helps to relieve sinus pain and empty the infected mucus from the sinuses.

Table 6.2

The Physical and Environmental Health Components of the *Sinus Survival Program* for Preventing and Treating *Sinusitis* and Preventing *Allergies* and *Colds*

	PREVENTIVE MAINTENANCE FOR SINUSITIS, ALLERGIES, AND COLDS	TREATING A SINUS INFECTION
★ Sleep	7–9 hrs/day; no alarm clock	8–10+ hrs/day
★ Negative ions or air cleaner	Continuous operation; use ions especially with air-conditioning.	Continuous operation
★★ Room humidifier, warm mist; and ★★★ central humidifier	Use during dry conditions, especially in winter if heat is on and in summer if air conditioner is on.	Continuous operation
★ Saline nasal spray (SS spray) (p. 135)	Use daily, especially with dirty and/or dry air.	Use daily, every 2–3 hrs.
★ Steam Inhaler (p. 134)	Use as needed with dirty and/or dry air.	Use daily, 2–4×/day; add VVAX (eucalyptus oil).
★ Nasal Irrigation (p. 136)	Use as needed with dirty and/or dry air.	Use daily, 2–4×/day after steam.
★ Water, bottled or filtered (p. 131)	Drink 1/2 oz./lb. body weight; with exercise, drink 2/3 oz/lb.	1/2 to 2/3 oz/lb of body weight
★ Diet (p. 140)	↑ Fresh fruit, vegetables, whole grains, fiber ↓ sugar, dairy, caffeine, alcohol	No sugar, dairy
★ Exercise, preferably aerobic	Minimum 20–30 min, 3–5×/week; avoid outdoors if high pollution and/or pollen, and extremely cold temperatures.	No aerobic; moderate walking OK. Avoid outdoors if high pollution and/or pollen, and cold temperatures.

Table 6.3

Vitamins and Supplements for Preventing and Treating *Sinusitis*, and Preventing *Allergies* and *Colds*

	ADULTS		CHILDREN (Over 3 Yrs of Age)		PREGNANCY	
	①PREVENTIVE MAINTENANCE FOR SINUSITIS, ALLERGIES, AND COLDS	TREATING A SINUS INFECTION	PREVENTION	TREATING A SINUS INFECTION	PREVENTION	TREATING A SINUS INFECTION
★ Vitamin C (polyascorbate or ester C)	1,000–2,000 mg 3×/day	3,000–5,000 mg 3×/day	100–200 mg 3×/day	500–1,000 mg 3×/day	1,000 mg 2×/day	1,000 mg 4×/day
★★ Beta carotene	25,000 IU 1 or 2×/d	②25,000 IU 3×/d	5,000 IU 1 or 2×/d	10,000 IU 2×/d	25,000 IU 1×/d	25,000 IU 2×/d
★ Vitamin E	400 IU 1 or 2×/d	400 IU 2×/d	50 IU 1 or 2×/d	200 IU 2×/d	200 IU 1×/d	200 IU 2×/d
★ Proanthocyanidin (grape-seed extract)	100 mg 1 or 2×/d (on an empty stomach)	100 mg 3×/d (on an empty stomach)	—	100 mg 1×/d	—	100 mg 1×/d
★★★ Vitamin B$_6$	50 mg 2×/d	200 mg 2×/d	10 mg 1×/d	25 mg 1×/d	25 mg 1×/d	25 mg 2×/d
③Multivitamin	1 to 3×/d	1 to 3×/d	Pediatric multivitamin		Prenatal multivitamin with 800 mg folic acid	
★★ Selenium	100–200 mcg/d	200 mcg/d	—	100 mcg/d	25 mcg/d	100 mcg 2×/d
★★ Zinc picolinate	20–40 mg/d	40–60 mg/d	10 mg/d	10 mg 2×/d	25 mg/d	40 mg/d
★★ Magnesium citrate, aspartate, or glycinate	500 mg/d	500 mg/d	150–250 mg/d	300 mg/d	500 mg/d	500 mg/d
★★ Calcium (citrate or hydroxyapatite)	1,000 mg/d; menopause: 1,500 mg/d	1,000 mg/d; menopause: 1,500 mg/d	600–800 mg/d from diet		1,200 mg/d	1,200 mg/d

	ADULTS		CHILDREN (Over 3 Yrs of Age)		PREGNANCY	
	*1 PREVENTIVE MAINTENANCE FOR SINUSITIS, ALLERGIES, AND COLDS	TREATING A SINUS INFECTION	PREVENTION	TREATING A SINUS INFECTION	PREVENTION	TREATING A SINUS INFECTION
*** Chromium picolinate	200 mcg/day	200 mcg/day	—	—	in prenatal multi-vitamin	
* Garlic	1,200 mg/d	1,200–2,000 mg 3×/d	—	1,000 mg 3×/d	—	1,200 mg 3×/d
* Echinacea	200 mg 2×/d or 25 drops 2–3×/d (allergy prevention)	200 mg 3×/d or 25 drops 4–5×/d	—	100 mg 3×/d or 7–10 drops 3×/d	—	200mcg 3×/d or 25 drops 4×/d
** Berberis or ⊛⁴Goldenseal	—	200 mg 3×/d or 20 drops 4–5×/d	—	100 mg 3×/d or 7–10 drops 3×/d	—	—
*** Bee propolis	—	500 mg 3×/d	—	200 mg 3×/d or 500 mg 1×/d	—	500 mg 3×/d
* Grapefruit- (citrus) seed extract	—	100 mg 3×/d or 10 drops in water 3×/d	—	4 drops in water 2×/d	—	100 mg 3×/d or 10 drops in water 3×/d
*** Flaxseed oil (or Omega -3 fatty acids in fish oil)	2 tbsp/d	2 tbsp/d	1 tbsp/d	1 tbsp/d	2 tbsp/d	2 tbsp/d
⊛⁵Antibiotics						

Key to Tables 6.1 and 6.2

*¹Use the higher dosage on days of higher stress, less sleep, and increased air pollution.

*²Use this dosage for a maximum of 1 month.

*³Dosage depends on brand.

*⁴Avoid with ragweed allergy.

*⁵Antibiotics—an option for sinusitis if taken infrequently, i.e., 1 or 2×/year, or if no improvement with this Program after 2 weeks.

* Stage One—begin the Program with these.

** Stage Two—take these after 3 weeks into the Program, or earlier if you choose.

*** Stage Three—start these 6 weeks into the Program, or sooner if you're comfortable with doing so.

Table 6.4

Allergy Treatment

These recommendations should be followed *in addition* to those listed in tables 1.1 and 1.2 in the *preventive maintenance* column.

	ADULTS	CHILDREN (Over 3 Yrs of Age)	PREGNANCY
★ Grape seed (empty stomach)	★¹ 100 to 200 mg 3×/day	50 mg 3×/day	100 mg 2×/day
★ Nettles, freeze-dried	300 mg 1–3×/d	—	—
★ Quercetin + Bromelain (empty stomach)	1,000–2,000 mg/d (into 3–6 doses/d)	250–500 mg 1–2×/d	—
★ Echinacea	200 mg 3×/day or 25 drops 3–4×/day	—	—
★ ★² Ephedra or Ma huang	12.5–25 mg 2 or 3×/d	5 mg 2×/d	—
★★ ★³ Licorice (Glycyrrhiza glabra)	★⁴ 10–20 drops 3×/d	5–10 drops 2–3×/d	—
★★ Pantothenic acid	500 mg 3×/d (after meals)	50 mg 2–3×/d	—
★★ Hydrochloric acid	1 or 2 after protein-based meals	—	—
★⁵ Antihistamines	OTC or Rx	OTC or Rx	OTC or Rx
★⁵ Corticosteroid nasal spray	Rx	Rx	Rx
Allergy desensitization injections	Physician supervised		

Key to Table 6.4

★¹ Use the higher dosage of grape seed (200 mg 3×/day) only during the peak of your pollen allergy season.

★² Use only if nasal congestion is a primary symptom, but do not use with high blood pressure.

★³ Do not use with high blood pressure or an enlarged prostate.

★⁴ Watch for low potassium with long-term use.

★⁵ OK to use both antihistamines and steroid nasal spray at the outset of allergy treatment program, or wait and see outcome of taking the supplements. They can safely be taken along with the supplements.

★Stage One—begin allergy treatment with these.

★★Stage Two—if after 4 or 5 days you still have uncomfortable allergy symptoms, then begin taking these.

Table 6.5

Natural Quick-Fix Symptom Treatment

Cough
Gargle, then drink lemon juice and honey (1:1) with a tablespoon of
vodka or a pinch of cayenne pepper.
Ginger tea
Wild cherry bark syrup
Bronchial drops (a homeopathic)
Sinus Survival Cough Syrup (with elderberry)

Fatigue
Ginseng
Antioxidants, especially vitamin C
Folic acid
Vitamin B_{12} 500 mcg 2x/day
Vitamin B_6 75 to 100 mg/day
Pantothenic acid 500 mg 1 or 2x/day
Meditation
Exercise
Sleep
Pace yourself between activity and rest.
Rule out anemia.

Headache
Adequate water intake
Negative air ions
Steam
Eucalyptus oil
Acupressure/reflexology points
Hydrotherapy—alternate hot and cold shower
Garlic or horseradish (chew it)
Calcium/magnesium
Quercetin, 2 caps 3x/day
Fenu/Thyme (Nature's Way), 2 caps 3x/day
Ginkgo biloba, 40 mg 3x/day
Feverfew avena, 20 drops 3x/day

Runny Nose
Adequate water intake
Saline spray every 1 to 2 hours

Ephedra (not with high blood pressure)

Nettles, 1 cap 3x/day

Quercetin, 1000 mg, 2 tabs 3x/day (on an empty stomach)—take with bromelain

Vitamin C, 6,000 to 10,000 mg/day or higher—take as ascorbate or Ester C

Sneezing

Adequate water intake

Acupressure/reflexology points

Nettles, 2 caps 2 to 3x/day

Quercetin, 1000 mg, 2 tabs 3x/day (on an empty stomach)—take with bromelain

Sore Throat

Gargle with lemon juice and honey (1:1).

Gargle with pinch of cayenne + 1 tsp salt in 8 oz water.

Licorice-based tea (Long Life, Traditional Medicinals, or Throat Coat)

Lozenges (Zand Eucalyptus, Holistic brand Propolis)

Zinc picolinate, 30 mg 3x/day—begin with zinc gluconate lozenges for three days, then switch to picolinate

Garlic, 2 caps 3x/day

Zand Throat Spray

Stuffy Nose

Adequate water intake

Hot tea with lemon

Hot chicken soup

Steam

Hydrotherapy (hot water from shower) or hot compresses

Eucalyptus oil

Horseradish

Anger release, especially punching

Acupressure/reflexology points

Massage

Orgasm

Exercise

Garlic

Onions

Cayenne pepper

Breathe Right™—External Nasal Dilator
No ice-cold drinks
No dairy
No gluten (wheat, rye, oats, barley)
Ephedra, 20 to 30 drops 4x/day for 2–3 days (max.)
Rule out allergies.
Papaya enzyme, 1 or 2 tablets 4x/day (dissolved in mouth)—use also
  for ear congestion, sinus congestion, and sinus pain
Sinupret, or Quanterra Sinus Defense (a combination of five herbs)

Another option for relieving pressure and draining mucus is to mix radishes and apples in a juicer to create a "sinus juice." It is suggested that you not use too many radishes since it may cause stomach irritation.

A reader from Canada found a local product called Intra, a liquid blend of 23 herbs that kept her free of sinusitis for over a year, after she'd suffered with chronic problems for nearly ten years.

I've heard similar claims about Argyrol or Colloidal Silver, silver solutions used as anti-infective drops in the nose; and Icthyol at 20 percent in glycerin, applied as a nasal packing to open the ostia and sinus ducts and draw infected mucus out of the sinuses.

I was also intrigued with the following remedy for allergies that I found in *Prevention* magazine: Find a fresh horseradish root and cut a slice out of the middle about the size of a thick potato chip; chop it up very finely. Put it in a blender with about two or three tablespoons of apple cider vinegar. Blend for about 30 seconds. Next, take a full tablespoon of the mixture, put it in your mouth, and hold it there for about two minutes, and then swallow it. Not the greatest taste, but the author claims fantastic results. He followed this procedure for two consecutive mornings and one evening and was totally cured of his allergies for five years, at which time he took a "booster" and is still fine four years later.

In recent years I know several holistic practitioners who have been successfully treating allergies using NAET (Nambudripad

Allergy Elimination Technique). This method utilizes chiropractic, acupuncture, and kinesiology to permanently desensitize a person to an allergen. It can be highly effective in treating both airborne and food allergies as well as asthma. A comprehensive presentation of this revolutionary technique can be found in the book *Winning the War Against Asthma & Allergies* by Ellen W. Cutler, D.C.

PROFESSIONAL CARE THERAPIES

Sinus Survival is a book and a holistic treatment program with a self-care orientation. However, there are instances in which therapies administered by a physician, conventional or holistic, are needed. These situations may include a sinus infection that has not improved after two weeks of steaming, irrigating, and taking the recommended vitamins, antioxidants, and medicinal herbs; nasal polyps, mucocele, or a cyst obstructing the sinus ducts (ostia); or an abscess or cancer in a sinus cavity. It is also perfectly acceptable and not uncommon for an individual with sinusitis or allergies to choose to enhance the results of the Sinus Survival Program with a complementary therapy administered by a physician or health care practitioner. The discipline of holistic medicine facilitates self-care while also including the prudent use of both conventional medicine and professional care alternatives, such as **Ayurveda, acupuncture, behavioral medicine, Chinese medicine, chiropractic, energy medicine, environmental medicine, homeopathy, naturopathic medicine, nutritional medicine,** and **osteopathic medicine.** Each of these practices offers treatment options for both sinusitis and allergies. Nutritional and environmental medicine have been presented earlier in this chapter, while behavioral medicine is the subject of the next chapter.

Since chronic sinusitis is a much greater challenge for conventional medicine than allergies, I will focus attention in the following discussion on the professional care therapies for treating sinusitis. I will present only those with which I'm most familiar—osteopathic medicine, naturopathic medicine, Chinese medicine, and homeopathy.

Osteopathic Medicine

Osteopathic medicine is holistic medicine. It was founded and developed by Andrew Taylor Still, M.D., in 1874. The D.O. degree stands for Doctor of Osteopathic medicine, and D.O.'s are fully licensed physicians with unlimited rights and privileges to practice in all fifty states in the U.S. D.O.'s who have graduated from an osteopathic medical school have completed at a minimum a four-year undergraduate degree, four years of osteopathic medical education at one of the eighteen accredited osteopathic medical schools, and several years of residency training, depending upon their specialty and area of expertise. D.O.'s practice in all medical and surgical specialties with the greatest percentage of practitioners being in primary care—family practice, pediatrics, and internal medicine.

Andrew Taylor Still was a fourth-generation M.D. who, after losing four of his own children one winter to an epidemic of meningitis, began to question the completeness of his medical training. He also suffered from terrible headaches for which he had found no solution in the medical model of his day. In the truly Hippocratic tradition, he became a seeker of answers to his own challenging medical problem. He became widely known for his effective, non-invasive, hands-on approach, and was referred to as a "bonesetter." Dr. Still was unsuccessful in his attempts to have his ideas and methods incorporated into the traditional medical model. Since his apprentices (seven-year apprenticeships were the accepted method of medical training in his day) were being taught medical "heresy," they were not granted the traditional M.D. degree. Instead, they were called D.O.'s—Doctors of Osteopathy. (The Latin root *osteo* means "bone," and *patheia* is Greek for "passion" or "suffering.")

When medical schools opened around the turn of the twentieth century, osteopathic students were still thought to be medical heretics, and thus began the two different forms of complete medical training, with two separate medical degrees—M.D. and D.O. Today, osteopathic medical schools have a very similar four-year curriculum to allopathic schools, with most of the same courses and textbooks but with several profound differences. Osteopathic medicine has at its core a holistic philosophy and highly developed system of manual diagnostics and treatment techniques that are designed to stimulate our own innate healing and homeostatic mechanisms. The holistic principles upon which osteopathic medicine was founded are as follows:

(1) **A person is a complete dynamic unit of function, comprising body, mind, and spirit.** Osteopathic medicine recognizes the importance and uniqueness of each of these three elements in every individual and their relationship to disease and optimal health.

(2) **The body possesses self-regulatory mechanisms that are self-healing in nature.** The primary objective of the osteopathic physician is to remove the obstacles to health, thereby enabling the body to seek its own path back toward health.

(3) **Structure and function are interrelated at all levels.** Therefore, if there is an asymmetry, restriction of motion, or tissue texture change present (these are called somatic dysfunctions by osteopathic physicians), one can predict a subsequent alteration in function of the same or referred regions.

(4) **Rational treatment is based on understanding and integrating the previous three principles.** Osteopathic medicine, in fact, offers a unique way of looking at a patient and his or her disease. It is based upon a whole-person perspective, an awareness that the body can heal itself and that its natural state is one of optimal health, combined with a scientific focus on understanding and treating the causes of disease.

Osteopathic manipulative treatment is as much an art as it is a science, and therefore each patient with chronic sinusitis may be treated a bit differently by an osteopathic physician. A thorough osteopathic structural exam from foot to head should precede any assumptions that all sinus problems have their origins in the sinuses or sinus regions. This means that because of the interconnectedness of the body, the sinuses could possibly manifest symptoms as a result of compensating for a primary structural problem elsewhere in the body. If other primary problem sites are not ruled out and/or diagnosed and treated appropriately, the sinuses could be treated repeatedly without significant improvement. This is often the case when one forgets that the body is a complete unit. Attempting to segment it often results in inadequate or unsuccessful treatment.

The two different types of osteopathic treatment that are highly effective for chronic sinusitis are **cranial osteopathy** and **sinus drainage and lymphatic pump** techniques.

Cranial osteopathy, also known as *osteopathy in the cranial field* or *craniosacral therapy,* is a system of diagnosis and treatment originally described and developed by William Garner Sutherland, D.O. He graduated from the American School of Osteopathy in 1900 and worked on developing what would become cranial osteopathy over the next fifty-plus years. His first publication on this subject was called the *Cranial Bowl* and was published in 1939. The underlying principles behind cranial osteopathy are the following:

(1) There is an inherent motion of the brain and spinal cord.
(2) There is regular fluctuation of the cerebrospinal fluid.
(3) There is inherent mobility of the intracranial and intraspinal membranes
(4) There is articular mobility of the cranial bones.
(5) There is involuntary mobility of the sacrum between the hipbones.

A practitioner of cranial osteopathy evaluates and treats the entire body of the patient but is particularly good at diagnosing and addressing structural alterations in the head. This can be of significant benefit to a sinus sufferer with a structural problem contributing to his or her sinusitis. Cranial technique is usually gentle and rarely induces pain. There are intra-oral (fingers in your mouth) techniques as well as techniques that are performed on the outside of the head. The sacrum (bone at the base of the spine) will be checked as well due to the strong connection between the sacrum and the skull via the dura mater (literally translated as "hard mother," it acts as a protective sheath covering the brain and spinal cord). Cranial manipulation can improve the way the sinuses function by eliminating obstruction, inflammation, and infection. Another very important benefit associated with cranial manipulation is that it tends to normalize autonomic nervous system imbalances. The autonomic nervous system is that part of the nervous system that controls "automatic" actions in the body, such as heart rate and breathing; it has been divided into a sympathetic and parasympathetic component—the sympathetic being associated with "fight-or-flight" stress responses, while the parasympathetic has to do with relaxation responses. Autonomic nervous system imbalances have been linked with many diseases, allergic hyperreactivity, and widespread effects influencing all parts of the body. As you can see, cranial osteopathy can be an extremely powerful tool for treating sinusitis, allergies, and many other disease conditions.

Sinus drainage and lymphatic pump techniques have been described by many individuals in the osteopathic community since their development in the 1920s. These techniques have proven to be just as useful today as they were in the days before antibiotics and antihistamines were available.

Like cranial osteopathy, most sinus drainage and lymphatic pump techniques are fairly gentle and are well tolerated even by the most pain-sensitive individuals. Osteopathic physicians may perform gentle kneading and milking of the soft tissues and muscles of the neck region to promote drainage of the cervical lymphatic chains. They may use circular type pressure over specific regions on the face and back of the head and then proceed to perform rhythmic impulses to the chest cavity. The actual techniques performed and their sequence is ultimately determined by the physician and the patient's needs at the time of treatment.

In treating sinusitis, it is especially helpful to combine the sinus drainage and lymphatic pump techniques with cranial osteopathy. Together they will enhance the drainage of the sinuses, expedite removal of excess mucus and toxins via the lymphatic and venous systems, and improve immune function so that sinus infections may be prevented in the future. The sinus drainage and lymphatic pump are fairly easy to perform and can be taught to family members, significant others, friends, or caretakers to be used regularly to help prevent recurrence of sinus problems and to promote the normal self-healing, self-regulating mechanisms each of us possess.

The importance of taking the whole person into consideration is essential to the practice of osteopathic medicine. Therefore, it is important to find a physician who is not only skilled in these techniques but will treat you holistically.

To help you find such a physician, a specialist in Osteopathic Manipulative Medicine, please contact the following organization:

American Academy of Osteopathy
3500 DePauw Blvd., Suite-1080
Indianapolis, IN 46268-1136
Phone: (317) 879-1881   Fax: (317) 879-0563
Web site: <http://www.academyofosteopathy.org>

The Cranial Academy
8202 Clearvista Parkway, Building #9, Suite-D
Indianapolis, IN 46256
Phone: (317) 594-0411   Fax: (317) 594-9299

Naturopathic Medicine

Naturopathic physicians (N.D.'s) are specialists in natural medicine. They are trained at four-year naturopathic medical colleges and are educated in the conventional medical sciences. They treat both acute and chronic disease, and their treatments are drawn from clinical nutrition, herbal or botanical medicine, homeopathy, traditional Chinese medicine, physical medicine, exercise therapy, counseling, acupuncture, and hydrotherapy. Some naturopaths combine several or all of these therapies, whereas others specialize in one specific area.

The basic principles of naturopathy are based on the concept that the body is a self-healing organism. The naturopathic physician enhances the body's own natural immune response through noninvasive measures and health promotion. Rather than treat the symptoms, naturopaths strive to uncover the underlying cause of patients' diseases, looking at physical, mental, and emotional factors. Health is seen not as the absence of symptoms but as the absence of the causes of symptoms. Prevention and wellness are vital principles in naturopathy. These physicians are trained to know which patients they can treat safely and which ones they need to refer to other health care practitioners. As teachers, naturopaths facilitate the growth of patients' responsibility for their own health and spark the enthusiasm and motivation patients need to make fundamental lifestyle changes. The origins of naturopathic philosophy extend as far back as Hippocrates, who set forth the principles "Do no harm" and "Let your food be your medicine, and your medicine be your food."

As a distinct American health care profession, naturopathic medicine is almost one hundred years old. Early in this century there were more than twenty naturopathic medical colleges. Today there are only four. In the 1940s and 1950s, with the advent of more technological medicine, the increased popularity of pharmaceutical drugs, and the belief that such drugs could eliminate all disease, naturopathy experienced a decline. During the past two decades, however, as more people have begun to seek alternatives to conventional medicine, it has seen a resurgence in popularity. N.D.'s are currently licensed to practice in fourteen states.

Naturopathy seems to be making its greatest contributions to the healing arts in the fields of immunology, clinical nutrition, and botanical medicine. Much of the vitamin and herbal regimen for the treatment of sinusitis and allergies and the strengthening of the immune system described in this chapter comes from naturopathic medicine.

Traditional Chinese Medicine

Traditional Chinese medicine is the primary health care system currently used by approximately 30 percent of the world's population. It is believed to be one of the oldest medical systems in existence, dating back almost 5,000 years. The practice of acupuncture (a method of using fine needles to stimulate invisible lines of energy running beneath the surface of the skin) is the component of Chinese medicine most familiar to Americans, but the system also includes Chinese herbology, moxibustion (the burning of an herb at acupuncture points), massage, diet, exercise, and meditation.

In ancient China, doctors were not paid if patients under their care became sick. The job of the physician was to keep patients healthy. Chinese medicine believes that a certain process happens before the body develops a problem or disease. A Chinese medicine practitioner (O.M.D., Doctor of Oriental Medicine) looks for this process or pattern of disharmony. Through questioning, observation, and palpation, a practitioner can determine a person's current state of health and the problems that individual will be at highest risk for developing in the future. In this way, Chinese medicine is an effective preventive therapy.

Traditional Chinese medicine is based on a history, philosophy, and sociology very different from those of the West. Over thousands of years it has developed a unique understanding of how the body works. Practitioners of Chinese medicine see disease as an imbalance between the body's nutritive substances, called yin, and the functional activity of the body, called yang. This imbalance causes a disruption of the flow of vital energy that circulates through pathways in the body known as meridians. This vital energy, called *qi* or *chi,* keeps the blood circulating, warms the body, and fights disease. The intimate connection between the organ systems of the body and the meridians enables the practice of acupuncture to intercede and rebalance the body's energy through stimulation of specific points along the meridians.

People who have used Chinese medicine for a particular physical symptom frequently experience improvement in seemingly unrelated problems. This occurs because the Chinese approach tends to restore the body to a greater degree of balance, thereby enhancing its capacity for self-healing. The entire person is treated, not just the symptom, and the relationship of body, mind, emotions, spirit, and environment are all taken into account.

The World Health Organization has published a list of over fifty diseases successfully treated with acupuncture. Included on the list are sinusitis, asthma, arthritis, the common cold, headaches (including migraine), constipation, diarrhea, sciatica, and lower back pain. Acupuncture has also been effective in the treatment of allergies, addictions, insomnia, stress, depression, infertility, and menstrual problems.

Chinese herbs are the most common element of Chinese medicine as it is currently practiced in China. The herbs are becoming more popular in the United States, but it is still much easier to find a licensed acupuncturist (L.Ac., C.A., R.Ac., Dipl. Ac.) than an O.M.D. who is knowledgeable about Chinese herbs as well as acupuncture. Since 1995, there has been national board certification in Chinese herbal medicine, offering the degree Dipl. C.H. As more schools of traditional Chinese medicine are established in this country, these licensed practitioners will be much easier to find.

Pharmaceutical drugs are usually made by synthetically producing the active ingredient of an herb. Medicinal plants differ from the isolated active ingredients in synthetic drugs because they contain associate substances that balance the medicinal effects. Uncomfortable side effects are generally the result of the removal of these associate substances. Chinese herbs are capable of regenerating, vitalizing, and balancing the vital energy, tissue, and organs of the body without harmful side effects. They can be taken in pill or powder form or as raw herbs made into tea.

Sinusitis and allergies can both be treated effectively with a combination of acupuncture and Chinese herbs. The herbs most commonly used for sinuses and allergies are: Bi Yan Pian, Pe Min Kan Wan, Seven Forests-Xanthium 12, and Pollen Allergy.

Although both of these conditions are commonly treated with Chinese medicine, only sinusitis lends itself to self-treatment with herbs. Allergies are considered to be a complex problem and should be treated by a qualified practitioner of traditional Chinese medicine, who can not only treat the acute attacks but also prevent flare-ups from occurring in between these crises.

Acupressure works according to the same principle as acupuncture, using the same points on the meridians, but with direct finger pressure used in place of needles to stimulate these points. Of the two techniques, acupuncture is generally more effective, but acupressure allows you to do it yourself. The two diagrams in Figure 6.5. illustrate the acupressure points you can use for sinusitis. Pressure should be applied gently with your index fingers; abrupt application detracts from the relaxing effects. According to Cathryn Bauer in her book *Acupressure for Everybody,* there are a few basic principles concerning how to press points sensitively.

(1) Your hands should be clean, warm, and dry. Start by holding your palm over the point for a moment. Then, using the tip of your index finger, probe the area gently until you feel a slight dip; this is the acupressure point.

(2) Press in lightly, holding your finger in this position until you feel the muscle relax. Increase the pressure very slowly. Stop pressing when you feel that you're forcing it; just hold the pressure steady. Pay close attention to the way the point feels. Acupressure points often become warm as muscle tension eases.

(3) Keep the pressure steady until the point is neither warm nor cool and pulses steadily. (The pulsation is not as strong as the

Sinus Acupressure Points

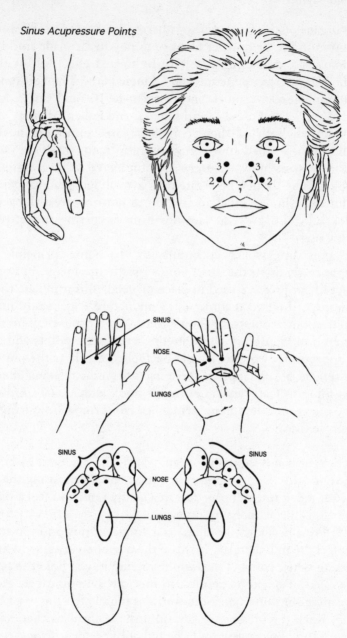

FIGURE 6.5.   *Finger acupressure.*

pulse in your wrists and neck.) This usually takes at least three minutes, and it may take ten minutes or longer to release tensions if your symptoms are acute.

(4) When the pulse is throbbing evenly, ease your fingertip off the point. An abrupt release can feel unpleasant.

Points 1, 2, and 3 are helpful for anyone with a sinus condition. Point 4 need only be used if it is sore to the touch (using mild pressure). Stimulating these acupressure points can help to relieve sinus pain and congestion, as well as the symptoms of nasal allergy. Keep in mind that symptom relief may not occur for up to thirty minutes. The points shown in Figure 6.5 are defined and described in the following material.

(1) LI (large intestine) 4—in the webbing between thumb and index finger. To locate the exact point, place your thumb beside your index finger; the hump, or "meatiest" part, of the web is the spot. Stimulate both hands. This point addresses problems anywhere in your head, such as a headache, toothache, or eye or vision problem.

(2) Extra bitong—along the edge of the nasal bone in the groove along the nose.

(3) LI 20—beside the nose at the midpoint of its widest part.

(4) ST (stomach) 2—in the tiny notch on the bony ridge below the eye, in line with the pupil.

Although not identical, *reflexology* is quite similar to acupressure both in philosophy and practice. It is a healing art that makes use of the reflex areas in the feet and hands that correspond to all of the glands, organs, and parts of the body. It employs a unique method of using the thumb and fingers on the reflex areas to relieve stress and tension, improve blood supply and promote the unblocking of nerve impulses, and help the body achieve homeostasis—a state of balance.

Figure 6.6 illustrates the sinus points on the hands and the feet as well as the nose and lung points. Both hands have identical points in the webbing between the fingers. They can be stimulated with the thumb and index finger or even with the eraser of a pencil. Apply the pressure for twenty to thirty seconds and with enough force to cause some discomfort. The sinus points are the same on the soles of both feet. There are also three other points—liver and ileocecal valve (both on the right foot) and spleen (on the left)—that are important in treating the sinuses. Try stimulating all of these points on a daily basis and see what happens. If nothing else, you will be giving your feet, one of our most abused body parts, some welcome attention.

If you are interested in adding this approach as a complement to the Sinus Survival Program, I recommend beginning with a visit to a reflexologist. See how it feels to have your feet worked on by a professional.

Homeopathic Medicine

Homeopathy is a form of treatment that gently nudges the body toward a healthier state. Its practice was begun in 1820 by Samuel Hahnemann, a German physician who believed that whatever caused disease would also cure it. The Latin phrase *similia similibus curantur* ("like shall be cured by like") is the cornerstone of homeopathic medicine. According to Hahnemann, the proper remedy for an illness that exhibits any set of symptoms in a sick person is that substance that would produce the same set of symptoms in a healthy person. This "law of similars" was not original with Hahnemann. The idea had been advanced by philosophers and physicians for thousands of years, and Hahnemann acknowledged his debt to Hippocrates, in whose writings the principle of "like cures like" appears. Hahnemann, however, was the first to build a consistent system based on this principle.

Homeopathy flourished in the 1800s and hasn't changed much since then. The Hahnemann School of Medicine in Philadelphia was originally a school of homeopathic medicine. The advent of rigorous scientific medicine in the United States during this century almost completely eliminated homeopathy.

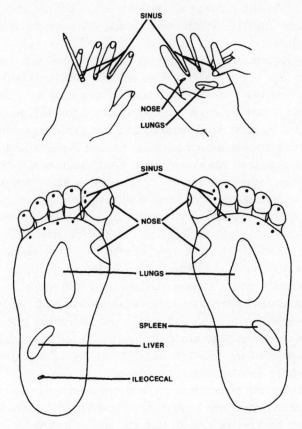

FIGURE 6.6. *Reflex points.*

Today this healing discipline is once again on the rise all over the world, including this country. The National Center for Homeopathic Medicine in Washington, DC, estimates that there are somewhere between one and two thousand practitioners in the United States and that about 300 of them are M.D.'s or D.O.'s. Homeopathy has fared much better in other parts of the world. One third of all French physicians practice it. In Britain, members of the royal family have been cared for by homeopathic physicians since the reign of Queen Victoria. Homeopathy is taught and used in hospitals and physicians' offices in Scotland, Germany, Austria, Switzerland, India, Mexico, Chile, Brazil, and Argentina.

Homeopathy uses infinitesimal or microdoses of natural materials—that is, mineral, plant, or animal. Some standard homeopathic solutions may be as weak as one part in a hundred thousand. These mixtures must be shaken vigorously (succussed) in a carefully prescribed manner in order to be activated. Only tiny amounts of a substance are used, but homeopaths believe that the treatment works because even if the substance were reduced to a single molecule, or lost altogether, its "pattern" would remain in the liquid and could produce an effect. Scientific support for this theory was contained in a 1988 issue of the prestigious British journal *Nature*. The publication described a study from a French laboratory headed by a well-known medical research scientist in the fields of allergy and immunology. The research team demonstrated that a solution that had contained a human antibody, yet was so diluted that not a molecule of it was left, had produced a response in human blood cells. Science cannot explain precisely how this could happen, but the reasons why many pharmaceutical drugs, including aspirin, are effective are also still largely a mystery.

Homeopathic medicines are not required to meet the safe and effective standards of the Food and Drug Administration. They are sold by mail, in drugstores, and in health food stores. Most are nonprescription and legally can be advertised as remedies only for self-limiting conditions, such as colds. Prescription homeopathic substances can be dispensed only by someone licensed to prescribe drugs.

Many patients who seek the care of a homeopathic practitioner have a chronic condition considered incurable by conventional medicine. A homeopathic nasal spray that works quite well is called Euphorbium Nasal Spray, which is manufactured in Germany and distributed by Biological Homeopathic Industries in Albuquerque, New Mexico. A double-blind study published in the journal *Biological Therapy* in January 1995 showed Euphorbium to be effective in relieving the symptoms of nasal congestion and headaches in people with chronic sinusitis. The study took place over a five-month period, during which time the patients were instructed to spray twice in each nostril four times a day. This product can be found in many health food stores.

With the most recent of the three sinus infections I've suffered during the past twelve years, I added a homeopathic treatment to the standard Sinus Survival Program. I took Kali bichromium 30 c three times a day and Kali sulphuricum 30 c three times a day, but not at the same time, and always on an empty stomach. I continued them both until the infection was completely gone. A healing process that has usually taken seven to ten days in the past took only *four* days this time! Now that's a quick fix. Both of these homeopathic remedies are available in most health food stores.

CANDIDA

If you've been diligently doing all of the assigned "homework" from the previous sections of this chapter and listening attentively to your body but the message is that there is still something basically wrong, then you may be one of the many millions of Americans who are unknowingly suffering from too much yeast.

Yeast is an integral part of life. It is a hardy fungus found in food, air, and on the exposed surfaces of most objects. There are more than 250 species of yeast organisms, and more than 150 of them can be found as harmless parasites in the human body. The most prevalent type of yeast found in and on our bodies is *Candida albicans.* It is an innocuous single-cell fungus and a normal inhabitant of our intestines primarily, and the mouth and vagina as well. Although not well documented, it is believed that its only function is to help absorb the B vitamins.

Candida is kept under control by the good bacteria that also make their home in the human gastrointestinal, respiratory, and genital tracts. A large percentage of the millions of these friendly bacteria are lactobacillus and bifidus. Similar to the bacteria in yogurt or in raw fermented foods, the lactobacilli make enzymes and vitamins, help fight undesirable bacteria, and lower cholesterol levels. While assisting us in keeping our bowel function and digestion normal, these friendly bacteria, also referred to as acidophilus bacteria, regard candida as their food. Since they are the chief "predator" of candida, they are critical to maintaining a "balance of nature" in our intestines. As long as this homeostatic relationship is maintained, candida poses no problem.

Causes

However, to an increasing extent, massive overgrowth of candida is resulting in a condition medically known as candidiasis, candida-related complex, or candida toxicity syndrome. *The most frequent cause of this imbalance is the recurrent or extended use of antibiotics,* which kill the "good" bacteria along with those causing the infection for which the antibiotic is being taken. The more broad-spectrum the antibiotic, the broader the range of bacteria it will eliminate, therefore killing more of the lactobacilli. Millions of women are familiar with vaginal yeast infections, which develop when or just after using antibiotics. What I have repeatedly observed in my practice is that *the vast majority of people with chronic sinusitus, who have taken three or more ten-day to two-week courses of antibiotics within a six-month period, probably have some degree of candidiasis.* Since most antibiotics are given by mouth, the friendly bacteria of the intestines are particularly vulnerable to these medications.

A 1999 Mayo Clinic study that I referred to in the introduction to this book reported that **an immune system response to fungus rather than bacterial infection is the cause of most cases of chronic sinusitis.** The investigators reached this conclusion after studying 210 patients with chronic sinusitis and discovered 40 different kinds of fungus, including candida, in the mucus of 96 percent of them. In a control group of normal healthy volunteers they found very similar organisms. They therefore concluded that the immune system response to these fungi in patients with chronic sinusitis is markedly different than in healthy people, and this unusual immune reaction is responsible for the chronic inflammation, pain, and swelling of the mucous membrane associated with sinusitis.

The primary goals of the Sinus Survival Program are:

(1) To heal the mucous membrane
(2) To strengthen the immune system
(3) In people with candidiasis, to reduce the level of candida and fungal organisms in the respiratory and gastrointestinal tracts

These objectives are certainly compatible with the findings of this study. However, the study omits one critical factor. I strongly believe that the **cause** of this immune system reaction is that repeated courses of antibiotics have destroyed most of the good bacteria living in the mucous membrane. This has created an imbalance with the candida and other fungal organisms, which in turn triggers the immune response observed in this study. Whether or not this theory (shared by a growing number of physicians) is fully accepted by the medical and scientific community, I'm thrilled that medical science has now found objective evidence supporting the treatment of most cases of type 1 (most severe) chronic sinusitis with antifungal medication. However, as you'll soon learn in this section, the drugs for killing candida and the other fungi are only part of the treatment. Although they can make a dramatic difference, there's no quick fix for curing this condition.

In March 2000, in collaboration with William Silvers, M.D., a Denver allergist, the first Sinus Survival Study was completed. Each of the participants was a patient of Dr. Silvers with a long-term history of moderate to severe (types 1 and 2) chronic sinusitis. Every one of these patients scored above 180 on the Candida Questionnaire and Score Sheet (p. 218), and each was treated with Diflucan, a powerful antifungal drug, in addition to the rest of the Sinus Survival Program. After four months on the Program, including six weeks on Diflucan, all but one of the participants (he had severe asthma and had to take a course of antibiotic and prednisone during the study) experienced a very signficant improvement in their condition. The majority reported feeling better than they had in years. (For more information about the Sinus Survival Study refer to page 349.)

Hormones, especially progesterone, and birth control pills can also contribute to causing candidiasis, which is why the overgrowth of candida is more prevalent in women than in men, children, or nonmenstruating women. Progesterone, found in most birth control pills and also secreted at high levels during the ten to fourteen days prior to menstruation, has been shown to stimulate the growth of candida. The combination of high progesterone levels just prior to menstruation and an existing excess of candida can contribute to particularly severe symptoms of PMS (Premenstrual Syndrome). As you will see in Table 6.8 on page 214, many of the symptoms of candidiasis are also present with PMS. Pregnancy is also favorable for candida, since it is accompanied by continuous high levels of progesterone.

Anything that weakens the immune system can contribute to yeast overgrowth or help to trigger the immune response to candida and fungi observed in the Mayo Clinic study. Cortisone medications, such as prednisone and prednisolone, often used to treat chronic diseases such as asthma, arthritis, lupus, and colitis, are well-known immune system suppressants. (To an increasing extent, they're also being used to treat chronic sinusitis.) They, too, have the potential for stimulating candidiasis, and can actually aggravate the disease the cortisone was treating. Chemotherapy and radiation treatments given to cancer patients can also weaken immunity and open the door to candida.

Any medication that can potentially cause gastrointestinal ulcerations or inflammation and weaken the lining of the gut can allow candida to gain a stronger and deeper foothold. These drugs may include aspirin, cortisone, and nonsteroidal anti-inflammatories such as Feldene, Naprosyn, Anaprox, Motrin, Advil, and Nuprin. Medicines given to ulcer patients, such as Tagamet or Zantac, can reduce acidity and raise pH levels high enough for yeast to grow. Candida thrive in a pH of 4 to 5, and normal stomach acidity is 2 to 3.

Environmental toxins and chemicals such as pesticides, herbicides, solvents, paints, formaldehyde, pentachlorophenol, combustion products of natural gas and coal (sulfur and nitrous oxide), petrochemicals (exhausts), and heavy metals such as lead, cadmium, arsenic, mercury, aluminum, and nickel can also weaken the immune system. People with occupational exposure to these substances are at highest risk for candidiasis, but as you've already learned, most of us in urban America live in such a toxic environment that we are all probably receiving significant exposure.

Other conditions that diminish immune function and can thereby potentially allow yeast overgrowth to occur are: allergies to inhalants, foods, or chemicals; viral infections such as Epstein-Barr virus (EBV), cytomegalovirus (CMV), human immunodeficiency virus (HIV), chronic or recurring flu illnesses; intestinal parasitic infections brought on by amoeba, giardia, or ascaris; hypothyroidism; nutrient deficiencies due to a poor diet or digestive problems (hydrochloric acid, pancreatic enzymes, and bile); major surgery; and emotional stress. The more severe the condition, the greater the potential for candidiasis.

Once the scale has been tipped and the overgrowth begins, it is fueled by the staple of the typical American diet—sugar. Like most of us, yeast consider sugar to be their favorite food. While candida thrive on it, sugar weakens our immune system. It decreases the ability of white blood cells, phagocytes in particular, to engulf unwanted organisms. It is therefore no surprise that diabetes, a chronic condition of high blood sugar, is also a major predisposing factor to candidiasis.

Obviously there are a multitude of causes that can contribute to creating the condition of candidiasis and/or trigger the un-

Table 6.7

Factors Tipping the Balance in Favor of Yeast

Antibiotics, primarily from medicines, also from commercial meats
   and poultry
Birth control pills
Pregnancy
Cortisone and other immunosuppressant drugs
Sugar
Alcohol
Typical American diet (high fat, high sugar, nutrient-poor)
Environmental chemicals
Chemotherapy and radiation
Free radicals
Food and other allergies
Malabsorption of nutrients
Deficiencies of hydrochloric acid, pancreatic enzymes, and bile
Undiagnosed hypothyroidism
Chronic viral infections
Occult parasitic infections, especially giardia and amoeba
Diabetes
Anti-inflammatory and other medications that produce gastrointesti-
   nal ulcerations
Acid antagonists (ulcer medications)
Major surgery
Physical trauma
Emotional trauma
Poor coping mechanisms to life's stresses
Diarrhea
Adrenal dysfunction—increased cortisol and decreased DHEA

(Reprinted with permission from *Optimal Wellness* by Ralph T. Golan, M.D.,
Ballantine Books, 1995)

usual immune response to fungi. In most instances it is the combination of several factors occurring simultaneously that actually precipitates the overgrowth of yeast and the atypical immune reaction. Typically in patients with chronic sinusitis, the primary causes are: (1) repeated broad-spectrum antibiotics, along with (2) a sugar-filled diet and (3) significant emotional stress. As a general rule in medicine, as in life, there is rarely just one cause for anything. However, in my experience, *in almost every instance of a particularly resistant case of chronic sinusitis, candida is a primary cause.*

Symptoms

Once the overgrowth occurs, the yeast invade the tissues of the gastrointestinal tract by growing in a plantlike form and sending roots into the walls of the small intestine. These roots can eventually bore holes in the intestinal wall, causing a condition known as "leaky gut syndrome." This means that the damage to the wall is allowing candida, bacteria, food, pollen, environmental pollutants, and other material to enter the bloodstream. It's almost as if your intestine has become a superabsorbent sponge. Candida often travel through the rectum and anus to the vagina and urinary tract and can subsequently enter the bloodstream via this more indirect route. Candida are then carried throughout the body and take up residence in those parts of the body with the most favorable environment for their growth—moist mucous membranes, especially those of the sinuses and lungs. In whatever tissue the candida have colonized, they cause inflammation and subsequent physical discomfort, such as sinus pain, muscle aches, joint pain, and itchy anus or vagina. There is still great controversy on this point: Are the candida organisms themselves traveling through the bloodstream and causing these symptoms throughout the body, or is it the toxins that have been released from candida?

As a result of widespread inflammation in the small bowel from the direct toxicity of candida, symptoms of the gastrointestinal tract are usually noticed first. Due to incomplete digestion and poor absorption of nutrients, these symptoms may include bloating, a feeling of fullness, diarrhea, constipation, alternating diarrhea and constipation, rectal itching, gas, and cramping. If the inflammation is severe and/or long-standing, it may be another contributing factor to causing leaky gut syndrome. As a result of this condition, large undigested particles of food, especially proteins, pass into the bloodstream and trigger multiple food allergies and sensitivities.

But the greatest health risks presented by candida result from the toxins they release (79 different ones have been identified), which can damage tissues directly or circulate throughout the bloodstream and cause problems in distant organs. These toxins can also significantly weaken the immune system by inhibiting the function of suppressor T-cells. These white blood cells, a type of lymphocyte, are responsible for modulating antibody production. When they are not working, there is a resulting excess of antibodies. The combination of this overabundance of antibodies along with the absorption of incompletely digested protein helps to explain the exaggerated sensitivities and *multiple adult-onset allergies,* both airborne and food, experienced by many people suffering "systemic" (whole body) candidiasis. The immune system sees the protein particles as antigens or foreign invaders of the body, and initiates a powerful "attack," resulting in an allergic reaction.

A yeast-impaired immune system also has less than the normal tolerance for ordinarily safe levels of common chemical odors such as gas and oil fumes, cleaning fluids, chlorine, perfume, etc. An increasing number of people with candidiasis have become so allergic that almost every odor, all clothing except cotton, almost all foods, or anything in their immediate environment has become a major health problem. This condition has several names: multiple chemical sensitivity, environmental or ecological illness, or the universal reactor phenomenon. The immune system weakened by candida can also produce antibodies to the body's own tissues, especially the ovaries and thyroid, resulting in PMS and hypothyroid symptoms. These symptoms may include fatigue, irritability, sugar craving, headache, depression, and constipation.

One of the major toxins produced by yeast is acetaldehyde. Its multiple effects can be devastating. It is converted by the liver into alcohol, depleting the body of magnesium and potassium, reducing cell energy, and causing symptoms of intoxication—disorientation, dizziness, or mental confusion. The *spaciness* or *mental fog,* as it's often described by patients, is one of the most frequent symptoms of candidiasis. Patients relate a detached state of mind, poor concentration, faulty memory, and difficulty making decisions. The longer this condition persists, the more likely it is that depression will be added to the list of symptoms. The less oxygen in the body, the worse these symptoms are. Exercise, which supplies more oxygen, becomes more difficult to do because of this low-energy state. Energy is also depleted because *acetaldehyde interferes with glucose metabolism—a key component of energy production.* Along with other yeast toxins, *acetaldehyde reduces the absorption of protein and minerals, which in turn diminishes the production of enzymes and hormones needed for energy.* The combination of these multiple factors explains why **excessive fatigue** is the chief complaint of people with candidiasis. It usually comes on gradually but is most noticeable after a night's rest, after eating, and in mid- to late afternoon. If you eventually seek medical attention for extreme fatigue, a physical exam and lab tests will most likely be normal. You may even be told, "It's all in your head!" And if you weren't depressed before, you could begin to feel that way now.

The specific organ, tissue, or system damaged by candida will determine which symptoms occur. Table 6.8 is a comprehensive list of the possible symptoms of candidiasis. Many of them have other causes as well. However, if you have several, in addition to a history that is compatible with a yeast overgrowth, you can be relatively certain of the diagnosis.

Table 6.8

Possible Symptoms of Candidiasis

(I have italicized symptoms that are most common.)

Brain and neurological

Fatigue and lethargy, lack of mental or physical stamina, *depression,* crying, *mood swings,* anxiety, nervousness, agitation, restlessness, grumpiness, explosive *irritability,* hostility, suicidal thoughts, *loss of ability to concentrate,* decreased intellectual functioning, behavior and learning problems, hyperactivity/poor attention span, tantrums, *memory impairment,* increasing lack of self-confidence, impaired ability to reason, *"spacey"* or unreal feeling, *foggy/fuzzy/thick-minded,* drunk feeling (without alcohol consumption), *headaches* (all varieties, including migraines), dizziness, light-headedness, clumsiness/incoordination, shaking, *insomnia,* "schizophrenia," catatonia, autism, manic-depressive syndrome, psychosis, multiple sclerosis, myasthenia gravis

Urogenital

Women: *vaginal itching, burning,* and/or discharge, vulvar itching and inflammation, vaginal or pelvic pain, painful intercourse, infertility. **Men:** impotence, *recurrent prostatitis* or inflammation of the prostate. **Both men and women:** *recurrent urethritis/cystitis* (bladder infection), bladder irritations, *burning on urination,* having to urinate too frequently, bladder "cramping," loss of sex drive

Skin

Rough, dry, or *scaly skin, acne,* hives, *generalized itching,* eczema, chronic or recurrent fungal infections of the skin/nails, psoriasis, easy bruising, recurrent staph infections of the skin, folliculitis, rosacea, tingling, burning, numbness, and electrical feelings on the skin

Ear

Ringing in the ear, stuffed or clogged ear, itching ears, *recurrent ear infections, ear pain, diminished hearing*

Musculoskeletal

Arthritis, arthralgia, *joint pain,* joint stiffness, joint swelling, *muscle pain/aching/*discomfort, muscle weakness, muscle swelling, fatigue

Gastrointestinal and bowel

Constipation, *diarrhea, cramping,* excessive gas, *bloating and distention,* intestinal "growling," mucousy or bloody stools, colitis, Crohn's disease, enteritis, irritable bowel syndrome, spastic colon, esophagitis, *indigestion,* heartburn, itchy anus, decreased appetite, oral thrush, canker sore, coated tongue, cracked/fissured tongue, chronic gum inflammation

Respiratory

Chronic stuffy or runny nose, congested or allergic sinuses, chronic sneezing or coughing, asthma, shortness of breath/difficulty getting deep breath, recurrent or chronic sore throat, *itchy throat,* snoring, recurrent colds and flu, *recurrent infections: sinusitis,* tonsillitis, bronchitis, pneumonia, ear infections

Menstrual/female

Premenstrual symptoms: depression, emotional fragility, irritability, *anxiety,* fluid retention (including puffy face and fingers), breast tenderness, abdominal bloating, nausea, headaches, etc. Delayed periods, *irregular periods,* bleeding between periods, scanty or profuse bleeding, passing clots, *painful periods, decreased libido (sexual desire), endometriosis,* infertility, miscarriages, fibrocystic breast disease, under-normal breast development

Multiple allergies to foods; cravings for sweets, alcohol, bread, and cheese; intolerance or allergy to beverages and foods containing dietary yeasts and molds

Alcoholic beverages, aged cheeses, vinegar, soy sauce, peanuts, bread, brewer's yeast, B vitamins with yeast, mushrooms, bread and other yeast-raised baked items

Chemical sensitivities

Cigarette smoke, exhaust fumes, perfumes, gasoline odor, new carpets, marking pens, paints, solvents, cleaning agents, etc.

Inhalant allergies

Mold, mildew (overall worsening condition in damp, cold season), "hay fever," dust, etc.

Heart/circulatory system

Rapid heartbeat, mitral valve prolapse, cold hands and feet

Senses

Disturbances of smell, taste, vision and hearing (i.e., increased sensitivity to noise or light, deafness), salty or metallic taste, *blurred vision, watery eyes*

Autoimmune

Rheumatoid arthritis, multiple diseases: sclerosis, systemic lupus erythematosus, myasthenia gravis, autoimmune hemolytic anemia, scleroderma, thyroiditis

Other

Intolerance to heat and cold, hot and cold sweats, underweight, *overweight,* feeling sick all over, fluid retention/edema, anorexia nervosa, tendency to bleed easily/slow clotting

This list is reprinted from *Optimal Wellness* by Ralph T. Golan, M.D., Ballantine Books, 1995.

Diagnosis

The most reliable way to make the diagnosis of candida is by compiling a thorough history and reviewing symptoms. If you are experiencing several of the possible symptoms and have a story compatible with causing candidiasis, there are few laboratory tests that are as dependable as this combination for establishing the diagnosis. However, further confirmation could also attained through the results of the treatment for yeast or a clinical evaluation by a physician knowledgeable about yeast-related illness. He or she may also employ laboratory techniques such as stool cultures for candida and measurements of antibody levels for candida or candida antigens in the blood (see page 223 for further details). However, while these laboratory exams are useful aids, they should not be used to confirm the diagnosis. In other words, the diagnosis is best made by evaluation of a person's history and clinical picture.

In his book *The Yeast Connection,* William Crook, M.D., has formalized the symptom and history information into the Candida Questionnaire and Score Sheet, which can be ordered separately from Professional Books, P.O. Box 3494, Jackson, TN 38301. In his book, Dr. Crook says that yeast are especially apt to play a role in causing health problems in patients who:

(1) Feel bad "all over," yet the cause can't be identified and treatment of many kinds hasn't helped
(2) Have taken prolonged courses of broad-spectrum antibiotics, including tetracycline, ampicillin, amoxicillin, Keflex, Ceclor, Septra, and Bactrim
(3) Have consumed diets containing a lot of yeast and sugar
(4) Crave sweets
(5) Crave other carbohydrates, especially breads and pizza
(6) Notice that sweets make symptoms worse or give a "pickup," followed by a "letdown"
(7) Crave alcohol
(8) Have taken birth control pills, cortisone, or other corticosteroid drugs
(9) Have had multiple pregnancies
(10) Have been troubled by recurrent problems related to reproductive organs, including abdominal pain, vaginal infection or discomfort, premenstrual tension, menstrual irregularities, prostatitis, or impotence
(11) Are bothered by persistent or recurrent symptoms involving the digestive and nervous systems
(12) Have been bothered by athlete's foot, fungus infection of the nails, or jock itch
(13) Feel bad on damp days or in moldy places
(14) Are made ill when exposed to perfumes, tobacco smoke, and other chemicals

The following is a modification of Dr. Crook's score sheet that can be used to reliably diagnose an overgrowth of candida.

Candida Questionnaire and Score Sheet

This questionnaire is designed for adults and the scoring system isn't appropriate for children. It lists factors in your medical history that promote the growth of *Candida albicans* (Section A), and symptoms commonly found in individuals with yeast-connected illness (sections B and C).

For each "Yes" answer in Section A, circle the point score in the box at the end of the section. Then move on to sections B and C and score as directed.

Filling out and scoring the questionnaire should help you and your doctor evaluate the possible role of candida in contributing to your health problems. Yet, it will not provide an automatic "Yes" or "No" answer.

SECTION A: HISTORY   POINT SCORE: _____

(1) Have you taken tetracyclines (Sumycin™, Panmycin™, Vibramycin™, Minocin™, etc.) or other antibiotics for acne for one month or longer?   25

(2) Have you, at any time in your life, taken other "broad spectrum" antibiotics★ for respiratory, urinary, or other infections for 2 months or longer or in shorter courses 4 or more times in a 1-year period?   20

(3) Have you taken a broad spectrum antibiotic★—even in a single course?   6

(4) Have you, at any time in your life, been bothered by persistent prostatitis, vaginitis, or other problems affecting your reproductive organs?   25

(5) Have you been pregnant
   2 or more times?   5
   1 time?   3

(6) Have you taken birth control pills
   For more than 2 years?   15
   For 6 months to 2 years?   8

(7) Have you taken prednisone, Decadron or other cortisone-type drugs, by injection or inhalation
   For more than 2 weeks?   15
   For 2 weeks or less?   6

(8) Does exposure to perfumes, insecticides, fabric shop odors and other chemicals provoke

Moderate to severe symptoms?	20
Mild symptoms?	5

(9) Are your symptoms worse on damp, muggy days or in moldy places?   20

(10) Have you had athlete's foot, ringworm, jock itch or other chronic fungus infections of the skin or nails? Have such infections been

Severe or persistent?	20
Mild to moderate?	10

(11) Do you crave sugar?   10

(12) Do you crave breads?   10

(13) Do you crave alcoholic beverages?   10

(14) Does tobacco smoke really bother you?   10

TOTAL SCORE, SECTION A: _____

*Including Keflex, ampicillin, amoxicillin, Ceclor, Bactrim, and Septra. Such antibiotics kill off "good germs" while they are killing off those which cause infection.

SECTION B: HISTORY   POINT SCORE: _____

For each of your symptoms, enter the appropriate figure in the point score column:

Not at all	0 points
Occasional or mild	3 points
Frequent and/or moderately severe	6 points
Severe and/or disabling	9 points

Add total score and record it in the box at the end of this section.

POINT SCORE: _____

(1) Fatigue or lethargy   ____

(2) Feeling of being "drained"   ____

(3) Poor memory or concentration   ____

(4) Feeling "spacey" or "unreal"   ____

(5) Depression   ____

(6) Numbness, burning, or tingling   ____

(7) Muscle aches   _____

(8) Muscle weakness or paralysis   _____

(9) Pain and/or swelling in joints   _____

(10) Abdominal pain   _____

(11) Constipation   _____

(12) Diarrhea   _____

(13) Bloating   _____

(14) Troublesome vaginal discharge   _____

(15) Persistent vaginal burning or itching   _____

(16) Prostatitis   _____

(17) Impotence   _____

(18) Loss of sexual desire   _____

(19) Endometriosis or infertility   _____

(20) Cramps and/or other menstrual irregularities   _____

(21) Premenstrual tension   _____

(22) Spots in front of the eyes   _____

(23) Erratic vision   _____

TOTAL SCORE, SECTION B: _____

SECTION C: OTHER SYMPTOMS

For each of your symptoms, enter the appropriate figure in the point score column:

Not at all	0 points
Occasional or mild	1 point
Frequent and/or moderately severe	2 points
Severe and/or disabling	3 points

Add total score and record it in the box at the end of this section.

POINT SCORE: _____

(1) Drowsiness   _____

(2) Irritability or jitteriness   _____

(3) Incoordination   _____

(4) Inability to concentrate   _____

(5) Frequent mood swings   _____

(6) Headache   _____

(7) Dizziness/loss of balance   _____

(8) Pressure above ears, feeling of head swelling and tingling   _____

(9) Itching   ____
(10) Other rashes   ____
(11) Heartburn   ____
(12) Indigestion   ____
(13) Belching and intestinal gas   ____
(14) Mucus in stools   ____
(15) Hemorrhoids   ____
(16) Dry mouth   ____
(17) Rash or blisters in mouth   ____
(18) Bad breath   ____
(19) Joint swelling or arthritis   ____
(20) Nasal congestion or discharge   ____
(21) Postnasal drip   ____
(22) Nasal itching   ____
(23) Sore or dry throat   ____
(24) Cough   ____
(25) Pain or tightness in chest   ____
(26) Wheezing or shortness of breath   ____
(27) Urinary urgency or frequency   ____
(28) Burning on urination   ____
(29) Failing vision   ____
(30) Burning or tearing of eyes   ____
(31) Recurrent infections or fluid in ears   ____
(32) Ear pain or deafness   ____

TOTAL SCORE, SECTION C: _____

TOTAL SCORE, SECTION A: _____

TOTAL SCORE, SECTION B: _____

GRAND SCORE: _____

The Grand Total Score will help you and your doctor decide if your health problems are yeast-connected. Scores in women will run higher as 7 items in the questionnaire apply exclusively to women, while only 2 apply exclusively to men.

IF YOUR SCORE IS:	SYMPTOMS ARE:
180 (women) 140 (men) $\longrightarrow$	almost certainly yeast-connected
120 (women) 80 (men) $\longrightarrow$	probably yeast-connected
60 (women) 40 (men) $\longrightarrow$	possibly yeast-connected
Less than 60 (women) 40 (men) $\longrightarrow$	probably not yeast-connected

Much of the original research on candida was performed by C. Orian Truss, M.D., who wrote *The Missing Diagnosis.* In that book he states that the diagnosis of systemic candidiasis should be suspected in any individual with chronic sinus and upper respiratory conditions and allergies, runny nose, postnasal drip, mucus in the throat, itchy ears, or chronic sore throat. The current laboratory tests that have been most often used to diagnose candida are:

The Comprehensive Digestive Stool Analysis (CDSA)

Rather than simply culture a stool sample for the presence of *Candida albicans,* the CDSA is more clinically useful. This battery of integrated diagnostic laboratory tests evaluates digestion, intestinal function, intestinal environment (amount of beneficial and bad bacteria), and absorption by carefully examining the stool. It is a very useful tool in determining the digestive disturbance that is likely to be the underlying factor responsible for candida overgrowth. When the candida can be cultured, then the lab can assess which natural and prescription antifungal medications are most likely to be effective. In addition, the CDSA may determine that the symptoms are not related to candida overgrowth but rather to conditions such as small intestine bacterial overgrowth, food allergies (sensitivities) and/or the "leaky gut" syndrome. A physician, chiropractor, or naturopathic doctor can order this test for you. (For more information, see the Resource Guide.)

Candida Antibody and Antigen Levels

Another laboratory method to confirm the presence of candida overgrowth is measuring the level of antibodies to candida or the level of antigens in the blood. The newer candida antibody testing indicates four different responses of the body to candida: (1) whether the person has ever had a candida infection; (2) whether the infection is likely to be currently present; (3) whether the infection has invaded mucous membranes; and (4) how significantly the person is reacting to the antibodies. Usually these tests are not needed, as the results typically only confirm what the patient history, physical examination, and CDSA reveal. Hence, the test does not usually change the course of action. Nonetheless, some patients and physicians may desire confirmation that *Candida albicans* is a responsible factor in the patient's health status. In that situation, these blood tests can be quite helpful and can also be used as a way of monitoring treatment.

Although these laboratory tests are improving, they have not met the current high scientific standards expected for medical diagnosis. This is primarily the reason that the majority of physicians fail to recognize the existence of systemic candidiasis, and many have become antagonistic even to the suggestion of that diagnosis. Unfortunately this lack of acknowledgment prevents most physicians from ever treating the condition. Although they're not perfect, these tests—especially the CDSA—can still be helpful in the diagnosis of candida. Ultimately, regardless of the test results, a trial candida treatment program has been the best diagnostic test we've had. If there's a definite improvement in your symptoms within four weeks or even sooner, then you probably have candidiasis.

Treatment

Although similar in its holistic scope, the comprehensive treatment program for systemic candidiasis is more challenging than
the regimen for simple chronic sinusitis (i.e., without candida).
Treatment depends upon the degree of yeast overgrowth and to
what extent immune function has been diminished. If yeast
symptoms are confined only to the gastrointestinal tract or
vagina, the program is shorter and much less involved than if the
yeast toxins have spread throughout the body and are causing recurrent sinus infections along with other problems. In the latter
case, which is most often the situation with my patients, it can
take from six to nine months to cure candidiasis.

The treatment program for systemic candidiasis consists of
four components*, and for the best results you should start with
phases I and II before progressing to III and IV:

Phase I: Kill the overgrowth of candida.
Phase II: Eliminate the fuel for the growth of candida
through diet.
Phase III: Restore normal bacterial flora in the bowel.
Phase IV: Strengthen the immune system.

*Phases I, II, and III are summarized in Table 1.5 on page 18.

Phase I

In my experience, the most effective means of killing candida is
through the use of the prescription antifungal drugs Diflucan,
Sporanox, and Nizoral. I know of some physicians who have
used Lamisil with good results. Although they're all expensive
(200 mg of Diflucan can cost as much as $13 per tablet; 200 mg
of Nizoral averages about $3) and have potentially harmful side
effects, nothing else works as well. They're usually prescribed at
200 mg per day for at least one month. Diflucan is recommended daily for six weeks, and I will often reduce Nizoral to
one every other day for a second month. Many physicians are
reluctant to prescribe these, especially Nizoral, because of pos-

sible liver toxicity. Diflucan, Sporanox, and Lamisil are all potentially less harmful to the liver and seem to work a little better than Nizoral. However, during the seven to eight years that I have prescribed it, I have seen only two patients develop the symptoms of hepatitis (inflammation of the liver) from Nizoral, and both resolved quickly after stopping the drug. A blood test for liver enzymes before starting on Nizoral would be helpful in minimizing this risk, as well as taking silymarin (milk-thistle extract), which protects the liver. The recommended dose is two tablets twice a day. A more probable side effect in using these drugs is die-off, or Herxheimer's reaction, which usually occurs during the first two weeks of treatment and typically lasts for two days to one week. These medications are so powerful in killing yeast that as the organisms die they release a "flood" of toxins into the bloodstream that can cause fatigue, headaches, nausea, loose stools, flulike aches and pains, and any other symptom that yeast are known to produce. Distilled water, both drunk and used as an enema, vitamin C, and ibuprofen can all help to relieve these die-off symptoms. Although it's possible that for a short time you may feel worse than you did before, you may also choose to look at the "regression" resulting from die-off as a confirmation of your diagnosis of candida, as well as a hopeful sign that you are eliminating yeast and will be feeling much better very soon. Following die-off, most patients experience a level of health significantly greater than they had prior to treating candida. The other prescription drug that's been around far longer than the others I've mentioned is nystatin, available in tablets and powder. It kills candida very well in the bowel, but seems to be ineffective for the rest of the body. When a person has a severe case of candida or grows out candida in their stool and has antibodies in their blood, another option is to take nystatin for three to five months and add Diflucan, Sporanax, or Nizoral in addition for four to six weeks. That way the candida can be eradicated in the intestine and genital tracts and then the rest of the body. This is a powerful combination and I recommend you must be followed closely by your physician. I have seen a few patients require even slightly longer treatments. These prescription drugs are not the whole answer, however: You must be prepared to adhere to dietary recommendations and continue to nurture yourself or it may not be worth the risk of these powerful medications.

If you are not able to obtain or cannot take a prescription antifungal drug, there are other available options that work, although they are not quite as effective in quickly reducing candida. Three homeopathic remedies that I'm familiar with are Aqua Flora and Candida-Away (available in health food stores) and Mycocan Combo, available only through health care practitioners. I've used Mycocan with many patients and have seen good results. It's sold, along with a few other similar products, through Mountain States Health Care Products. Metagenics has recently created a highly effective candida-fighting product called CandiBactin-AR. For a stronger combination, the homeopathics can also be used in conjunction with nystatin. There are a variety of products available in health food stores that can help to eliminate candida. Most contain caprylic acid, garlic, pau d'arco, plant tannins, grapefruit-seed extract, and other herbs that act directly on candida or indirectly by strengthening the immune system. However, most of these are weak substitutes for prescription drugs or professional products. I would suggest asking a health care practitioner for a recommendation. These anti-yeast products, however, can be helpful following drug therapy as a method of preventing candida from "rebounding."

Another product that I always use in my practice to kill candida is Flora Balance. It is a unique strain of bacteria called *Bacillus laterosporus B.O.D.*, which is available in health food stores or through physicians as Latero-Flora. It has been tested extensively and found to be extremely effective for gastrointestinal dysfunction, food sensitivities, and candidiasis. It is suggested that two capsules be taken twenty minutes before breakfast. I usually continue that dose for about two to three months before reducing it to one daily capsule for several more months.

An herbal combination (made up of more than twenty herbs) that I frequently use as part of my candida elimination program is Intestinalis. It is an excellent remedy for any intestinal infection. In addition to treating candida, it can be used to treat or even prevent giardia (a parasite frequently found in untreated water), other internal parasites, and traveler's diarrhea. Two years ago a woman I was treating for chronic sinusitis and candidiasis went on a group tour to Egypt. Upon her return she was so pleased to report to me that she was the only member of the forty-person group who did not get diarrhea. I'd guess that she was also the only one on the tour taking Intestinalis every day.

In recent years there have been reports of dramatic results in eliminating candida using 35 percent food-grade hydrogen peroxide. (Store-bought hydrogen peroxide is a 3-percent solution.) It can be taken orally or intravenously. I have had no personal experience with this method, but I have read about Dr. Kurt Donsbach's success using this treatment at his holistic center, Hospital Santa Monica in Rosarito Beach, Baja California, Mexico.

The average American diet can cause a thick coat of mucus and impacted food residue to form on the walls of the large intestine. Not only can this encrusted matter affect colon function and contribute to disease by preventing absorption of vital nutrients, it also provides an ideal environment for yeast to thrive. That's why colonic treatments provide another rapid method of removing excess candida from the bowel as well as mitigating die-off effects. Much more effective than an enema, they are best done on a weekly basis in conjunction with taking an antifungal drug. They can cleanse the bowel of candida, toxins, and dead yeast organisms while also helping the inflamed lining of the bowel to begin the healing process. These treatments need to be performed by trained colon hydrotherapists, and in most cities they are not that easy to find. Look for them through the office of a chiropractor or naturopath.

Although not as fast (it can take several months), it is possible to clean the colon by following a candida-control diet, drinking plenty of water, getting regular exercise, taking caprylic acid to kill candida, and using two natural agents that eliminate colon toxicity—psyllium and bentonite. Mix one heaping teaspoon of psyllium plus two tablespoons of liquid bentonite with 8 to 10 ounces of water or diluted juice twice a day (morning and night). If there is bloating, cut the above dosages in half but still take it two times a day.

Phase II

Eliminating the fuel for candida through diet, while at the same time strengthening your immune system, is the foundation of any treatment program. Since each of us has a unique body chemistry, no two candida-control diets will be exactly the same. Also, every physician who treats candidiasis has somewhat different dietary recommendations. But there are some basic principles that apply to almost anyone for a *Candida and Hypoallergenic Diet:*

(1) The diet consists primarily of protein and fresh organic vegetables and a limited amount of complex carbohydrates and fat-containing foods, along with a small amount of fresh fruit.

(2) Sugar and concentrated sweets are always to be avoided.

(3) Three to six months is a minimum time frame for maintaining the diet, although it can be less restrictive the longer you're on it.

(4) It's best to rotate the acceptable foods and not eat a particular food more than once every three or four days. This is especially true for grains.

(5) Changing one's diet can be a challenge. The more involved you are in the process—planning, shopping, and cooking—the easier and more rewarding it will be.

The following diet is a composite from the two naturopathic physicians with whom I work closely on treating candida, Todd

Nelson and Sylvia Flesner, and my holistic medical colleague Ralph Golan, M.D.

Note: The first 21 days, avoid starch, high sugar foods, including fruit. Also avoid yeast and mold foods.

Foods to Include

Vegetables   Eat freely; 50 to 60 percent of total diet; raw or lightly steamed; organic and clean (wash well); high-water content and low-starch vegetables are best (refer to tables 6.9 and 6.10, Glycemic Index and Carbohydrate Classification of Fruits and Vegetables, pp. 233–235):

- **Green leafy:** all lettuce, spinach, parsley, cabbage, kale, collard greens, watercress, beet greens, mustard greens, bok choy, sprouts
- **Other low-starch vegetables:** celery, zucchini, summer squash, crookneck squash, green beans, broccoli, cauliflower, brussels sprouts, radish, bell pepper (green, red, yellow), asparagus, cucumber, tomato, onion, leek, garlic, kohlrabi
- **Moderately low starch:** carrot, beet, rutabaga, turnip, parsnip, eggplant, artichoke, avocado, water chestnuts, peas (green, snow peas), okra

Protein   Emphasis at breakfast and lunch with no less than 60 grams per day; meats should be antibiotic- and hormone-free; fish should be fresh deep-water ocean fish; seeds and nuts should be raw organic. Acceptable proteins include: fish, canned fish (salmon and tuna—okay occasionally), turkey, ground turkey, chicken, lamb, wild game, Cornish hens, eggs (limit two to four per week), seeds and nuts—almonds, cashews, pecans, filberts, pine nuts, Brazil nuts, walnuts, pistachios, sunflower seeds, sesame seeds (raw or dry roasted), pumpkin seeds.

Complex carbohydrates   Starchy vegetables, legumes (introduce after the first 21 days), and whole grains; eat only enough to maintain your energy (try to limit yourself to one serving a day or less); restriction varies according to food allergy, which can be determined with food rotation.

- **Starchy vegetables:** new and red potatoes, sweet potatoes, yams, winter squash (acorn, butternut), pumpkin
- **Legumes:** lentils, split peas, black-eyed peas, beans (kidney, garbanzo, black, navy, pinto, lima, adzuki)
- **Non-gluten grains:** brown rice, millet, quinoa, and amaranth: eat sprouted or cooked; organic and clean; available in bulk at health food stores; rotate grains every four days; tasty as breakfast cereals, in salads and soups, in casseroles and stir-frys; store away from light and heat in airtight containers; other whole grains that should be eaten in only limited amounts include barley, spelt, wild rice, corn, buckwheat, oats, cornmeal, bulgur, and couscous.

Flaxseed oil   1 to 2 tablespoons daily; use on grains or vegetables or as a salad dressing; do *not* heat or cook with; keep refrigerated and away from light; other acceptable oils (cold-pressed)—extra virgin olive oil, canola, walnut. Use within six weeks of opening.

After 21 Days

Fruits   Introduce fruits into your diet slowly, limiting yourself to one serving per day until you are sure they do not make your symptoms worse. Start with melons, berries—blueberries, raspberries, huckleberries, blackberries, lemon and grapefruit (only after first 21 days of the diet); then choose from among most other fresh fruits, all of which are generally sweeter than the first group. These include apple, pear, peach, orange, nectarine, apricot, cherry, and pineapple. Fruit juices should be very diluted, at least 1:1 with water. Freshly squeezed is best. Avoid full-strength fruit juices, canned fruit juices, and all dried fruits.

Yeast and mold-containing foods   These are allowable only if you're not allergic. However, I would introduce them very gradually (eat a particular food no more than once every three to four days) and not begin until you have been on the diet for at least three weeks. These foods include: fermented dairy products such as yogurt, kefir, buttermilk, low-fat cottage cheese, and sour cream; fermented foods such as tofu, tempeh, miso, soy sauce; raw almond butter and raw sesame tahini.

Foods to Avoid

- Refined sugar and sugar-containing foods: cakes, cookies, candy, doughnuts, pastries, ice cream, pudding, soft drinks, pies, etc.; anything containing sucrose (table sugar), fructose, maltose, lactose, glucose, dextrose, corn sweetener, corn syrup, sorbitol, and manitol; honey; molasses; maple syrup; date sugar; barley malt; rice syrup; NutraSweet; and saccharine; table salt (often contains sugar; use sea salt)
- **To diminish sugar cravings, use chromium picolinate, 200 mcg 2 ×/day; biotin, 500–1,000 mcg 2 ×/day; and a yeast-free B complex, 50 mg 2 ×/day. Four days without any sugar will also usually eliminate this craving.**
- Milk and dairy products—all cheeses; (unsweetened soy milk is okay and so is butter, but not in excess)
- Bread and other yeast-raised baked items, including cakes, cookies, and crackers; whole grain cereals; pastas; tortillas; waffles; and muffins
- Beef and pork
- Mushrooms—all types
- Rye and wheat (avoid for first three weeks)
- Grapes, plums, bananas, dried fruit, canned fruit, and canned vegetables
- Alcoholic beverages
- Caffeine—both tea and coffee (herbal tea and green tea are okay)
- White or refined flour products, packaged/processed and refined foods
- Fried foods, fast foods, sausage, and hot dogs
- Vinegar, mustard, ketchup, sauerkraut, olives, and pickles

- Margarine, preservatives (check frozen vegetables), artificial sweeteners
- Refined and hydrogenated oils
- Leftovers—freeze them for a later date
- Rice milk (high carbohydrate content)

This diet is meant to be a guide. The responses to it will vary greatly depending upon the severity of the candidiasis, food allergies, and the type of medication (if any) you're taking to eliminate candida. The majority of people who closely adhere to it will experience a significant improvement within one month. But suppose you follow it for three to four weeks in addition to taking medication and you see no improvement. Then I'd recommend going back to the basic vegetable (low-starch) and protein diet and be suspicious of food allergy. The food you're allergic to is often something you eat every day and have developed a craving for. If you reintroduce new foods very gradually, every three to four days, then you should be able to detect the offending food from the symptoms that arise after eating it.

Initially many people complain, "There's nothing to eat on this diet," and it's not unusual to lose eight to ten pounds during the first month. However, there are in fact a multitude of nutritious and tasty choices, and the weight loss will usually subside. A key factor in successfully maintaining the diet lies in finding some recipes that you like. Candida cookbooks are relatively easy to locate in most health food stores. Gail Burton's *Candida Control Cookbook,* Dr. Crook's *The Yeast Connection Cook Book,* and Vicki Glassburn's *Who Killed Candida?* and Dr. B. Semon's *Feast Without Yeast* are all excellent resources. The menu and recipe suggestions that follow have been provided by Todd Nelson, N.D.

Menu Suggestions for a Candida Hypo-allergenic Diet

★ = Recipe included
★★ = At health food store

Table 6.9

Glycemic Index

Carbohydrates act like a powerful drug elevating insulin in the body. This in turn can increase fat deposits, LDL cholesterol (the unhealthy kind), and inflammation, while decreasing immunity. The amount of insulin the body produces is based on the amount of carbohydrates that actually enters the bloodstream as the simple sugar glucose. This is why you can consume a large amount of the 3-percent or 6-percent vegetables and fruits (refer to Table 6.10, Carbohydrate Classifications Table, p. 235) in comparison to the amount of grains, starches, breads, or pastas at any given meal.

Example: 1½ cups of broccoli, or any other 3-percent vegetable = ¼ cup pasta.

This is why it is best to focus on the low-density carbohydrates (3 percent and 6 percent). Not only can you eat more, but there are many other benefits, including high water content, high fiber content, vitamins, minerals and enzymes.

People are genetically designed to eat primarily fruits and vegetables as their major source of carbohydrates.

All carbohydrates, simple or complex, have to be broken down into simple sugars before being absorbed by the body and entering the bloodstream. The only simple sugar that can actually enter the bloodstream is glucose. The faster glucose enters the bloodstream, the more insulin you make. This is important for you to know when you are making your choice of carbohydrates. *The higher the glycemic index of carbohydrates, the faster it enters the bloodstream as sugar.*

Low Glycemic (Examples: 3-percent and 6-percent fruits and vegetables)
Fructose has to be converted into glucose via the liver, so fruits are lower glycemic index than grains and starches.

High Glycemic (Examples: bagel, pasta, cooked starches)
Cornflakes are pure glucose linked by chemical bonds. These bonds are easily broken in the stomach and glucose rushes into the bloodstream. Table sugar is one half glucose and one half fructose, so it actually enters the bloodstream slower than a bagel.

There are other factors involved that have an effect on how fast the carbohydrates are broken down into simple sugar. Fat and soluble fibers slow the entry of glucose. Soluble fiber is an important distinction. There are two types of fiber, soluble (pectin, apples) and insoluble (cellulose and bran cereal). And because fat slows down the entry of glucose into the bloodstream, the sugar in ice cream actually is absorbed more slowly than that of a bagel. High fiber in low glycemic foods is the slowest to release sugars.

The more the carbohydrates are cooked, the higher the glycemic index will be. This is because the cell structure is broken down by cooking and processing. The glycemic index is dramatically increased in instant foods like rice and potatoes. Therefore all bread has a high glycemic index.

Highest Glycemic Index Foods (Examples: puffed cereal and puffed rice cakes)

The body needs a constant intake of carbohydrates for optimal brain function. Too much carbohydrate and the body increases insulin secretion to drive down blood sugar. Too little and the brain will not function efficiently. High glycemic food should always be avoided with candida overgrowth.

Remember, protein stimulates glucagon, which reduces insulin secretion, while fat and fiber slow down the rate of entry of any carbohydrate.

Breakfast suggestions
- Non-gluten whole grain porridge★ (add nuts, seeds, or soy)
- Non-gluten whole grain hot cereal★ (add nuts—use stevia for sweetener)
- Steamed or lightly sautéed vegetables with poached eggs on top
- Fish and steamed vegetables with flaxseed oil
- 12 raw almonds, walnuts, filberts, pecans, or pine nuts
- Small handful of raw sunflower seeds or pumpkin seeds
- Ground raw sesame or flaxseeds sprinkled on hot cereal
- Nut butter or nut milk★
- Steamed vegetables
- Nut milk smoothie★

(Also refer to Non-Gluten Grains and Recipes, pp. 238–242.)

Table 6.10 *Carbohydrate Classifications of Fruits and Vegetables*
(According to Carbohydrate Content)

VEGETABLES

3%	6%	15%	20+%
asparagus	beans, string	artichoke	beans, dried
bean sprouts	beets	carrot	beans, lima
beet greens	brussels sprouts	oyster plant	corn
broccoli	chives	parsnip	potato, sweet
cabbage	collard greens	peas, green	potato, white
cauliflower	dandelion greens	squash	yam
celery	eggplant		
chard, swiss	kale		
cucumber	kohlrabi		
endive	leek		
lettuce	okra		
mustard greens	onion		
radish	parsley		
spinach	pepper, red		
watercress	pimento		
	pumpkin		
	rutabagas		
	turnip		

FRUITS

3%	6%	15%	20+%
cantaloupe	apricot (fresh only)	apple	banana
melons	blackberries	blueberries	figs
rhubarb	cranberries	cherries	prunes
strawberries	grapefruit	grapes	or any dried
tomato	guava	kumquats	fruit
watermelon	kiwi	loganberries	
	lemon	mango	
	lime	mulberries	
	melons	pear	
	orange	pineapple (fresh)	
	papaya	pomegranate	
	peach		
	plum		
	raspberries		
	tangerine		

Lunch suggestions: Protein/vegetable combinations
- Fresh green salad with raw nuts or seeds
- Fresh green salad with turkey, fish, lamb, beef, or chicken
- Fresh green salad with sprouted beans or cooked beans
- Steamed vegetables sprinkled with ground-up raw nuts or seeds
- Steamed vegetables and an animal protein
- Steamed vegetables or salad and bean, lentil, or pea soup★
- Vegetable and nut stir-fry (no rice)
- Vegetable and animal protein stir-fry (no rice)
- Fresh tuna salad with no mayo or almond mayo from health food store
- Vegetable and animal protein soup
- Vegetable and bean soup
- Vegetable soup or stew★
- Fresh vegetable sticks and nut butter for dip
- Fresh vegetables and hummus for dip★★
- Steamed asparagus wrapped in thinly sliced turkey breast
- Turkey or chicken drumsticks and vegetables

Dinner suggestions: Complex carbohydrate/vegetable combinations (refer to non-gluten grain recipes; add nuts and seeds or protein if needed)
- Vegetable and non-gluten whole grain casserole★
- Vegetable and non-gluten whole grain salad★
- Vegetable and non-gluten whole grain soup★
- Rice paper spring rolls with no sauce★★
- Vegetable nori rolls with no mustard★★
- Steamed vegetables or green salad with new red potatoes
- Vegetables and baked squash or sweet potatoes
- Vegetables with beans and rice
- Vegetable stir-fry with a non-gluten whole grain
- Non-gluten pasta salad
- Non-gluten pasta with dairy-free pesto sauce★★ and vegetables
- Mashed potatoes and vegetables with flax oil and herbs
- Stuffed peppers with a non-gluten whole grain and vegetables★

- dairy-free new red potato salad with vegetables
- vegetable sandwich on a non–gluten whole grain bread★

Note: Avoid pasta for the first 21 days.

Beverages
- Herb teas★★
- Fresh organic vegetable juice diluted 50 percent★★ (after 2 weeks on the diet)
- Pure water
- Fresh grated gingerroot tea

Flavorings
- Flaxseed oil for salad dressings or in place of butter on steamed vegetables or cooked grains
- Cold-pressed olive oil or sesame oil (Omega Nutrition)
- Bragg Liquid Amino Seasoning★★ as a salt substitute
- Fresh lemon, lime, in dressings or on steamed vegetables
- Fresh herbs: cilantro, mint, basil, dill, parsley, or rosemary to flavor salads and grains
- Fresh spices★★ (avoid table salt and black pepper)
- Use butter or ghee instead of margarine
- Garlic (great for candida diets)
- Gingerroot
- Nut butter for sauces and dressings
- Sea salt (use sparingly)

Snack suggestions
- Organic vegetable sticks
- Raw organic almonds, walnuts, filberts, pine nuts, sunflower seeds, or pumpkin seeds
- Non-yeast rye crackers or vegetable sticks with raw nut butter
- Nut milk★
- Hummus★★
- Nori roll★★
- Baked acorn squash
- Celery sticks stuffed with mayo free tuna salad

- Cup of bean soup
- Non-gluten waffle★★ toasted with almond butter

Non-Gluten Grains

Gluten is a protein found in some cereal grains, mainly wheat, oats, rye, triticale, barley, spelt, and buckwheat. It is responsible for making bread "springy." As the dough is kneaded, the gluten molecules join together forming long chains that make it elasticlike.

Gluten is the major source of protein for many people who live on a wheat-based diet. However, gluten does not agree with everyone. Some digestive problems have been found to be associated with an intolerance to gluten. Fortunately there are non-gluten grains that are tasty.

Grains marked with an asterisk (★) are not recommended for a strict detoxification cleansing diet, i.e., the first three to four weeks of the Candida diet.

Gluten-free grains: Amaranth, brown rice, coarse cornmeal★, millet, quinoa, wild rice.

Gluten-free flours: Arrowroot, amaranth, brown rice, garbanzo (chickpea), soybean, potato★, nut and seed, legume.

Gluten-free pasta: Corn★, quinoa, rice, soy.

Cooking Chart for Grains (in cups)

	GRAIN	WATER	COOK TIME
Amaranth	1	2–2¼	20–25 min
Brown rice★	1	1¾–2¼	50–55 min
Buckwheat	1	2	15–20 min
Millet	1	2½	35–40 min
Quinoa	1	2	15–20 min
Teff	½	2	15–20 min
Wild rice	1	3¼	50–60 min

★Short, medium or long grain: For softer rice use more water; for firmer rice, use less water.

Rice

If you think of a white, gummy, tasteless dish when you think of rice, think again! Whole brown rice has a pleasant, mild flavor—a somewhat chewy and satisfying texture. Rice may well be one of the easiest whole grains to introduce into your new, healthier lifestyle. Rice is extremely versatile and comes in many shapes and sizes. Here is a list to help you choose wisely.

Instant rice: Pre-cooked rice that has had the outer coating totally removed. It lacks protein, 75 percent of its original mineral content, and most of its vitamin B.

Polished white rice: Very white, milled rice with the hull, bran, germ, and endosperm removed.

Converted rice: Rice that has been soaked and steamed before milling, to retain more of the vitamins and nutrients.

Brown rice: Rice that has had its outer husk removed. Much of its nutritional qualities has been retained.

White rice flour: Made from polished white rice, so it has little taste and low nutritional value.

Brown rice flour: Faint taste and more nutritious than white rice flour.

Rice polishings: The bran and other materials have been removed from brown rice to make polished rice.

Wild rice: Actually from the *grass* family and not a true rice. It is commonly found growing wild in the Great Lakes region. It is a nutritious, tasty, and expensive food product.

BASIC STEAMED RICE
> 1 cup raw brown rice
> 2 cups pure water
> ½ tsp sea salt (optional)

If the rice looks dusty; wash it by letting water run over it in a colander or sieve. (Brown rice has a little debris left when you buy it.) Bring the water to a boil. Add the rice and allow the water to resume boiling. If you choose to, add the salt. As soon as the water is boiling, turn the heat low and simmer the rice with the lid tightly in place. Allow the rice to cook this way for about 45 minutes. Remember, by lifting the lid, steam is allowed to escape and that may disrupt the water/grain ratio.

YIELD: 3–4 SERVINGS

RICE WITH SNOW PEAS
The rice for this dish is cooked separately from the vegetables and the two are mixed together just before serving.

> 1 cup uncooked brown rice cooked in 2 cups of water or 3 cups of cooked brown rice
> 2 tbsp olive oil
> 2 cups fresh snow peas, strings removed
> 4 scallions, thinly sliced
> ½ cup thinly sliced fresh zucchini
> ¼ cup slivered almonds or sesame seeds
> ¼ tsp sea salt
> Dill, basil or oregano to taste

Cook rice. Heat oil in a skillet. Stir-fry vegetables for 3 to 5 minutes until onions are barely tender. Season with herbs, salt and pepper. Stir hot rice into vegetables. Add almonds or sesame seeds.

YIELD: 3–4 SERVINGS

GOOD MORNIN' RICE
> 2 cups cooked rice
> ½ tsp cinnamon
> 2 tbsp sunflower seeds
> Flaxseed oil

Place everything except the flax oil in a small baking dish, mixing gently. Bake for 15–20 minutes in a 350° oven. Top with a splash of flaxseed oil and enjoy.

YIELD: 3 SERVINGS

GARDEN RICE
> 1 tbsp olive oil
> 1 small onion, chopped
> 1 clove garlic, chopped

1 small carrot, chopped
½ cup cauliflorets
1 cup green beans cut in 1″ segments
½ cup bean sprouts (optional)
¾ cup uncooked brown rice
1¼ cups water
2 tbsp tamari (wheat-free)
1 bay leaf
½ tsp sea salt

Heat oil in a 3-quart pot and sauté onion and garlic for about 5 minutes until tender. Add vegetables and sauté 5 minutes longer. Add sprouts, rice, water, tamari, salt, and bay leaf. Place cover on pot and cook until tender, about 40 minutes.   YIELD: 3–4 SERVINGS

WILD RICE

1 cup wild rice
⅓ cup brown rice
4 cups stock or water
2 large stalks celery
6 green onions
1 carrot
2 tbsp olive oil
1 tsp marjoram
¼ tsp rosemary
¼ tsp thyme
1 tsp sea salt
Garlic to taste
½ cup almonds or sesame seeds raw

Chop celery and carrots in ¼″ cubes. Chop green onions and sauté in olive oil. Add water and bring to a boil. Stir in remaining ingredients (except almonds). Bring to a boil, cover, reduce heat and cool for an hour or more, until rice is tender. Add chopped almonds or sesame seeds.   YIELD: 3–4 SERVINGS

CREAMY TAHINI RICE
  2 tbsp water
  ½ tbsp olive oil
  1 medium onion, chopped fine
  1 cup mixed seeds (sunflower, sesame and pumpkin)
  3 cups cooked brown rice
  1 tbsp tamari
  ⅓ cup tahini (ground sesame seeds)
  ⅓ cup water

Heat water and oil in a large skillet. Add onions and seeds and simmer for about 5 minutes or until seeds are lightly browned. Then stir in rice, tamari sauce, tahini, and water. Cook until heated through and sauce is thick and creamy around the rice. You can add 1 tbsp of flaxseed oil before serving.   YIELD: 4 SERVINGS

Millet

The birds of North America eat a lot more millet than do we humans. Millet is among the least familiar of the grains in our country and it's time to change that as it is more than birdseed. Millet is a delicious, mild-flavored, yellow-colored grain. Its protein, calcium, magnesium, iron, and lecithin levels are of significant value and its versatility in recipes is exceptional.

BASIC MILLET
  1 cup millet raw
  3 cups water (less 2 tbsp for a fluffier millet)

Bring the water to a boil. While you wait for the water to boil, rinse the millet well using a sieve. Add the millet and bring the mixture to a boil once again. Quickly lower the heat to a slow simmer, cover the pot and simmer for 30–45 minutes.

YIELD: 4 SERVINGS

MILLET AND VEGETABLES
  1 cup millet
  1 carrot or parsnip, sliced

1 cup cabbage, sliced or try shredded zucchini
1 cup cauliflower or broccoli pieces
1 tsp olive oil
½ tsp sea salt
½ tsp tamari (wheat-free)

Cook the millet as in "Basic Millet" until all the water is absorbed, about 25 minutes. Add the vegetables and cook for another 5–10 minutes. Add the oil and salt, and season with the tamari sauce. Serve with a green salad and flax oil dressing. For additional flavor you may add a bay leaf or some oregano to the cooking water.   YIELD: 4 SERVINGS

MILLET CROQUETTES
2 cups millet, cooked
½ cup celery, finely diced with the leaves
¼ cup carrots, finely grated
½ cup onion, diced
½ cup rice flour
¼ cup parsley, chopped
½ cup water
½ tsp dill
½ tsp oregano
Dash sea salt

Mix the millet and vegetables in a large bowl. Slowly add the salt, flour, and herbs; mix well. Add the water and mix once more. Form into small balls or patties and place on a lightly oiled (sesame or olive) baking sheet. Bake in a 350°F oven for 25 minutes. To make the patties crispy, brush the tops with the same kind of oil after they have been baked for 10 minutes. Serve with steamed vegetables.   YIELD: 4 SERVINGS

MILLET PILAF
⅔ cups millet raw
1 tsp olive oil
½ onion sliced (if intolerant, substitute zucchini)

½ tsp sea salt or salt substitute
Dash oregano
1½ cups water

Sauté the onions in a small amount of water; when the onions are transparent, add the oil and simmer until soft. Add the seasonings and millet. Sauté for 3 minutes. Add the water and bring to a boil. Cover, reduce the heat, and simmer for 20 minutes. Serve with a vegetable almond stir-fry.   YIELD: 4 SERVINGS

Quinoa

This interesting grain comes from the Andes Mountains and was one of the several staple foods upon which the great Inca civilization dined. Quinoa has an unusually high protein profile and expanding qualities (cooked quinoa expands almost five times its original size). It is often a favorite with children and its appearance is rather unique. As a cooked grain it is almost transparent, with little white "o" rings in the center. It can be substituted for just about any grain in recipes and has a light yet satisfying quality.

BASIC QUINOA
   2 cups water
   1 cup quinoa

Rinse quinoa thoroughly, either by using a strainer or by running fresh water over the quinoa in a pot. Drain excess water. Place quinoa and water in a 1½-quart saucepan and bring to a boil. Reduce to a simmer, cover, and cook until all of the water is absorbed (15 minutes). You will know that the quinoa is done when all the grains have turned from light beige to transparent with little white rings. Please note: Most varieties of quinoa have a naturally occurring bitter coating that helps prevent insect and bird damage. This coating is usually removed before it is shipped, but a small amount of bitter residue may occasionally remain. This can be removed simply by rinsing the quinoa before cooking. Serve with vegetables and salad for a meal.

YIELD: 3–4 SERVINGS

CURRIED QUINOA
 2 tbsp olive oil
 1 clove garlic, pressed
 1 small onion, minced
 ¼ tsp curry powder (or to taste)
 ½ tsp sea salt
 4 cups water
 2 cups quinoa

Heat a 2-quart soup pot. Add the oil and sauté garlic, onion, and then pepper. Add curry and salt. Cover and cook for a few minutes. Add water, cover, and bring to a rapid boil. Add quinoa to boiling water. Cover, reduce heat, and simmer 15 minutes. With a damp wooden spoon, mix from top to bottom. Cover and allow to rest for an additional 5 minutes.

YIELD: 5 SERVINGS

QUINOA TABOULI
 2 cups quinoa, cooked
 1 cup parsley, chopped
 ½ cup scallions, chopped
 2 tbsp fresh mint (or 1 tsp dried mint)
 1 clove garlic, pressed
 ½ tsp basil
 ½ cup lemon juice
 ¼ cup olive oil
 Dash sea salt
 Lettuce leaves (whole)

Place all ingredients except lettuce in a mixing bowl and toss together lightly. Chill for 1 hour or more to allow flavors to blend. Line a salad bowl with lettuce leaves and add the tabouli. Serve as a main dish salad.

YIELD: 3–4 SERVINGS

QUINOA AND PEA CHOWDER
   2 cups water
   ¼ cup quinoa, rinsed
   ½ cup zucchini
   ¼ cup onion, chopped
   1½ cups peas, fresh or frozen
   2 cups water
   ½ tsp sea salt
   ¼ cup parsley, chopped

Simmer the quinoa and vegetables in 2 cups of water until tender (15 minutes). Add the second batch of water and bring to a slow boil. Season to taste. Garnish with parsley.   YIELD: 4–5 SERVINGS

Amaranth

There is a story told that when the Spaniards invaded the Aztec people, a Spanish adviser suggested that if they wanted to crush this mighty culture, they needed to first destroy its staff of life. This happened to be the unique and exceptionally nutritious amaranth. A decree was delivered that the cultivation of amaranth was forbidden. The ultimate demise of the Aztecs is outlined in history books. The amazing survival of amaranth, though, is a much different story. Much to the Spaniards' annoyance and amaranth's good fortune, isolated mountain villagers kept the grain alive. The grain was rediscovered and has recently made it to North American health food stores. The tiny grain has an unusual flavor and texture. Unlike other grains, it remains fairly sticky rather than fluffing up like rice. If you are a cooked-cereal fan, this grain is for you! The grain is often ground into flour and can be added to any recipe.

BASIC AMARANTH
   1 cup amaranth
   2 cups water

Bring the water to a boil. Add the amaranth, cover, and simmer over low heat for 20 minutes. For a different taste, add any spice, (cinnamon, nutmeg, or cloves) or any herb (dill, basil, oregano, or curry). For a savory switch, lightly toast amaranth in 1–2 tbsp of sesame oil. Heat the oil and add the amaranth while stirring constantly over medium heat. The tiny grain will actually "pop" slightly. When this happens, add the correct amount of water and cook as above.

PUFFED AMARANTH

To puff or pop amaranth, preheat a dry skillet over medium heat. Sprinkle 2 tbsp whole amaranth into the skillet. Gently stir the grain for a few seconds until it pops (amaranth doesn't pop like corn, but it does become enlarged and light golden). Quickly transfer the amaranth to a bowl and begin popping another 2 tbsp in the skillet.

Recipes for a Candida Hypoallergenic Diet

WHOLE GRAIN PORRIDGE

Use leftover (already cooked) non–gluten grains: brown rice, millet, amaranth, or quinoa. Place the cold grain in the blender with water or nut milk. The amount of liquid determines how thick the porridge will be. Blend together to desired consistency. Heat the porridge. Add flaxseed oil to taste. Be creative, and after the first 21 days on the diet, try other flavorings such as cinnamon, almond butter, banana, ground flaxseeds, raisins, applesauce, or almond slivers. No two porridges are alike.

WHOLE GRAIN HOT CEREAL

If you like Cream of Wheat, why not try Cream of Millet, Cream of Amaranth, or Cream of Quinoa? Pick any non-gluten grain and grind up ½ cup in a coffee grinder. Add the grain very gradually to 1½ cups boiling water or apple juice, stirring constantly. Simmer for five minutes. Top it off with nut milk and flax oil. Also try nuts and seeds, cinnamon, apple sauce, or banana slices. Quick, easy, and delicious!

Nut Milk

Place ½ cup raw almonds, sunflower seeds, sesame seeds, or cashews and two cups of water in the blender. Blend until smooth and creamy. Strain milk through a cheesecloth. Flavor with cinnamon, dash of stevia powder, and/or alcohol-free vanilla flavoring. Delicious hot or cold, and a great milk substitute for baking.

Poached Eggs over Steamed Vegetables
   ¼ cup thin sliced leak
   ¼ cup chopped celery or bok choy
   ¼ cup diced green, yellow or red pepper
   ¼ cup chopped broccoli, asparagus, or zucchini
   1 large handful of leafy greens (spinach, kale, chard, etc.)

Place harder vegetables in bottom of steamer, steam for about 3 to 5 minutes, then add softer vegetable or leafy greens and turn burner off. Poach 2 eggs over easy to over medium and serve over vegetables. Sprinkle with Bragg liquid amino seasoning or sea salt.

Smoothie
   1 cup nut milk
   1 tablespoon organic brown rice protein powder
   1 tablespoon ground flaxseeds
   Dash of stevia powder
   Dash of alcohol-free vanilla

After the first 21 days on the diet, you can begin to add other ingredients, i.e., ½ banana, ½ cup frozen berries, carob powder, etc. Be creative. Blend with ice or make a hot carob drink.

Sprouted Grains

Soak a non-gluten grain for 12–24 hours, rinsing twice daily until tiny, ¼" sprouts begin to appear. At this point, spread the sprouts on a towel and allow to dry for 1–4 hours. Do not allow them to wither and harden. Place in refrigerator and they will last three to ten days. To serve, warm the sprouts very carefully in a pan with melted butter or soak in hot tap water for a minute or so. Eat them for breakfast or in place of cooked grains at other meals.

Sprouts are high in fiber; the enzymes in the grains have not been destroyed by the heat, and they are often less allergenic than cooked grains.

Acorn Squash

Cut squash in half and steam facedown for 20–30 minutes. Set in an oven dish and fill with 1 teaspoon butter or ghee. Place in 350° oven for 10 minutes. Also delicious with flax oil, but do not add until after baking. (Avoid maple syrup or honey.)

Vegetable Soup

In large saucepan, sauté diced celery, carrot, zucchini, broccoli, cauliflower, cabbage, onion, and garlic in a little pure water. Cover with water and add 1 teaspoon oregano, 1 tablespoon basil, and cayenne to taste. Simmer ½ hour. Serve, then add Bragg liquid amino seasoning or sea salt to taste. Also try this soup with diced new potatoes or sweet potatoes.

Split Pea Soup

Dice and sauté carrots, celery, and onion. Boil 1 cup green split peas in ½ to 1 quart water. Add vegetables after 20 minutes. Add ¼ teaspoon thyme.

Clean Casserole

Steam zucchini and celery for 5 minutes. Turn off burner, add a good portion of mung bean sprouts, and let sit for 5 minutes. Place ½ inch of cooked rice in bottom of buttered casserole dish. Pour vegetables on top of rice and sprinkle with sunflower seeds. Bake at 350° for 20 minutes. Allow to cool slightly, then add 1 to 2 tablespoons butter or flax oil and sprinkle with Bragg liquid amino seasoning.

Curry Rice

Sauté mushrooms, onion, and green peppers in butter. Add cooked brown rice, a little Bragg liquid amino seasoning, and curry powder to taste. Garnish with fresh chopped parsley. Serve with sautéed vegetables and a side of raisins and/or coconut.

Quinoa Salad

¾ cups pure water
1cup quinoa, rinsed 2 or 3 times
½ cup finely diced cucumber or celery
4 stems green onion, diced finely
¼ cup finely diced fresh cilantro
3 tablespoons fresh lime juice
2 tsp fresh lime juice
2 tsp flax oil
Sea salt to taste
Cayenne pepper to taste

Bring water to boil in a 1-quart pot, then add quinoa. Reduce heat and simmer, covered, for 15 minutes, stirring occasionally until grain is tender. Remove from heat and let cool, uncovered. Toss cucumber, green onion, and cilantro with cooked quinoa. Combine the lime juice, oil, salt, and cayenne, and add to quinoa. Stir thoroughly with a fork to coat the grains and vegetables.

Veggie Sandwich

Pile high on a non-gluten bread any or all of the following: grated carrot, cucumber, green pepper, onion, sprouts, lettuce, avocado. Sprinkle with your favorite herbs and spices.

Rose's Sauce

Mix together 1–2 tablespoons flax oil, 1–2 tablespoons raw sesame tahini, 2 teaspoons Bragg liquid amino seasoning, and fresh lemon juice to taste. Top steamed vegetables (cabbage, onion, zucchini, and red pepper make a great combination) and wild rice. Serve hot. This also makes a great salad dressing if you decrease the tahini and increase the lemon juice. Add your favorite herbs and spices.

CANIDIDA DIET SALAD DRESSING
  ¼ cup fresh-squeezed lemon juice
  ½ cup flaxseed oil (may substitute or mix with other oil—olive, sesame, or canola)
  ⅛ cup pure water
  ⅛ tsp sea salt

OPTIONAL INGREDIENTS
  Fresh or dried herbs (i.e., basil, oregano, thyme)
  Curry powder
  Crushed garlic
  Onion powder
  Sesame tahini, 1–2 tsp (will make it smooth and creamy)
  Bragg liquid amino seasoning or wheat-free tamari.

Phase III

The best way to restore normal bacterial flora in the bowel is through the administration of acidophilus bacteria. This should be done after Phase I and during Phase II (diet) of the treatment program. The good bacteria cannot grow back fully until the yeast overgrowth in the bowel has been greatly diminished. A reasonable time to begin Phase III is about six weeks into the Program.

The friendly intestinal bacteria can be restored through a multitude of *Lactobacillus acidophilus* and *bifidus* products available in health food stores. These can be found in liquids, powders, capsules, and tablets. There are new and better strains being developed on a regular basis, with a wide variety of potency. While there are many brands of acidophilus and bifidus sold in health food stores, most of these actually contain only a small amount of *living* organisms because these products lack the nutrients necessary for survival. Even freeze-dried types usually contain insufficient amounts of acidophilus at the time of use, despite the billions-of-organisms-per-gram content at the time of bottling. To assure potency, follow these guidelines:

(1) Buy only refrigerated brands that clearly state an expiration date between one and ten months from the date the item is purchased.
(2) Buy either liquid cultures (such as yogurt culture) or powdered forms containing whey (dairy) or nondairy varieties. Lactobacilli are living organisms and only these forms provide an ample food supply with which to sustain the fragile acidophilus bacteria.

Be aware that many yogurt products do not contain a high amount of viable organisms by the time they reach the consumer. This is especially true of highly processed ones and those with many additional ingredients. People who are sensitive to dairy products, as well as those with chronic respiratory disease, should not use yogurt as a consistent source of friendly bacteria. Remember to avoid those brands of yogurt that have added sweeteners.

Phase IV
Strengthening the immune system is a vital aspect of treating candidiasis. Phases I, II, and III can all contribute in varying degrees to a stronger immune system. In addition to the complete vitamin, mineral, and herbal regimen described earlier in this chapter, I recommend:

- Biotin, 300–1,000 mcg three times a day
- Flaxseed oil (already a part of the candida diet) or other essential fatty acids found in primrose or black currant oils
- Amino acid supplements
- Adrenal-enhancing supplements (I use a product called Adrenal Complex, available only through practitioners)

The remainder of the physical health recommendations in this chapter—a whole-foods diet (not as restrictive as the candida diet), adequate water intake, and regular exercise—as well as the guidelines concerning mental, emotional, social, and spiritual health found in chapters 7 and 8, will all contribute to a powerful immune system.

If you are highly suspicious that you have candidiasis, have followed this treatment plan for one to three months, and still experience little or no improvement, there are other options available to you. If you have not already done so, I recommend consulting with your physician about the possibility of taking one of the antifungal prescription drugs—Diflucan, Sporanox, or Nizoral. If you've already completed a full course of one of these medications with no improvement, then I'd be most suspicious of food allergy and leaky gut syndrome. This condition can take close to a year to completely resolve, even using some of the new and highly effective dietary supplements formulated to treat this challenging problem. Another way to assess food allergies or sensitivities is a blood antibody test to check for delayed antibody response (IgG-mediated) by the Great Smokies Lab. This test checks for 96 different foods and can be ordered and interpreted by a physician, chiropractor or naturopathic doctor. It is not a perfect test, but can be a helpful guide in some people. This lab also has testing for the leaky-gut syndrome. (See Resources Section for Great Smokies Laboratory.) Ultra Clear® is the product I've used for leaky-gut syndrome with excellent results. It was formulated and developed by Jeffrey S. Bland, Ph.D., a clinical biochemist and internationally known authority on therapeutic nutrition. It helps to detoxify the body, feed the good bacteria, and assist in healing the "leaky" intestinal lining. It is available through Metagenics (see Resource Guide).

The other possible but less likely coexisting conditions that may be preventing improvement are: intestinal parasites (especially giardia), hypochlorhydria, pancreatic enzyme deficiency (all of which can be assessed by the Comprehensive Digestive Stool Analysis [CDSA] performed by Great Smokies Laboratory), helicobacter pylori, inhalant mold allergy, hypothy-roidism, adrenal exhaustion, chronic viral infections/chronic fatigue syndrome, chemical injury or hypersensitivity, heavy metal poisoning (especially mercury toxicity from silver mercury amalgam dental fillings), and hormone hypersensitivity (particularly to progesterone). Obviously you will need to work with your physician to investigate these possible diagnoses. You may also be getting reinfected with candida from your regular sexual partner. Men, particularly, may transmit candida without being symptomatic themselves, although it is possible for women to be the asymptomatic transmitters.

You will know when you have completely recovered from candidiasis because you'll probably feel better than you have in years. You may want to review your initial list of symptoms just to make sure, but most people have no trouble determining that the candida overgrowth is resolved. Don't allow this hard-earned victory over a tenacious foe to be short-lived. Try to maintain a healthy diet without reverting back to excess sugar and alcohol. Remember: *moderation*. Continue to nurture yourself in body, mind, and spirit, and your immune system will afford you excellent health with no concern about the recurrence of candida.

Chapter 7

HEALING YOUR MIND

"The greatest discovery of any generation is that human beings can alter their lives by altering the attitudes of their minds."

ALBERT SCHWEITZER

COMPONENTS OF OPTIMAL MENTAL HEALTH
Peace of mind and contentment
A job that you love doing
Optimism
A sense of humor
Financial well-being
Living your life vision

COMPONENTS OF OPTIMAL EMOTIONAL HEALTH
Self-acceptance and high self-esteem
Capacity to identify, express, experience, and accept all of your
    feelings, both painful and joyful
Awareness of the intimate connection between your physical
    and emotional bodies
Confronting your greatest fears
Fulfilling your capacity to play
Peak experiences on a regular basis

One of the most exciting developments in the field of medicine in recent decades has been the scientific verification that our physical health is directly influenced by our thoughts and emotions. The reverse is also true: Overwhelming evidence now exists showing that our physiology has a direct correlation to the ways we habitually think and feel. While Eastern systems of medicine, such as traditional Chinese medicine and Ayurveda, have for centuries recognized these facts and stressed the importance of a harmonious connection between body and mind, in the West this mind–body connection did not begin to be acknowledged until research conducted in the 1970s and 1980s conclusively revealed the ability of thoughts, emotions, and attitudes to influence our bodies' immune functions. In fact, many of the scientists exploring this relatively new field have concluded that *there is no separation between mind and body.*

In order to heal our minds and emotions, it helps to know what we mean by the term *mental health.* From the perspective of holistic medicine, the essence of mental health is peace of mind and feelings of contentment. Being mentally healthy means that you recognize the ways in which your thoughts, beliefs, mental imagery, and attitudes affect your well-being and limit or expand your ability to enjoy your life. It also means knowing that you always have choices about what you think and believe and are aware of your gifts, are practicing your special talents, working at a job that you enjoy, and being clear about your priorities, values, and goals. People who have made a commitment to their mental health live their lives with rich reserves of humor and optimism. They have chosen a nurturing set of beliefs and attitudes that fills them with peace and hope. Most people who buy this book do so with the belief, however minimal, that they do not have to suffer with sinusitis and allergies for the rest of their lives. Having read to this point and begun practicing the physical and environmental components of the Sinus Survival Program, that belief has probably been strengthened considerably. You can determine your own state of mental health by referring to the appropriate section of the Wellness Self-Test in Chapter 2 and then use the information in this chapter to improve the areas you may need to work on.

The term *mental health* can be interpreted to include not only our thoughts and beliefs but also our feelings. However, when your focus is specifically on "feelings," that is the realm of *emo-*

tional health. These aspects of ourselves—**mental** and **emotional**—are for the most part inextricably related and together form the "**mind**" aspect of holistic health. As your healing journey progresses, you will increasingly come to recognize how your own distorted or illogical thoughts are the underlying cause of feelings such as anger, depression, anxiety, fear, and unfounded guilt. Learning how to free yourself from such distorted thinking patterns is the goal of this chapter, and of behavioral medicine, the aspect of holistic medicine that deals with this interconnectedness among physical, mental, and emotional health. Behavioral medicine includes professional treatment approaches such as *psychotherapy, mind/body medicine, guided imagery and visualization, biofeedback therapy, hypnotherapy, neurolinguistic programming (NLP), orthomolecular medicine* (the use of nutritional supplements to treat chronic mental dis-ease), *flower essences,* and *body-centered therapies like Rolfing, massage therapy,* and *Hellerwork.* The focus in this chapter, however (with the exception of psychotherapy), is on proven self-care approaches that you can begin using immediately to heal the mind along with your nose and sinuses. They include creating new *beliefs and establishing clear goals, affirmations, breathwork, guided imagery, visualization, meditation, dreamwork, journaling,* and your approaches to both *work* and *play.* Each of these methods can help you become more aware of your habitual thoughts, emotions, and beliefs—both pleasurable and painful—in order to create a mind-set conducive to experiencing optimal health and more effectively meeting your professional goals and personal desires, including freeing yourself from the misery of sinusitis and allergies.

THE BODY-MIND CONNECTION

Growing numbers of Western scientists and physicians now recognize that *body* and *mind* are not separate aspects of our being but interrelated expressions of the same experience. Their view is based on the findings of researchers working in the field of *psychoneuroimmunology (PNI),* also referred to as *neuroscience,* which for the past three decades has shown us that our thoughts, emotions, and attitudes can directly influence immune and hormone function. In light of such research, scientists now commonly speak of the mind's ability to control the body. In large part this perspective is due to the scientific discovery of "messenger" molecules known as *neuropeptides,* chemicals that communicate our thoughts, emotions, attitudes, and beliefs to every cell in our body. In practical terms, this means that all of us are capable of both weakening or strengthening our immune system according to how we think and feel. Moreover, scientists have also proven that these messages can originate not only in the brain but in every cell in the body. As a result of such studies, scientists now conclude that the immune system actually functions as a "circulating nervous system" that is actively and acutely attuned to our every thought and emotion.

Among the discoveries which have occurred in the field of PNI are the following:

- Feelings of loss and self-rejection can diminish immune function and contribute to a number of chronic disease conditions, including heart disease.
- Feelings of exhilaration and joy produce measurable levels of a neuropeptide identical to interleukin-2, a powerful anti-cancer drug that costs many thousands of dollars per injection.
- Feelings of peace and calm produce a chemical very similar to Valium, a popular tranquilizer.
- Depressive states negatively impact the immune system and increase the likelihood of illness.
- Chronic grief or a sense of loss can increase the likelihood of cancer.
- Anxiety and fear can trigger high blood pressure.
- Feelings of hostility, grief, depression, hopelessness, and isolation greatly increase the risk of heart attack.
- Repressed anger is a factor in causing many chronic ailments, including sinusitis, bronchitis, headaches, and candidiasis.

- Acknowledgment and expression of feelings strengthens immune responses.
- Anger decreases immunoglobulin A (a protective antibody) in saliva, while caring, compassion, humor, and laughter increase it.
- Chronic stress has a broad suppressive effect on immunity, including the depression of natural killer cells, which attack cancer cells.

As exciting as these discoveries are, the studies that had the greatest impact on me were performed on multiple-personality patients at the NIH. Scientists found that in one personality an individual could have the strongest possible skin reaction to an allergen or be severely nearsighted, but after shifting to another personality (an unconscious process in the *same* body) there was *no skin reaction* to the same allergen and perfectly normal *20/20 vision!* Science is just beginning to understand the depth and power of the connection between mind and body.

The implications of these discoveries are enormous and are producing a paradigm shift in physicians' approaches to treating chronic disease. They play an essential role in the Sinus Survival Program: If emotions and attitudes can contribute to causing heart disease and cancer, it isn't too difficult to appreciate how they can also trigger sinus infections and allergies. They are also tremendously empowering for anyone committed to holistic health. Once you accept the fact that there is an ongoing, instant, and intimate communication occurring between your mind and your body via the mechanisms of neuropeptides, you can also see that the person best qualified to direct that communication in your own life is you. Learning how to do so effectively can enable you to become your own 24-hour-a-day healer by becoming more conscious of your thoughts and emotions and managing them better to improve all areas of your health. The first step in this process is acknowledging that you can no longer afford to continue feeding yourself the same limiting messages you most likely have been conditioned to accept since early childhood. Scientists now estimate that the average person has approximately 50,000 thoughts each day; yet 95 percent of them are the same as the ones he or she had the day before. Typically such thoughts are not only unconscious but often critical and limiting. For example, "Why did I say (or do) that? I should have said (or done) it this way." Or: "I'll never be able to overcome this sinus problem (or any chronic condition). I'm going to have to live with this pain and suffering for the rest of my life." When you're hearing messages like these repeated many times during the course of a typical day, it's easy to understand why for most people with a chronic condition like sinusitis, **fear, anger, hopelessness, sadness,** and **depression** might become their predominant feelings. You've just read that these painful emotions can be associated with weakening the immune system while also contributing to a myriad of physical problems. Sinus disease is no exception. However, *by consciously taking control of your thoughts and recognizing how they govern your behavior and impact your body, you can dramatically change your life and heal your dis-ease.* You will gain the freedom to think, unimpeded, feel, and believe as you choose, thereby flooding your body's cells with positive, life-affirming messages capable of producing optimal health. I've described this condition as the free flow of life force energy through your body, mind, and spirit. The remainder of this chapter provides a variety of approaches to enhance this flow of energy through your mind.

PSYCHOTHERAPY

The field of psychotherapy, an outgrowth of the theories and discoveries of Sigmund Freud, continues to evolve more than a hundred years since its inception. In addition to the mental and emotional benefits commonly attributed to psychotherapy, a growing body of research has documented that physical benefits can also occur. For example, in a study conducted at the UCLA

School of Medicine by the late Norman Cousins, a group of cancer patients receiving psychotherapy for 90 minutes a week showed dramatic improvement in their immune systems after only six weeks. During that same period, the control group of other cancer patients who received no counseling showed no change in immune function whatsoever.

Psychotherapy, by its very nature, is not a self-care protocol, but can be extremely valuable for individuals struggling with deeply rooted mental and emotional problems. *The most popular forms of psychotherapy are classical or Freudian psychoanalysis, Jungian psychoanalysis, family therapy, cognitive/behavioral therapy, brief/ solution-focused therapy, and humanistic/existential therapy. Though they all share the same goal of helping patients achieve mental health, their approaches can vary widely.*

If you feel that psychotherapy may help you, you will gain the most benefit by choosing the approach best suited to your specific needs and objectives. In addition, be aware that the work of psychotherapy is increasingly being conducted by nonpsychiatrists, including psychologists, social workers, and pastoral counselors. One of the reasons for this, perhaps, lies in the fact that many of today's patients seeing psychiatrists are given a psychiatric diagnosis (depression, manic-depressive, obsessive-compulsive, etc.) and then treated with drugs, such as the antidepressant Prozac. This trend within psychiatry, a departure away from counseling toward greater drug therapy, makes it a less desirable choice for someone interested in a holistic and self-care approach. While psychotherapeutic drugs can be effective at times, especially over the short term, each of the drugs commonly prescribed by psychiatrists has the potential to cause unpleasant side effects. Equally important, by focusing on treating psychological symptoms with drugs, many psychiatrists are depriving their patients of the opportunity to change their attitudes and behavior and to learn how to understand and grow from their emotional pain. Finally, whichever type of psychotherapist you choose, make sure that he or she is someone with whom you are comfortable. Psychotherapy can only be effective in a situation of trust, so you may wish to interview a number of therapists before making your choice.

BELIEFS, AFFIRMATIONS, AND GOALS

In his classic treatise *The Science of Mind,* noted spiritual teacher Ernest Holmes wrote: "Health and sickness are largely externalizations of our dominant mental and spiritual states. . . . A normal healthy mind reflects itself in a healthy body, and conversely, an abnormal mental state expresses its corresponding condition in some physical condition." At the time Holmes wrote those words, in the mid-1920s, modern science was far behind him in understanding how *our thoughts directly influence our physical health.* But today a growing body of evidence not only verifies this fact but also indicates that it is our predominant, habitual beliefs that determine the thoughts we primarily think. Socrates stated that the unexamined life was not worth living. Based on today's research in the field of behavioral medicine, we might paraphrase his statement to say: *The unexamined belief is not worth believing in.* Yet, most of us have never taken the time to actually examine the beliefs we hold and therefore remain unaware of how they may be influencing our well-being.

The importance of beliefs in the overall scheme of human functioning is confirmed by placebo studies. A placebo is a dummy medication or procedure possessing no therapeutic properties that works only because of our belief in it. Detailed analysis of 13 placebo studies from 1940 to 1979, including 1,200 patients, found an 82 percent improvement resulting from the use of medications or procedures that subsequently proved to be placebos.

Changing your beliefs is essential to your success with the Sinus Survival Program. Most patients who come to see me have already sought help from one or even several physicians. Their doctors have told them, "You're going to have to live with your sinus problem"; "You must take an antibiotic for your sinus infection"; "Your back/sinus/knee requires surgery"; or "There's nothing more that can be done for it" (the majority of diseases). These statements are, however, only beliefs. The beliefs are based on the limitations of modern medical science, a highly scientific and technologically advanced approach to the treatment of disease, and they are delivered to the patient by a highly educated individual in a society that defers to expertise. These pronouncements, which are in some cases death sentences, are quickly accepted by most patients and become a part of their own belief system. The vast majority of people with terminal diseases who accept whatever their doctors tell them (these patients are called "compliant") die very close to their predicted life expectancy. Patients who challenge prognoses tend to live longer. In *Love, Medicine and Miracles,* Bernie Siegel, M.D., vividly describes how the beliefs and attitudes of many of his cancer patients affected the outcome of their disease.

Most of the beliefs held by Americans have been defined by the standards, or norms, of our society, but how well does the norm fit you, a unique individual? If all of us attempted to conform, the world would be a boring place, devoid of creativity and innovation. We certainly wouldn't be enjoying the ease of living that technology has provided us were it not for the adventurous few who deviated from the conventional belief system.

Unfortunately, in every culture there is great pressure to conform. It isn't easy, to say the least, to hold beliefs that run counter to prevalent attitudes. Society, friends, and family all tell us we have strayed with phrases such as "You should . . ." "You ought to . . ." or—if your belief has caused them a lot of discomfort—"You're crazy!" Most of the time we respond to this pressure by giving up our unreasonable, or even outrageous, beliefs. Ultimately all of us would prefer to be accepted and loved by others; besides, we tell ourselves, "It wasn't that big a deal anyway."

Your belief system has a profound impact on your life: what you eat and think; how you dress and behave; what you do for a living; whom you choose to marry, befriend, or live with; how you spend your leisure time; what your values and goals are; and how you define health and quality of life. It also determines the nature of the silent messages you give yourself every day. All of us talk to ourselves, and this internal dialogue has a great deal to do with our state of mental health. These messages may be generally self-critical ("You stupid . . ." "Why did I say that?" "Why did I do that?" "How could I . . . ?" "I should've/could've . . ."); limiting ("I'll never be able to . . ."); or accepting and supportive ("Good job!" "That's fine" "I did the best I could"). Almost all of my patients are very hard on themselves. They are self-critical and put themselves under a great deal of unnecessary pressure, while at the same time, most are high achievers.

As human beings we are imperfect; all of us make mistakes. The way we respond to these failings is what creates more, or lessens, stress in our lives. Our pattern of response is one we probably have been repeating since childhood. One way to change the pattern is through the use of verbal *affirmations,* positive statements that you repeat to yourself as often as possible during the day. Affirmations should be in the present tense, contain only positive words, and serve as a response to an often-heard negative message or as an expression of a goal.

For example, if some of the previous critical messages sound familiar to you, two affirmations that would help counteract them are: "I love and approve of myself" and "I am always doing the best I can." When people begin repeating affirmations, they usually don't believe what they're saying (that's why they're saying them), although they would like to. Using affirmations is like reprogramming a computer. Your subconscious mind is the computer that has been receiving the same message for years; now you are going to change the input.

Most computers have a total capacity for processing information far beyond the ability of the majority of computer operators to access it. Similarly, neuroscientists believe that the average person uses only 5 to 10 percent of his or her total brain capacity. This average person has about 50,000 thoughts every day, and it is estimated that 95 percent of them are the same ones he or she had the day before. Your brain hears the same "program" repeated over and over again. It's no wonder you are able to realize only a small fraction of your (and your brain's) full potential. *Mental health will help to develop your creativity—you'll be re-creating yourself—while allowing you greater access to the parts of your brain that have been dormant.*

The best time to say your affirmation is immediately following the negative message you give yourself. I remember feeling so frustrated with my sinus headaches or congestion that I would think to myself, "This will never go away." After I began affirmations, I followed my hopeless comments with an immediate "My sinuses are now completely healed." This affirmation always made me feel a little better and gave me some hope. As my condition improved I began to believe it more and more until it was actually true. Louise Hay has written a wonderful book on self-healing called *You Can Heal Your Life,* in which she focuses on the healing potential of affirmations as a means of learning to love yourself. Her book contains a list of medical conditions, each with a corresponding affirmation. The one for sinusitis is: "I declare peace and harmony are within me and surround me at all times; all is well." I used that one, too, to help cure my sinus disease. For allergies she suggests: "The world is safe and friendly. I am safe. I am at peace with life." And for colds: "I allow my mind to relax and be at peace. Clarity and harmony are within me and around me."

You can use affirmations to help change any belief that doesn't feel good to you, to help you achieve any goal, or to create the life of your dreams. Most of my patients have come in because of one or more chronic physical or mental problems. Their objectives are clear: to stop having sinus infections, to get rid of allergies, to stop living with chronic pain, to have more energy, to suffer less anxiety, and so forth. After they have begun to see a definite improvement in their physical condition, which is usually after they have been working on the physical and environmental aspects of the Sinus Survival Program for about one to two months, I recommend that they create a "wish list" in the form of affirmations. The following is a powerful exercise for transforming your life and creating optimal mental health.

- List your greatest talents and gifts. You have several. These are things that are most special about you, or that you do better than most other people. Ask yourself, "What do I most appreciate about myself?"
- Next, list the things you most enjoy—both activities and states of being, e.g., "I really enjoy just being in the mountains, or on a beach." There will be some overlap with your first list. Many of the activities you enjoy doing are the things you're best at.
- After you have identified your talents and what you enjoy, list the things that have the most meaning for you. This is important, because if your goal doesn't meaningfully encompass more than one area of your life, or have benefit to others in some way, more than likely it is incomplete, and you will lack the passion necessary to commit to it. As you list the meaningful things in your life, you will more easily recognize the talents and activities you enjoy that are most worth your while.
- Now make a wish list of all your goals or objectives in every realm of your life—physical/environmental, mental, emotional, social, and spiritual. Physical and environmental goals can include recovering from illnesses or ailments, engaging in or mastering a particular physical activity (anything you've ever considered doing), or living or working in a certain place. Mental goals might address career plans, financial objectives, and any limiting beliefs that you'd like to change. Emotional goals have to do with feelings and self-esteem. Social goals are about your relationships with other people, while spiritual objectives have to do with your relationship with God or Spirit. As you do this part of the exercise, ask yourself, "What does my ideal life look like?" "Where do I see myself five or ten years from now?" "What is my purpose—what am I here to do?" Do *not* give yourself a time frame within which to attain any of these goals, and remember, it is *not* necessary to have a plan for getting there.
- Next, reword all of your goals into affirmations. Keep them short and simple, and no longer than two brief sentences. For

example, a goal might be "I'd like to cure my sinusitis." The affirmation could then be "My sinuses are now completely healed" or "My sinuses are getting better every day."

- Compile a list of about ten affirmations that includes your most important goals, desires, and any limiting beliefs that you'd like to change.
- Schedule a time each day to do your affirmations, and adhere to it. Doing something regularly at the same time each day adds to the momentum of what you are trying to achieve and eventually will become a positive, effortless habit.
- Recite this entire list at least once a day, and whenever you hear a negative, limiting, or critical message, recite the one affirmation that corresponds to that message. You can also choose to write them all down, reciting each one as you write, and then visualize each one. Or you can record them onto a cassette and listen to them in your own voice. I've found that writing, reciting, and then visualizing your affirmations is the most effective method for manifesting your desires.

I learned this technique from a patient, a man who owns an oil company and works part-time as a psychotherapist. He had a terrible case of chronic sinusitis. On our second session, one month into the Sinus Survival Program, I presented this idea of changing some of his limiting, critical, or negative beliefs and clarifying his goals and objectives as a foundation of greater mental health. Shortly after this visit, he formulated a lengthy list of affirmations and goals. Once each day he recited every one of his new beliefs, then wrote them down on a sheet of paper, and after each one he closed his eyes and visualized what that desire or goal would look or feel like. When I next saw him, just over two months later, he told me that he had been repeating this procedure of reciting, writing, and visualizing for sixty consecutive days. He was thrilled to report to me that at least half of his affirmations and goals had already become a reality, including healthy sinuses! He continues to practice this method (using new affirmations) along with the physical and environ-

Sinus Survival

mental health recommendations that he had implemented at the outset of the Program. It is now more than seven years since my third session with him. During that time he has had only two sinus infections, and his chronic sinusitis remains cured.

My patients' affirmation/goal lists provide a blueprint of our work together. The lists also become their personal vision and give direction to their own self-healing process.

You must be able to clarify your desires to have any chance of obtaining them, and as you do this exercise, try to be as specific as possible. The next step is to believe, however minimally, that it is possible for you to meet these goals. The more you repeat the affirmations, the stronger your belief will become.

The third step in this formula for self-realization is expectation. The stronger your belief and the more objectives you have already reached, the higher will be your level of expectation. After my chronic sinusitis was cured, I developed the belief that anything is possible, one that has helped me to realize other dreams. Whatever it is that you *desire,* as long as you *believe* it's possible, you can *expect* it to happen. It is not necessary to know how, or to have a definite plan. Just be patient and flexible and be willing to accept the result, even if the "package" in which it arrives is different from what you had envisioned. If your objectives are clear, your intuition will help you make the right decisions to get what you want. Remember that you can always choose what to believe. Rather than continuing with the attitude "I'll believe it when I see it," why not try "When I believe it, then I'll see it."

I've repeatedly seen this technique change lives in a variety of ways other than disease. My favorite example is a woman from Tennessee whom I was treating for chronic fatigue, allergies, and sinusitis. In the early years of my holistic practice, I worked with a number of patients long-distance over the phone, never actually meeting them in person. An RN in her fifties, she taught in a nursing school in a small town and had never married, although she wanted to. She had resisted putting marriage on her goal list because, as she explained to me, "I know all the

268

eligible men in town and in my church, and there aren't any possible candidates." I convinced her to include it on her goal list, and her affirmation read simply, "I am happily married." Within a few months, she received a letter from a former professor of hers with whom she had a friendship years earlier. His wife had died the year before, and he wanted to visit his former student. Within months they were engaged, and a year after beginning her affirmation she was happily married. Her tears of joy over the phone and her gratitude left me in tears as well. We both felt as if we had experienced a miracle.

How you choose to see your sinus condition or any other chronic illness can play a vital role in the way the disease affects you and whether or not it goes away. Some of the early reactions to a chronic or life-threatening disease are denial ("There must be some mistake"), anger and frustration ("Why me?" "What terrible luck"), self-pity ("I'll never be able to enjoy life again"), and resignation ("I'll just have to put up with it and continue to live this way for the rest of my life"). All of these are quite normal and understandable responses to something as devastating as a chronic illness. However, if you are interested in healing yourself, it is important to get beyond this point and look at your disease in a different light. According to Bernie Siegel, who contributed the following material to the book *Chop Wood, Carry Water,* you have several choices:

- Accept your illness. Being resigned to an illness can be destructive and can allow the illness to run your life, but accepting it allows energy to be freed for other things in your life.
- See the illness as a source of growth. If you begin to grow psychologically in response to the loss the illness has created in your life, then you don't need to have a physical illness anymore.
- View your illness as a positive redirection in your life. This means that you don't have to judge anything that happens to you. If you get fired from a job, for example, assume that you

are being redirected toward something else you are supposed to be doing. Your entire life changes when you say that something is just a redirection. You are then at peace. Everything is okay and you go on your way, knowing that the new direction is the one that is intrinsically right for you. After a while you begin to *feel* that this is true.

- Death or recurrence of illness is no longer seen as synonymous with failure after the aforementioned steps are accomplished, but simply as further choices or steps. If staying alive were your sole goal, you would have to be a failure because you do have to die someday. However, when you begin to accept the inevitability of death and see that you have only a limited time, you begin to realize that you might as well enjoy the present to the best of your ability.

- Learn self-love and peace of mind, and the body responds. Your body gets "live" or "energy" messages when you say "I love myself." That's not the ego talking, it's self-esteem. It's as if someone else is loving you, saying that you are a worthwhile person, believing in you, and telling you that you are here to give something to the world. When you do that, your immune system says, "This person likes living; let's fight for his or her life."

- Don't make physical change your sole goal. Seek peace of mind, acceptance, and forgiveness. Learn to love. In the process, the disease won't be totally overlooked—it will be seen as one of the problems you are having, and perhaps one of your fears. If you learn about hope, love, acceptance, forgiveness, and peace of mind, the disease may go away in the process.

- Achieve immortality through love. The only way you can live forever is to love somebody. Then you can really leave a gift behind. When you live that way, as many people with physical illnesses do, it is even possible to decide when you die. You can say, "Thank you, I've used my body to its limit. I have loved as much as I possibly can, and I'm leaving at two o'clock today." And you go. Then maybe you have spent half an hour dying and the rest of your life living; but when these things are not done, you may spend a lot of your life dying, and only a little living.

I realize that most of you do not have a terminal disease, just a case of good old chronic sinusitis or allergies, but each of these options for looking at physical illness can work for you as a form of preventive medicine. In my experience, chronic pain and imminent death have provided the greatest motivation for people to change, but why wait until you have reached that point of crisis?

GUIDED IMAGERY AND VISUALIZATION

Visualization is a skill all of us have and one that we use every day. Most of the time, however, we do so unconsciously, as when we daydream. The 50,000 thoughts we have each and every day are often accompanied by inner pictures, or imagery, with corresponding emotions. Since the 1970s, researchers, physicians, and other health care professionals have been examining how to harness these mental images in order to use them consciously to create improved states of well-being. Due to their continued work, thousands of individuals nationwide are learning how to use visualization and guided imagery to enhance their health. In many cases their results have been astounding. Since 1971, radiation oncologist O. Carl Simonton, M.D., for instance, has been a pioneer in developing imagery as a self-care tool for cancer patients to use to bolster their response rate to traditional cancer treatments, with remarkable success. The first patient to whom he taught his techniques was a 61-year-old man who had been diagnosed with a "hopeless" case of throat cancer. In conjunction with his radiation treatments, the man spent five to fifteen minutes three times a day imagining himself healthy. Within two months he was completely cancer-free.

A similarly remarkable case is that of Garrett Porter, a patient of Patricia Norris, Ph.D., another leader in the field of guided imagery. Garrett, who was nine, had been diagnosed with an inoperable brain tumor. Using biofeedback techniques in conjunction with imagery based on his favorite TV show, *Star Trek* (he pictured missiles striking and destroying his tumor), Garrett was able to completely reverse his condition within a year, with brain scans confirming his tumor's disappearance. Numerous studies also confirm the health benefits of imagery and visualization. For example, college volunteers who practiced imagery twice daily for six weeks experienced a marked increase in salivary immunoglobulin A as compared to a control group who did not practice imagery. In another study, the well-known drop in helper T-immune cells in students facing the stress of final examinations was greatly reduced in a group utilizing relaxation and imagery each day for a month before exams. And patients scheduled for gallbladder surgery who listened to imagery tapes before and after their operations had less wound inflammation, lower cortisone levels, and less anxiety, compared to controls who were treated with comparable periods of quiet only.

Like most of the other therapies outlined in this chapter, one of the most exciting things about guided imagery and visualization is that both techniques are powerful self-healing tools that can be used to create positive change in almost any area of your life. Besides physical health, imagery can help you feel more peaceful and relaxed, assist you in further developing your creative talents, create more fulfillment in your relationships, improve your ability to achieve career goals, and dissolve negative habit patterns. All that is necessary is a commitment to practice the techniques on a regular basis.

Guided imagery and visualization work to improve and maintain health because of their ability to directly affect our bodies at a cellular level, particularly with regard to neuropeptides. In addition, the use of imagery can often provide greater insight about causes and treatment for chronic conditions, guiding us toward the most personalized and effective solutions for our particular health problem. This occurs because our mental images are so deeply connected to our emotions, which are usually interconnected with the events in our lives. By using imagery, you can become better aware of what emotional issues may lie beneath the surface of your life and begin the process of healing them.

There are two types of guided imagery and visualization: preconceived or preselected images employed by you or your health care professional in order to address a specific problem and achieve a specific outcome, and imagery that occurs spontaneously as you sit comfortably, eyes closed and breathing freely. Both forms have value, so try them both and see which works best for you. What follows are two techniques you can use to make imagery a part of your Sinus Survival Program. The first is a form of guided imagery, while the latter is conducive for allowing spontaneous imagery to occur on its own.

The Remembrance Technique   This exercise can be adapted to improve issues or conditions in any area of your life. It's called the Remembrance Technique because in our core selves we are already whole. In many respects, healing is simply a remembrance of that state in order to reconnect with it. Begin this exercise by sitting comfortably in a chair or lying down in bed. Select a time and place when you will not be disturbed. Close your eyes and focus on your breathing. Take a few deep, unforced breaths to help yourself relax. With each inhalation, imagine that soothing, relaxing energy is flowing through all areas of your body. As you exhale, visualize the cares and concerns of the day gradually disappearing. Do this for two or three minutes, allowing your breath to carry you to a place of calm relaxation.

Now choose the issue you want to focus on for the rest of the exercise, and recall a time when the outcome you desire was something you already experienced. For example, if you have a sinus infection, remember a time when you felt healthy and energetic and could breathe freely. Allow yourself to reexperience that time, using all of your senses to make what you are imagining as vivid as possible. Once you have reconnected to the experience, bring it into the present *as if it were actually happening now.* Stay with the experience for at least five more minutes, mentally affirming that you are experiencing the state you desire here in the present.

Spontaneous imagery   In this exercise, instead of preselecting a specific outcome, you are going to allow your own unconscious to communicate with you through imagery about whatever situation in your life you choose to focus on. As in the preceding exercise, sit or lie down comfortably in a quiet place, close your eyes, and focus on your breath until you feel yourself settling into a deeper state of relaxation. Now focus on the physical problem you'd like to heal or the area in your life into which you desire to gain greater insight, allowing thoughts and images to freely and spontaneously emerge. You may be surprised by what you experience, but don't judge it. Trust that your unconscious knows what you most need to understand, and allow your imagery to lead you to that answer. Continue this exercise for five to ten minutes, and when you complete it, write down what you experienced so that you can contemplate it for possible further insight. As a variation of this exercise, you can first ask a question of yourself, such as "Why do I have sinusitis?" or "What do I have to learn from my sinusitis?" and then see what image appears. From there, you may find yourself engaged in a dialogue between yourself and your unconscious that results in answers and solutions you did not know were possible.

My most memorable experience with spontaneous imagery was associated with treating a sinus infection. Without having received any formal training in the method, I sat in a straight-backed chair and focused on deep, relaxed breathing for about twenty minutes. The following vision appeared to me: I saw a large sphere completely covered with a slimy, moldy, greenish-gray crud—terrible-looking stuff! At the top of this globe (if you picture the earth, this would be the North Pole) were a group of about ten little workmen clothed in overalls and caps, each holding a high-powered hose and a long-handled push broom. I watched as they methodically began to work their way down the sides of this sphere, hosing and sweeping away the green slime. Underneath was revealed the brightest and healthiest-looking orange I had ever seen. After the orange was completely uncovered, I got up from my chair and at that moment felt the largest clump of postnasal mucus I'd ever had in the back of my throat. As I marveled at the size of the greenish-yellow mass I had then spit into the sink, I could sense that my sinus infection was almost completely resolved. It never returned. Needless to say, I remain impressed with the power of mental imagery to treat physical ailments, although it is not the only therapy I used to cure my sinus disease. Another image you can use preventively for sinuses is to begin each day seeing yourself surrounded by several layers of bright, multicolored light. This light can act as a protective shield or as your own personal air filter removing air pollutants before they can enter your nose and sinuses. A very handy image indeed, especially in badly polluted environments.

When you first begin to practice mental imagery techniques, don't be discouraged if at first "nothing seems to be happening." Like any new skill, achieving results in imagery takes time. Remember that the language of your unconscious, like the symbolism of your dreams, is usually not literal or rational. It may take some time before you are able to grasp the messages of the images you perceive. Keeping a written log of your experience can make learning this new "language" easier.

OPTIMISM AND HUMOR

In the Bible it is written, "A cheerful heart is good medicine, but a downcast spirit dries up the bones" (Proverbs 17:22). Science is now beginning to verify this ancient truth, revealing that optimism and humor are integral factors in one's overall health, providing both physical and mental benefits. One of the most famous anecdotes illustrating this point concerns Norman Cousins, who in his book *Anatomy of an Illness* attributed his recovery from ankylosing spondylitis (a potentially crippling arthritic condition of the spine) to the many hours he spent watching Marx Brothers movies and reruns of *Candid Camera* while taking megadoses of vitamin C. The more he laughed, the more his pain diminished, until eventually his illness completely disappeared, never to return. Based on his experience with humor, Cousins went on to explore mind/body medicine at UCLA. Today a number of institutions are studying the healing potential of humor, such as the appropriately named Gesundheit Institute in Arlington, Virginia, founded and directed by Patch Adams, M.D.

Some of the most in-depth research in this area has been conducted by Robert Ornstein, Ph.D., and David Sobel, M.D., who presented their findings in their book *Healthy Pleasures.* They discovered that the people who are optimally healthy also tend to be optimistic and happy and possess the belief that things will work out no matter what their difficulties may be. Such people maintain a vital sense of humor about life and enjoy a good laugh, often at their own expense. According to Ornstein and Sobel, they also expect good things of life, including being liked and respected by others, and experience pleasure in most of what they do. They usually look at stressful situations as temporary setbacks, specific to the immediate circumstance, and due largely to external causes. Pessimists, on the other hand, when faced with life-challenging events, tend to think it will be permanent ("It's going to last forever"), generalize the problem to their whole life ("It's going to spoil everything"), and blame themselves ("It's my fault"). Recent research at the Mayo Clinic suggests that pessimism is a significant risk factor for early death. Over 800 patients were given a personality test that categorized them as optimistic, mixed, or pessimistic. After their health status was evaluated thirty years later, the pessimists had a significantly higher-than-expected death rate.

Optimistic people also tend to laugh a lot, something that most likely plays an important role in their health. Studies have shown that laughter can strengthen the immune system. One study, for instance, found that test subjects who watched videotapes of the comedian Richard Pryor produced increased levels of antibodies in their saliva. Furthermore, subjects in the study who said they frequently used humor to cope with life stress had consistently higher baseline levels of those antibodies that help to combat infections such as colds.

Hearty laughter is actually a form of gentle exercise, or "inner jogging." Describing the physiological effects of laughter, Ornstein and Sobel write:

> A robust laugh gives the muscles of your face, shoulders, diaphragm, and abdomen a good workout. With convulsive or side-splitting laughter, even your arm and leg muscles come into play. Your heart rate and blood pressure temporarily rise, breathing becomes faster and deeper, and oxygen surges through your bloodstream. A vigorous laugh can burn up as many calories per hour as brisk walking or cycling. . . . The afterglow of a hearty laugh is positively relaxing. Blood pressure may temporarily fall, your muscles go limp, and you bask in a mild euphoria. Some researchers speculate that laughter triggers the release of endorphins, the brain's own opiates; this may account for the pain relief and euphoria that accompany laughter.

In short, laughter's benefits are many and profound. When the questions posed to octogenarians is "If you had your life to live over again, what would you do differently?" The answer often is "I'd take life much less seriously." Comedian George Burns, who lived to be 100, wrote the book *Wisdom of the 90s* at the age of 95. He attributed his ability to laugh at himself as well as loving what he did for a living as the most important factors in his longevity.

Both optimism and a sense of humor are directly related to our beliefs. If you wish to become more optimistic and experience more humor and fun in your life, practice the exercises outlined in this chapter. It may take time before you achieve the results you desire, but your commitment will prove well worth it, and will impact your mood, mental health, and even survival. Nothing quite epitomizes the free flow of life force energy as laughter, and all of us can stand to laugh even more than we do. Be advised, however. There is one side effect to this powerful form of self-healing—more pleasure.

EMOTIONAL HEALTH

The emotionally fit are able to identify their feelings and can express, fully experience, and accept them as well. I have heard contemporary American culture referred to as the "no-feeling" society. The feelings are certainly present, but as a result of our lifestyle we have constructed such formidable protective barriers around ourselves that to a great extent we have become unconscious of our feelings, especially the more uncomfortable ones.

There are those who believe there are only two basic human emotions: love and fear. The so-called negative or painful emotions, such as anger, anxiety, depression, envy, guilt, hatred, hostility, jealousy, loneliness, shame, and worry, are all expressions of fear. The feelings of acceptance, intimacy, joy, power, and peacefulness are all aspects of love. The greater our degree of fear, the less capable we are of experiencing love.

There are other mental health professionals who consider four basic emotions: love or joy, sadness, anger, and fear. So at any given moment, you're feeling either glad, sad, mad, or scared, or some combination of these. In our culture it is not socially acceptable to express most of the "negative" emotions, and men especially are not supposed to show signs of weakness or insecurity or to cry ("Big boys don't cry"). The majority of us have learned to repress these feelings until we are unaware that we even have them. Society has helped us suppress our painful (negative) feelings by perpetuating the myth of an emotionally pain-free existence. The numerous ads in the media for analgesics to treat tension headaches and the common use of alcohol or drugs to dull the pain of an awkward social situation or personal crisis give us the relentless message that not only is pain a bad thing, but life can be pain-free.

If we spent less time avoiding emotional pain, but instead focused our attention on it, accepted it, and relaxed into it, the pain would diminish or even disappear. ***If we continue to ignore and repress it, it often manifests itself as physical pain, illness, or disease.*** Redford Williams, M.D., a researcher in behavioral medicine at the Duke University Medical Center, has gathered a wealth of data suggesting that chronic anger is so damaging to the body that it ranks with, or even exceeds, cigarette smoking, obesity, and a high-fat diet as a powerful risk factor for early death. Williams reported that people who scored high on a hostility scale as teenagers were much more likely than their more cheerful peers to have elevated cholesterol levels as adults, suggesting a link between unremitting anger and heart disease.

In another recent study, Dr. Mara Julius, an epidemiologist at the University of Michigan, analyzed the effects of chronic anger on women over a period of eighteen years. She found that women who had answered initial test questions with obvious signs of long-term, suppressed anger were three times more likely to have died during the study than those women who did not harbor such hostile feelings. In fact, chronic sinusitis is usually associated with a tremendous amount of unexpressed anger. *I've found it to be the primary trigger for most sinus infections.*

Clyde Reid is director of the Center for New Beginnings in Denver. In his insightful book *Celebrate the Temporary,* he says, "Leaning into life's pain can also be a lifestyle, and is far more satisfying than the avoidance style. It requires small doses of plain courage to look pain in the eye, but it prepares you for more serious pain when it comes. In the meantime, all the energy expended to avoid pain is now available for the business of living."

I am not advocating that you seek out painful experiences, nor am I proposing that you endure prolonged or persistent pain. That is called suffering. Health and happiness do not have prerequisites that require you to suffer. Life is to be enjoyed, but the notion that it can be lived entirely without painful feelings is an unhealthy belief. Pain and joy are intertwined, and ***the more***

you allow yourself to accept, embrace, and feel both joy and pain, the greater will be your sense of emotional health.

Of the mental-emotional connection, Albert Ellis a psychologist and founder of the Institute for Rational-Emotive Therapy in New York City, has said that "virtually all 'emotionally disturbed' individuals actually think crookedly, magically, dogmatically, and unrealistically." David D. Burns, M.D., a psychiatrist and author of *The Feeling Good Handbook: Using the New Mood Therapy in Everyday Life,* writes:

> Certain kinds of negative thoughts make people unhappy. In fact, I believe that unhealthy, negative emotions—depression, anxiety, excessive anger, inappropriate guilt, etc.—are *always* caused by illogical, distorted thoughts, even if those thoughts may seem absolutely valid at the time. By learning to look at things more realistically, by getting rid of your distorted thinking patterns, you can break out of a bad mood, often in a short period of time, without having to rely on medication or prolonged psychotherapy.

Burns offers the following list of thought distortions:

- All-or-nothing thinking. You classify things into absolute, black-and-white categories.
- Overgeneralization. You view a single negative situation as a never-ending pattern of defeat.
- Mental filtering. You dwell on negatives and overlook positives.
- Discounting the positive. You insist your accomplishments or positive qualities "don't count."
- Magnification or minimization. You blow things out of proportion or shrink their importance inappropriately.
- Making "should" statements. You criticize yourself and others by using the terms *should, shouldn't, must, ought,* and *have to.*
- Emotional reasoning. You reason from how you feel. If you feel like an idiot, you assume you must be one. If you don't feel like doing something, you put it off.

- Jumping to conclusions. You "mind read," assuming, without definite evidence of it, that people are reacting negatively to you. Or you "fortune tell," arbitrarily predicting bad outcomes.
- Labeling. You identify with your shortcomings. Instead of saying, "I made a mistake," you tell yourself, "I'm such a jerk . . . a real loser."
- Personalization and blame. You blame yourself for something you weren't entirely responsible for, or you blame others and ignore the impact of your own attitudes or behavior.

As I've already said, negative thoughts and the feelings they engender contribute to physical illness. The high-achieving perfectionism found in many people with chronic sinusitis is often associated with several of the above thought distortions. These repeated thoughts will usually trigger anger (ultimately with ourselves), which, if it's not expressed, will often result in a sinus infection. Many of these same critical and limiting messages are also preventing you from achieving you goals and seeing your "wish list" become a reality. These theories of Drs. Ellis and Burns comprise the foundation of *cognitive psychotherapy*—the form of counseling I've found to be highly effective for many of my patients.

EMOTIONAL CAUSES OF DIS-EASE

Every disease has multiple causes. There is often a genetic predisposition to developing a chronic ailment that is inherited from parents and grandparents. The risk of contracting cancer or heart disease is increased significantly if one or both parents has it. My father and one of my daughters had chronic sinusitis. Allergies also commonly run in families.

As you've learned in Chapter 6, environmental and dietary factors also play important roles in the disease process. But before an acute illness can continue to progress into a chronic condition, there must be an accompanying diminished function of the immune system. After being sick for a short time with a cold or sinus infection, in most people with normal immune function, the body is quickly restored to its original state of good health.

In the vast majority of cases, the primary cause of chronically depressed immunity is emotional stress. *Stress* is a broad and ubiquitous term in our "stressed out" society—stress management, stress reduction, stressful. Most of us recognize that stress doesn't feel good if there's too much of it, but what actually causes it? The answer to that question is different for each of us. But how many of us are able to identify the specific emotion most responsible for our feelings of stress? Are you depressed, angry, ashamed, guilty, afraid, or sad?

Holistic physicians and researchers in behavioral medicine and psychoneuroimmunology are just beginning to connect consistent emotional and behavioral patterns with predictable dis-ease responses. With chronic respiratory disease, I have mentioned the critical role of repressed anger in causing chronic sinusitis. Many of my sinus patients are high achievers with a strong need for control. Anger is often a result of their perceived loss of control or the need to be right. I also now believe that a deep sadness exists in most of these patients. The many tears that have not been shed can result in congestion of the tear glands, which surround the eyes and are in close proximity to the sinuses as well. Perhaps this swelling and congestion is also a contributor to congested sinuses.

Besides the skin tests and a scientific investigation of their environment to determine the cause of hay fever, people with allergies would do well to ask themselves who or what situation or circumstance they are "allergic" to or have some anxiety about. For several years I have been increasingly aware of the intimate connection between sneezing spells and disturbing thoughts or images. One patient in particular, who was having marital problems, would start to sneeze whenever I mentioned her husband. Yes, of course the pollen count or cat dander are certainly contributors. But even with those factors being present, symptoms can be minimal or nonexistent until a disturbing thought or situation occurs. Then the feeling of stress arises, and the allergy attack begins. The next time you experience a sudden onset of allergy symptoms, I would suggest looking back to your thoughts and feelings that were present just prior to the allergic reaction. Your sneezing, itching, congestion, and wheezing can become an emotional "barometer" that helps you to identify the deeper and hidden causes of allergic rhinitis.

I recognize that I have made a generalization regarding the emotional causes of sinusitis and allergies, and that they do not apply to everyone with these conditions. But before promptly dismissing them as not pertaining to you, please give it some thought and try to identify what it is you are feeling.

Another method you might use to help identify the emotional causes of your illness is to consider the possible benefits or secondary gain resulting from being sick. This is most easily seen with colds, which usually occur during a period when you've often been working too hard or doing too much. The cold might necessitate staying home in bed, missing a day of work, and receiving a lot more nurturing—all of which were sorely needed. Since you did not respond preventively, in order to meet those unconscious needs, your body created an illness. Whether it's more attention, a need to be cared for, job dissatisfaction, or school phobia, I believe there are always secondary gains associated with every chronic disease. If these not-so-subtle benefits can be understood and you become more aware of what your needs are, you can recognize the emotional causes of your physical problem. Once you have become aware of these emotions, you can then begin the process of accepting (knowing that it's okay to feel whatever you're feeling) and expressing all of your feelings and addressing the unmet needs your feelings bring up. This process will not only lead you to emotional health, it will help you practice preventative medicine, and will also take you a giant step closer to being completely free of your so-called "incurable" dis-ease. Remember, a basic tenet of mind-body medicine is that *your core issues are held in your tissues.*

BREATHWORK AND MEDITATION

The benefits of learning to breathe properly and consciously go far beyond the physical. Proper breathing can also improve your mood, make you mentally more alert, and help you to become more aware of deeply held and often painful feelings. Most importantly, by working with the breath, you can begin to heal the wounded, rejected, unacknowledged, and disowned parts of yourself and bring them into wholeness.

The primary reason so many of us breathe unconsciously and inefficiently lies in the fact that our breathing process began traumatically at birth. We were forcibly expelled from the security of the womb and compelled to take our first breath on our own when we encountered the outside world. Often that first breath came as a harsh and unexpected shock, accompanied by pain and confusion. In order to suppress such pain, newborns typically follow their first inhalation by pausing and holding their breath for a moment as they struggle to make sense of their new environment. Today a number of researchers in the field of mental health speculate that this first pause in our breath not only sets the stage for a lifetime of shallow, inefficient breathing but also conditions us to suppress our painful emotions instead of learning how to accept and relax into them. You can observe this pattern in yourself the next time you find yourself feeling shock, fear, pain, or worry. If you take a moment to observe yourself in the initial experience of such emotions, more than likely you will find that you are also holding your breath or breathing very shallowly.

Breathwork, also known as *breath therapy,* is a means of learning how to breathe consciously and fully in order to deal with emotional pain more effectively and healthfully. There are many approaches to breathwork, ranging from ancient breathing techniques found in the traditions of *yoga, tai chi,* and *chigong,* to modern-day methods such as *rebirthing* (also known as *conscious connected breathing*), developed by Leonard Orr, and *holotropic breathwork,* developed by Stanislav Grof. All of them have in common a focus on the breath and the ability to move energy through the body and connect you with suppressed emotions and limiting beliefs in order to heal them.

Most breathwork therapies use the technique of connected breathing, first pioneered by Leonard Orr. In connected breathing, each inhalation immediately follows the exhalation of the preceding breath without pause. (Typically we breathe unconsciously, pausing between inhalation and exhalation.) The pattern of respiration can vary according to the technique. Sometimes it is rapid; sometimes it is deep, slow, and full. In addition, some approaches recommend breathing in and out through the mouth, instead of the nose, and both abdominal and chest breathing can be used. In rebirthing, sometimes the therapy is performed in a tub or underwater with the use of a snorkel, although this usually does not occur until after the client has had a number of "dry" connected breathing sessions and has become comfortable with the movement of energy and the integration of emotions that commonly occur during the rebirthing process. Because of the emotional release that can result from breathwork, it is advisable to learn the techniques under the direction of a skilled breath therapist. Once you gain proficiency, however, you will have at your disposal a powerful self-healing technique that you can practice daily on your own.

Meditation   There are numerous meditation techniques, but all of them can be accurately described as conscious breathing methods. Meditation's many physiological benefits include improved immune function; reduced stress, including decreased levels of adrenaline, cortisone, and free radicals; increased oxygen intake; relief from chronic pain and headache; lower blood pressure and heart rate; and a reduction of core body temperature, which has been linked to increased longevity. Among the psychological benefits of meditation are greater relaxation, improved focus on the present instead of regrets and worries about the past and future, enhanced creativity and cognitive functioning, heightened spiritual awareness (including insights leading to the healing of past emotional trauma), improved awareness and management of beliefs and emotions, and a greater compassion and recognition of others and oneself as parts of a greater whole.

The following is a simple meditation technique that utilizes breathing to promote mental calm. Select a quiet place and sit in a chair, with your back straight and your feet on the floor. Close your eyes and begin abdominal breathing, inhaling and exhaling through your nose at a rate of three to four full breaths (inhale and exhale) per minute. The object of this exercise is to stay focused on your breath, allowing whatever thoughts you have to come and go without being absorbed by them. Should you find your attention wandering, bring it back to your breath. You can also enhance the process by silently repeating a short affirmation, or a positive phrase, such as *God, love,* or *peace,* on both the inhale and the exhale. At first try to do this exercise for five minutes once or twice a day, gradually working up to 20 minutes twice daily. Don't be discouraged if at first you find this exercise difficult to practice. For most Americans, sitting and breathing without thinking or external stimulation is not easy. With time and continued practice, especially in the morning and before you go to bed, you will begin to notice the benefits meditation affords. (For more on meditation, see Chapter 8.)

DEALING WITH ANGER

Unexpressed anger, or anger that is expressed inappropriately, is both harmful and extremely common in our society. Most of us were taught very early in life that anger was an unacceptable emotion. When it was expressed, it often elicited fear in us, and it was usually equated with bodily harm and loss of control ("He's really lost it" "He's out of control"). This inability to safely express anger has been shown to produce many serious health consequences, not the least of which is triggering sinus infections. Today many psychotherapists are combining sound and body movement techniques to help their patients deal with their anger, finding that such approaches can be far more effective than simply talking about it. The following techniques can be safely employed by anyone to release the highly charged emotional energy of anger. They are most effective when employed regularly as preventive measures, instead of allowing anger to build up into a state of chronic, health-impacting tension, much less explosive rage.

Screaming   This is the most common anger release technique due to the fact that all of us already know how to do it. In his novel *Tai Pan,* James Clavell wrote that the chieftains of ancient Scotland for centuries maintained the custom of the "screaming tree." From the time they entered adolescence, men of the clan were instructed to go into the forest and select a tree to which they could express their discontent. Then, whenever their troubles grew too great to otherwise deal with, they would go to the forest alone and scream with the tree as their witness until their emotions settled.

The value of screaming is no secret to young children, who commonly scream when they are greatly upset, only to exhibit a smiling face moments afterward. For adults, the biggest difficulty here is finding a place to scream in privacy. Screaming when you are home alone, in the basement or closet, in the car with the windows up, or in a secluded spot outdoors are all possibilities. To get the most benefit, take a deep abdominal breath before you scream, and then direct the scream from your diaphragm or deep within your chest cavity, as this will protect your vocal cords. As you scream, slowly move your upper body from side to side or up and down. Usually, after two or three screams in succession, you will begin to feel much better.

The angry letter (not sent)   This technique is increasingly employed by therapists to help their clients release their anger. It involves writing a letter to the person with whom you are angry, listing all the reasons why you are upset with them. As you write, allow yourself to express whatever comes to mind, no matter how harsh or offensive it might seem. Once the letter is written, read it over, and if anything else occurs to you that you wish to express, write that down too before signing it. Then either burn the letter or tear it up into small pieces.

Punching Punching a bag, pillow, or sofa is another effective method of dissipating anger. Remember to grunt or yell with each punch. A variation of this method is to take hold of a pillow and hit it against the floor, sofa, or wall. With either approach, it only takes a few moments before you will start to feel your anger transforming into satisfaction and even joy. Remember, anger in and of itself is not a negative emotion to be shunned. It's only when it remains bottled up inside of us unexpressed that it becomes unhealthy. Safely and appropriately expressing your anger in socially acceptable ways can dramatically improve the way you feel, both emotionally and physically.

As part of the Sinus Survival Program, I spent several years releasing anger on a daily basis through punching. I bought boxing gloves and hung a 70-pound punching bag from a wooden beam in my basement. After only a minute or less of vigorous punching, accompanied by yelling (with each punch), I felt much less stressed and surprisingly less sinus congestion too. When I finish, my breathing is always more relaxed and less restricted in both my head and chest.

However, simply venting anger doesn't do the whole job. In fact, one study in April 1999 concluded that punching to release anger actually tends to increase and prolong feelings of hostility. Although this finding runs counter to my personal experience and that of many of my patients who have benefited from this practice, there are several additional steps that can be taken to release anger. You can start by recognizing that your anger may be the result of unreasonable or even irrational demands you've made on yourself or someone else, and that by maintaining these demands you are hurting yourself with increased stress. It is therefore in your best interests to release the demands and let go of the anger.

Aerobic exercise This is another quick-fix method for dissipating anger and opening your nose and sinuses. However, if you're especially enraged about a particular incident or situation, wait at least twenty minutes and take some deep breaths before beginning a strenuous workout. There can be a greater risk of heart attack associated with exercise *immediately* following emotional trauma. Journaling, which I'll discuss in the next section, is also an effective means of releasing anger but not quite as fast as punching and exercise.

DREAMWORK AND JOURNALING

Dreams can play an important role in our healing journey. Serving as symbolic expressions of our inner emotional life, our dreams often provide the clues we need to better understand our mental and emotional states, as well as the guidance we may need to heal personal life situations. Dreams can also sometimes reveal how to heal physical disease conditions. This was illustrated in a dream of Alexander the Great recounted in Pliny's *Natural History.* One of Alexander's friends, Ptolemaus, was dying of a poisoned wound. Alexander dreamt of a dragon holding a plant in its mouth; the dragon said that the plant was the key to curing Ptolemaus. Upon awakening, Alexander dispatched soldiers to the place he had seen in his dream. They returned with the plant and, as the dream had predicted, Ptolemaus, as well as many others of Alexander's troops suffering from similar wounds, was cured.

In American society, dreams are often overlooked or ignored, although researchers like Stephen LaBarge, Ph.D., have in recent decades done much to scientifically demonstrate their importance. The two biggest obstacles that prevent us from getting the most benefit from our dreams are that we either do not remember or quickly forget them, or we do not know how to interpret the symbolism and imagery that dreams contain. Dream recall is a skill that anyone can develop with time and practice, however. One of the keys to dreamwork is to commit to focusing attention on your dreams. A deceptively simple way to do this is to tell yourself each night before you fall asleep that when you wake up you will remember what you dreamt during the night. At first you may not experience much success, but regular affirmation of this technique will instruct your unconscious to eventually make your dreams recallable.

As you start to remember your dreams, keep a pad and pencil or a tape recorder by your bed so that you can either write down or verbally record them immediately after you awaken. All of us dream an average of three or four times each night. With practice, many people who make the commitment to record and study their dreams are able to train themselves to spontaneously awaken after each dream cycle to record the gist of their dreams before settling back to sleep until after their next dream stage. Recording your dreams *immediately* after you awaken provides the best results, since dreams are quickly forgotten once you get out of bed and begin your day. At first, all you may recall are fragments of your dream experience. Don't be discouraged if this is the case. Over time, the regular recording of your dreams will begin to yield more details. In addition, after you have recorded your dreams for a few weeks or months, as you read over your dream diary, you will start to notice how certain symbols and events tend to recur. Pay attention to such common themes; usually they contain the most important messages that your dreams have for you.

Learning how to interpret the symbolism of your dreams takes time and practice. Certain psychotherapists, especially those with a background in Jungian theory, are skilled in dream interpretation and can help you, and a number of books on the subject can also guide you. Bear in mind, however, that your dreams are highly personal, and although many dream symbols do seem to be common to what Jung called the collective unconscious, there is no such thing as a standard for dream interpretation that will work for everyone. As the dreamer of your own life, you are ultimately the person best suited to appreciate your dreams and discern their deepest meanings. By taking the time to do so, you can improve your mental and emotional health immeasurably.

Journaling   Journaling is another simple but very effective way to become more conscious of your mental and emotional life and to help you better express your feelings. Studies have also shown that it can strengthen your immune system in addition to improving physical symptoms. The practice of journaling entails keeping a written record of your thoughts, emotions, and any other daily experiences that you would like to better understand. Instead of recording your dreams, you will be keeping a journal of your waking activities. When journaling is done on a regular basis, it usually results in increased self-knowledge, often with insights that are both enlightening and enlivening. In a very real sense, journaling can help you become your own therapist or best friend. Your journal becomes your own emotional diary.

Many people who begin the practice of journaling are amazed to discover how the simple act of writing out one's daily experiences can lead to sudden or deeper insights into what they are feeling. Journaling can also help you become better aware of your beliefs, providing you with the opportunity to recognize and change those that may be limiting you. As you use your journal, you will also start to take more control over what you are thinking and feeling, becoming less reactive to your life experiences and more creative in your approaches to dealing with them. Journaling also makes communicating with yourself easier and allows greater clarity, since you are free from judgment or criticism from others. Your journal is for you alone and isn't meant to be shared. Nor do you have to worry about spelling or grammar.

A number of researchers, including James W. Pennebaker, Ph.D., author of the book *Opening Up*, have documented the benefits that journaling can provide by writing about upsetting or traumatic experiences. For people who have difficulty in expressing their emotions, particularly those that are judged to be negative, such as anger or fear, journaling can be especially valuable as a tool for self-healing. The results of a recent study measuring the effects of writing about stressful experiences on symptom reduction in patients with asthma and arthritis were published in the Journal of the American Medical Association in April 1999. The subjects in the study were asked to write about the most stressful event of their lives for twenty minutes daily for three consecutive days. They changed nothing else in their treatment regimen. Four months later, researchers found a significant improvement in lung function in the asthmatics and a reduction in the severity of disease in the arthritics.

For best results with journaling, try to write in your journal at the same time each day. This will help you make journaling a healthy habit. Just before you go to bed can be an ideal time for journaling. You can express the emotions that you've been containing all day and provide resolution to the day's events prior to going to sleep. Journaling and dreamwork not only will help you to heal mentally and emotionally but can also open up new vistas of adventure that can last you a lifetime.

WORK AND PLAY

Do you enjoy your job? Does your work utilize your greatest talents? Is your job fulfilling and challenging? Sadly, for the majority of Americans the answer to these questions is no. Studies reveal that an alarmingly high proportion of our society—nearly 70 percent of us—do not experience satisfaction from our jobs. Unfortunately, there is a significant price to be paid, both physiologically and psychologically, for not loving your work. For example, in a study conducted by the Massachusetts Department of Health in the late 1980s, it was found that the two greatest risk factors for heart disease lie in one's self-happiness rating and one's level of job satisfaction. Low scores in these two areas were shown to be better indicators of the likelihood for developing heart disease than high cholesterol, high blood pressure, excess weight, and a sedentary lifestyle. No wonder, then, that in the United States more heart attacks occur on Monday morning around nine o'clock than at any other time of the week.

Your job is a vital aspect of your mental health. If you find yourself working at a job that you do not enjoy, chances are that you continue to do so due to one or more of the following limiting beliefs: *I don't have a choice; I need the money. I'll never be able to make enough money doing what I love. I have no idea what I'd enjoy doing or what my greatest talents are.* By using the techniques outlined in this chapter, especially in the section "Beliefs, Affirmations, and Goals," you can begin to liberate yourself from these unhealthy beliefs. You'll discover that you are not bound to your job for life, and you do have the ability to find a job for which you are better suited and which is more fulfilling. Every one of us is blessed with at least one God-given talent, and there is at least one activity that we enjoy doing that we do quite well. *That* is where you need to begin to investigate what your gifts are. Write down your talents as outlined in the goal-setting section on page 266, followed by a list of activities you truly enjoy. Then brainstorm all the possible ways you can think of in which you can earn a living combining your talents with each of the activities you wrote down. List every idea that occurs to you, regardless of how ridiculous it may seem. As you continue to practice this exercise, you will have a much clearer idea of new job options. At the same time, acknowledge that you are seeking a greater level of fulfillment, are willing to change and take a risk, and are committed to begin the exploration that will lead you to work that you love doing. In the process, you may discover that your capabilities are limitless.

Even if you are fortunate to have a job you do enjoy, you may still be prey to another modern-day dis-ease, *workaholism.* According to the Economic Policy Institute in Washington, DC, the majority of Americans are working longer and harder than they used to. Our yearly workload has increased by 158 hours compared to that of twenty years ago, including longer commuting times and a reduction of paid holidays and vacation time. That's the equivalent of an extra month's work per year. To counter this tendency, it is essential that you regularly engage in the counterbalance to work—*play.*

Many of us have unfortunately relegated play to childhood, yet play is a crucial aspect of mental health and is unrivaled as a means of expressing joy, passion, exhilaration, even ecstasy. The word *play* comes from the Dutch *pleien,* which means "to dance, leap for joy, and rejoice," all activities that suggest a vibrantly healthy mental state. Play has also been defined as any activity in which you lose track of time. Believing that play is not appropriate adult behavior is both limiting and unhealthy.

If your work involves your greatest talents and is something you truly enjoy doing, work and play for you can seem virtually indistinguishable. Even so, to optimize mental health, find at least one other activity to participate in, besides your work, that you can thoroughly enjoy. Such activities include sports, games, dance, and active creative pursuits, such as playing a musical instrument, acting, singing, painting, crafts, or gardening. Although many people derive great pleasure from playing cards, chess, and other board games, or stamp or coin collecting, all of these are mental pursuits. To create a healthier balance, select activities that utilize your body, allow you to better express your feelings and creativity, and perhaps even bring you to a greater level of spiritual attunement. Ideally the activity should be something so consuming and absorbing that it requires your total attention, providing a pleasurable escape from your normal tension, stress, and habitual thought patterns. Choose something that instinctively appeals to you and do it on a regular basis, for at least an hour three times a week. Be prepared to make mistakes and look silly. That's part of the risk, and the excitement, of doing something new. The more you commit to and practice whatever activity you choose, the better you'll become at it and the more you'll enjoy the benefits it provides.

We live in a society where work has become the greatest addiction, and the majority of us gauge our self-worth according to our achievements and net worth. For this reason alone the importance of play cannot be overemphasized. All of us, for a short time at least, need to regularly let go of that responsible, mature, working adult part of ourselves to reconnect with our woefully neglected playful "inner child."

SUMMARY

The biggest obstacles each of us must overcome in order to achieve optimal mental health are our largely unconscious denial and repression of emotional pain and our limiting thoughts, beliefs, and attitudes, which combine to create our unhealthy behaviors. The tools in this chapter will enable you to heighten your awareness, allowing you to consciously transform your life in harmony with your greatest needs and desires. The more you practice the methods outlined here, the more profound the impact you will have on your mental health, as well as your physical health. *You will become more conscious of your behavior and gain the freedom to choose how you wish to think, feel, and behave.* By letting go of your fear of experiencing life more fully, you can embrace and be more accepting of all your thoughts, beliefs, and emotions. This will allow you the joy of realizing your life's goals and the exhilaration of the unimpeded free flow of life force energy. Remember, only through fully experiencing *both pain and joy* can you truly use your unique gifts and talents to thrive and fulfill your life purpose. And *if you can't feel it, you can't heal it.* This holds true for sinusitis, allergies, or any other chronic dis-ease. Your underlying emotional pain will be mirrored back to you with the ill health of your body and/or your mind. But so, too, will vitality and happiness reflect a condition of radiant health.

Chapter 8

HEALING YOUR SPIRIT

"What profit does a man receive if he gains the whole world only to lose his soul?"

MATTHEW 16:26

COMPONENTS OF OPTIMAL SPIRITUAL HEALTH
Experience of unconditional love/absence of fear
Soul awareness and a personal relationship with God or Spirit
Trust in your intuition and a willingness to change
Gratitude
Creating a sacred space on a regular basis through prayer, meditation, walking in nature, observing a Sabbath day, or other rituals
Sense of purpose
Being present in every moment

The ultimate outcome of healing ourselves holistically is the recognition that we are truly spiritual beings, and the heightened awareness of the transcendent power known as God or Spirit. By making the commitment to become spiritually healthy, we open ourselves to the underlying life force energy to which all religions refer, known in holistic medicine as *unconditional love*. Learning to love yourself in body, mind, and spirit is also the simplest and most effective way to learn to love God. (Most religions teach that all human beings have been created in the image of God.) To heal yourself spiritually means developing a relationship with Spirit in your own life and attuning yourself to Its guidance in all aspects of your daily existence. By doing so, you will begin to experience a profound reduction in your feelings of fear and a greater capacity for loving yourself and others unconditionally. You will also become better able to identify your special talents and gifts and use them to fulfill your life's purpose, *while fully experiencing the power of the present moment.*

In the deepest sense, all *dis-ease* can be seen as a disconnection between ourselves and Spirit. From that perspective, spiritual health encompasses not only a conscious awareness of the Divine but also an intimate connection to ourselves and our families, friends, and communities. Just as mental health encompasses emotional health, spiritual health embraces social health. You cannot have one without the other. This truth is illustrated in the lives of the world's great spiritual teachers, including Moses, Jesus, Mohammed, Krishna, and Buddha, all of whom remained closely connected to their communities throughout the course of their ministry. Despite the apparent differences in their instructions to us, at their core, their messages are actually the same: *Place God first in all that you do, and love your neighbors as you love yourself.* As you reclaim your spiritual health, you fulfill their intention.

ACCESSING SPIRIT

"Every advance in knowledge brings us face to face with the mystery of our own being."

MAX PLANCK, FATHER OF QUANTUM PHYSICS

You may believe that you are incapable of experiencing Spirit in your life, but that is not the case. *Spirit is present in any moment when we feel profoundly alive.* During these special moments, our predominant emotions are exhilaration and joy. The Jesuit priest and scientist Teilhard de Chardin described *joy* as "the most infallible sign of the presence of God." Usually these fleeting moments surprise us: Our perception of reality is suddenly free of our normal judgments and concerns. Time seems to slow as we lose ourselves in *pure awareness*. Examples of these moments include experiencing the birth of your child, time spent with your beloved, being present at the death of someone you love, witnessing a sunset, entering "the zone" while playing sports, and being in the presence of inspirational works of art. Such peak experiences can also occur unexpectedly and spontaneously during the course of your normal routine, sparked by something as innocuous as hearing your favorite song on the radio. For most of us, these moments may seem to be accidental occurrences.

The purpose of this chapter is to help make your encounters with Spirit a more frequent and conscious part of your life. As you learn to master the techniques that follow, recognize that Spirit operates in much the same fashion as subatomic particles: Both can be identified without being directly observed. Most often, and especially at the beginning of your spiritual journey, Spirit will be identified by the traces it leaves behind as it flows through you. With time and attention, each of us can deepen our perception of Spirit in our lives. Among the ways of doing so are *prayer, meditation, gratitude, spiritual practices, reconnecting with nature, and working with spiritual counselors.*

Are We Spiritual Beings?
The Near-Death Experience

Most of us spend our lives deluded by the belief that our traits, habits, and actions are the sum total of who we are. In actuality these characteristic behaviors only constitute our conscious personality, or the sense of self that psychology refers to as the ego. Our ego is the source of our thoughts, judgments, and comparisons, which usually are based on past experience or future concerns. Largely fear-based, the ego diverts our attention from appreciating the reality that exists in the present moment. We live most of our waking hours in this ego state, yet our true self, the *soul* (the individualized expression of Spirit), extends well beyond the limits of comprehension of the human intellect.

Letting go of the ego entails a surrender of mind and body that most of us equate with death. The thought of our death can be overpoweringly frightful. Yet, it is also one of the surest methods for reconnecting with our true spiritual natures. Every experience we have of transcendence and Spirit is also one in which we feel exhilarated and access a dimension of being beyond body and mind. If death is the freeing of our deeper self, or soul, from the physical plane, isn't it possible that it, too, can be an exhilarating experience? Certainly that is the report given by the vast majority of people who have had near-death experiences. These episodes, also known as NDEs, involve people who were considered clinically dead in emergency or operating rooms, or at the scenes of accidents, and were subsequently resuscitated. In almost every case, these people report experiencing profound feelings of peace and unconditional love, as well as a reluctance to leave the spiritual dimension to return to their bodies.

The consistency of the reports of NDEs confirms the observation of many physicians and researchers who have scientifically studied the phenomena of death and dying that the soul remains intact beyond the death of the body. One of the leaders in this field, known as thanatology, is Elisabeth Kübler-Ross, M.D., who pioneered this investigation for most of her professional career. After nearly thirty years of scientific research, she has concluded, "Death does not exist . . . all that dies is a physical shell housing an immortal spirit." She also describes the time that we spend on earth as but a brief part of our total existence, and that *to live well while we are here means to learn to love*—which is an active recognition, engagement, and appreciation of Spirit in ourselves and others. In one of her studies of over two hundred people who had experienced a near-death experience, almost all reported that they went before God and were asked the question: "How have you expanded your ability to give and receive love while you were down there?"

Whether or not you choose to believe the data being gathered in the fields of thanatology and NDEs, there is mounting evidence strongly suggesting the existence of Spirit beyond the realms of mind and body. Choosing to believe this theory can heighten your creativity, enhance your healing capacity, free you to realize your life's purpose, diminish the level of fear in your life, and release the self-imposed limitations of past traumas. By becoming more aware of your soul—that part of yourself that does not die—you will be better able to take risks and pursue the dreams of your life.

Prayer

The most common form of spiritual exercise engaged in by most Americans is prayer. Nearly 90 percent of us pray, and 70 percent of us believe that prayer can lead to physical, emotional, or spiritual healing. Most people who pray have a greater sense of well-being than those who don't, and, when polled, the majority of people who pray say that through prayer they experience a sense of peace, receive answers to life issues, and have even felt divinely inspired or "led by God" to perform some specific action. Interestingly, people who experience a "sense of the Divine" during prayer also score the highest on ratings of general well-being and satisfaction with their lives.

In recent years a great deal of scientific study has focused on the beneficial effects of prayer. Among the studies is one by the National Institute of Mental Health (NIMH) in 1994, which examined nearly three thousand North Carolinians and found that those who attended church weekly had 29 percent less risk of alcoholism than those who attended less frequently. In the same study, the risk of alcoholism decreased by 42 percent among those who prayed and read the Bible regularly. Another NIMH study conducted in the same year found that frequent churchgoers also had lower rates of depression and other mental problems.

An examination of 212 medical studies examining the relationship between religious beliefs and health by Dale Matthews, M.D., associate professor of medicine at Georgetown University, found that 75 percent of the studies showed health benefits for those patients with "religious commitments." Among patients with hypertension, regular prayer reduced blood pressure in 50 percent of all cases.

Among the pioneers in the study of the physiological effects of prayer and meditation is Herbert Benson, M.D., a Harvard cardiologist. In 1968, Benson began studying people who regularly practiced transcendental meditation (TM). The subjects meditated by focusing on a mantra, such as *Om,* that had no apparent meaning to its user. Benson discovered that repetition of the mantra resulted in a lower metabolic rate, slower heart rate, lower blood pressure, and slower breathing. He dubbed this physiological effect the *relaxation response.* Benson then turned his attention to Christians and Jews who prayed instead of meditating, instructing them to repeat religious phrases such as the first line of the Lord's Prayer, "Hail Mary, full of grace," "The Lord is my shepherd," or "Shalom." He found that the phrases all produced the same relaxation response that is triggered by meditation, and that the degree of physiological benefit is determined by the degree of faith on the part of the person praying.

Since 1988, Benson and psychologist Jared Klass have been conducting a series of programs at the Mind/Body Medical Institute at New England Deaconess Hospital, inviting priests, rabbis, and ministers to investigate the spiritual and health implications of prayer. In their studies, a psychological scale developed by Benson and Klass for measuring spirituality is employed. People scoring high in spirituality—defined by Benson as a feeling that "there is more than just you" and as not necessarily religious—score higher in psychological health. They also:

- Were less likely to get sick, and were better able to cope if they did
- Had fewer stress-related symptoms
- Gained the most from meditation training
- Showed the greatest rise on a life-purpose index
- Exhibited the sharpest drop in pain

To begin the practice of prayer, start with any prayer you are comfortable with or recall from your religious training as a child. You can also use a favorite psalm or passage from the Bible or prayer book you find especially meaningful. In addition you can engage in personal prayer, talking to God as if you were speaking to your best friend. State your need or concern and ask for God's help. (It is more effective to pray for the peace that would result from having what you desire, than for the specific things themselves.) Whichever form of prayer you choose, try to establish a regular routine and repeat your prayer morning and night.

Meditation

In the West, meditation has primarily been studied for its mental, emotional, and physiological benefits, while in the East it has primarily been used for thousands of years to still the mind in order to heighten awareness and contact soul and Spirit. During meditation, practitioners enter into a neutral emotional state, becoming a witness to their passing thoughts and feelings as they move into a state of heightened attention that can ultimately result in pure awareness.

As with prayer, there are many ways to meditate. Meditation can be performed while sitting or in a supine position, or while on the move—walking, jogging, and even during sports. What all forms of meditation have in common is a focusing on the breath and an emptying of the mind of thought. With regular practice, meditators typically report increased feelings of calm and peace, improved mental functioning and enhanced powers of concentration, and a deeper connection to Spirit, which is often perceived as a quiet, inner voice guiding them in their actions. Other reported benefits include increased equanimity toward, and detachment from, life events; increased energy and joy; feelings of bliss and ecstasy; and increased dream recall.

Ideally it is best to learn meditation under the guidance of a qualified instructor, but a variety of books and audiotapes are also available on the subject. The simplest method of meditation is to sit in a quiet place, resting comfortably in a chair, with your spine erect and your feet flat on the floor. Close your eyes and begin focusing on your breathing, keeping your awareness on each inhalation and exhalation. To improve your concentration, you may wish to silently repeat the word *in* as you inhale, and *out* as you exhale. Or you can repeat a word or mantra, such as *love, peace, God, Om,* or *Hu* (the latter two are names for the Divine). Allow your thoughts to come and go, without lingering on them, as if your awareness is a running stream and your thoughts are simply leaves floating by. At first it may seem as if you are deluged with thoughts. Each time you find yourself distracted, simply bring your attention back to your breathing. Eventually you may notice longer periods of silence between each thought. It may take months to quiet your mind to this extent, but with consistent practice your meditation *will* become deeper and easier. Try to sit for at least ten minutes once or twice a day, gradually working up to two half-hour sessions per day. It's important to keep your practice regular and consistent, but don't force things. If you find yourself too distracted or pressed for time, end your session until the next time, instead of sitting restlessly.

Walking meditation is another form of meditation, which in recent years has been popularized by the Buddhist monk Thich Nhat Hanh. This form of meditation is often suited for active people who find it difficult to sit still. The goal is to focus your attention in the present by focusing on each step you take in tandem with your breathing. To enhance your experience, you can mentally repeat: *With each step I take I am fully present to my surroundings.* Over time, as you practice this form of meditation, don't be surprised if you find it becomes more difficult to hurry. The more you focus on the present, the less consequence time has, as you discover how profound even a simple act such as walking can be.

Gratitude

Most religious traditions prescribe specific prayers or grace before meals as a way of thanking God for our food and sustenance. As with other spiritual practices, there is something to be gained from these rituals, or they wouldn't have survived for thousands of years. A sense of gratitude for all the other areas of our lives can elicit similar life-enhancing benefits.

Gratitude has been called the Great Attitude. Although most of us tend to take our lives for granted, they are in fact a gift, and every day that we are alive, each of us receives many blessings. Even times of pain and adversity, such as suffering with chronic sinusitis, can be seen as opportunities for growth for which we can be grateful. By committing ourselves to becoming more aware of our blessings, we strengthen our connection with Spirit and are able to better recognize the wisdom and intelligence that underlies all of creation.

Once we allow ourselves to appreciate the lessons presented during times of struggle or life crises, the brunt of the pain subsides and a state of inner peace follows. This is especially true of most chronic diseases, which can be seen as external reflections of inner (emotional and/or spiritual) pain. Typically, when people choose to consciously focus on the positives in their lives and express gratitude for them, more positive things start to happen. For instance, while you're learning to live with your sinusitis, suppose you spent time each day focusing on the blessings and the many pleasures your body has provided you with in the past along with the multitude of basic functions for which it still serves you well. These include the ability to breathe, to enjoy lovemaking, eating, drinking, digesting, and eliminating. You may not have the energy to exercise as you once did, but you can still relish the peacefulness of a quiet walk in nature. You've still retained the capacity to choose your beliefs and attitudes, as well as to experience, express, and accept all of your feelings. In addition, this physical discomfort can serve as a powerful catalyst for becoming better acquainted with your soul and Spirit. You may have never recognized the spiritual being that you truly are or your purpose for being here, had you not been blessed with sinusitis. This may sound unreasonable or even irrational to you, but it was certainly helpful to me in curing my own sinusitis. For many years I suffered and felt as if I was cursed. I angrily asked of God, "Why me? What have I done to deserve this misery?" Yet now I can clearly see how this physical pain has so enriched my life. It's taught me how to give and receive love—to nurture my body, home and work environments, mind, emotional body, intimate relationships, and my soul. This is the essence of the work I came here to do and it has become my full-time job. I call it training to thrive, and at 53, I'm healthier and more fit physically, environmentally, mentally, emotionally, spiritually, and socially than I've ever been. Who knows what my life would've been like had I not been blessed with sinusitis? I am most grateful.

Gratitude can produce powerful feelings of joy and self-acceptance, and is an attitude that anyone can choose to have, just as you can choose to see the glass half full or half empty. By focusing on what you do have, instead of what you lack, you feel a sense of abundance that makes your problems seem much less acute, and you are better able to let go of negative thoughts and attitudes. This usually isn't easy to do, especially if you are feeling a great deal of fear or anger. But if you make the effort to release these painful emotions and *choose the attitude of gratitude,* even for a moment, wonderful things can happen.

Like any habit, that of recognizing and acknowledging the gifts in your life requires practice. One simple way to begin feeling grateful is the following visualization taught by Rabbi Mordecai Twerski, the spiritual leader of Denver's Hasidic community. As soon as you wake up each morning, before you get out of bed, close your eyes and picture a person, scene, or situation that made you happy to be alive and for which you are still grateful. You never would have had that experience if you weren't alive, and by allowing yourself to reexperience it, you open yourself up to the awareness that something equally wonderful can happen today. Create the habit of practicing this visualization each morning upon awakening and you will soon instill in yourself a new attitude of anticipation and appreciation for the day ahead.

Another way to cultivate feelings of gratitude is by making a *gratitude list.* This exercise is best performed before going to bed, as a way to detach from any concerns or problems you may have in order to appreciate the gifts and lessons that came your way during the day. Some people prefer to write out their list; others simply close their eyes and mentally review their day, making themselves aware of all the things that happened for which they feel grateful. Either way works well. Complete the exercise by praying silently, giving thanks for all that you experienced and learned that day.

By making gratitude a regular part of your daily experience, you set the stage for living more deeply connected to Spirit. In the process, your life will be transformed into an increasingly joyous adventure.

Intuition

As you progress in your healing journey, eventually you will find yourself being guided by your intuition, which is often experienced as an "inner nudge" or a "still, quiet voice" speaking from within. If you are not already aware of your intuitive messages, most likely it is because your intuition is having a tough time competing for your attention. Most of the inner messages you hear come from your ego and tend to be loud, self-centered, and fear-based. Intuitive messages, by contrast, come from the heart and are usually more subtle, compassionate, energizing, and enlivening.

In order to develop your sense of intuition, you will need to slow down, eliminate distractions, and do a lot less talking. The methods provided in this chapter can help you to do so. Slow, relaxing walks are another helpful way to make contact with this inner guidance. The next step is learning to recognize when your intuition is truly speaking to you and when it is not. Learning to discern the difference requires practice. One useful method for determining whether the "voice" you hear is indeed your intuition is to notice how it feels. Often intuitive messages occur accompanied by feelings of excitement or an unequivocal sense that acting upon them is "the right thing to do." People who haven't learned to trust their intuition often experience doubts or fears immediately following such feelings. "How can

I be sure this is true?" "What if I'm wrong?" These and similar questions can quickly quash your inner guidance if you haven't learned to trust it.

To help you know if the messages you receive are in your best interest, experiment with the following exercise. Out loud, tell yourself something that you know to be true. As you do so, notice how you feel. Now state aloud something you know to be false. Again notice how you feel. Usually people practicing this exercise experience feelings of discomfort, confusion, even pain, in their bodies when they make the false statement, whereas they feel in alignment with the statement that is true. (Often the sensations occur in the area of the solar plexus, with false statements provoking queasy feelings or tension.)

Allowing yourself to be guided by your intuition is ultimately an act of faith. At first, learning to trust and act on the intuitive messages you receive will involve risk. The more trust you bring to your practice, however, the easier it will be to take action. Realize, too, that sometimes the results of following your intuition may be painful. Such times are not necessarily mistakes. They can be seen as lessons teaching you how to listen more effectively. Or they may be necessary to facilitate your growth and help you to better understand the higher purpose toward which Spirit is guiding you.

Spiritual Counselors

Due to the many uncertainties that can be part of the spiritual journey, you may consider working with a spiritual counselor, especially if you haven't been in the habit of listening to your intuition or need help in "tuning in" to Spirit. Just as you would visit a doctor to heal your physical body, or a psychotherapist to heal mental and emotional issues, spiritual counselors can help connect you to your spiritual core. The most common resources for spiritual counseling are priests, rabbis, ministers, and other clergy. Spiritual psychotherapists, medical intuitives, clairvoyants, and spiritual healers or shamans can also be of assistance. What these healers have in common is an ability to see beyond the boundaries of the five senses. Their services may include helping you to identify your life purpose, pointing out opportunities for your spiritual growth, or scanning your body's bioenergy field to diagnose the underlying cause of a particular health condition. Their primary value, however, lies in the assistance they can provide in helping you appreciate the meaning and lessons of your daily life.

Because of the lack of certification in these areas, to find a spiritual counselor, you may need to rely on references from people you trust, experience some trial and error, and call upon your own intuition. Keep an open mind and see how you respond to the information provided. Some of these counselors are truly gifted and can provide you with information that can be a catalyst for transforming your life.

Spiritual Practices

Most of us have some sort of spiritual orientation, even if it is no more than rituals we were taught in childhood. Yet, we often fail to realize how much some of these practices can contribute to our health. The ritual observance of Sabbath, for instance, can be an enormously healing experience as it restores the sacred rhythm between work and rest. We're so busy *doing* in our society that we've forgotten how to just *be* and appreciate the delight of simply being alive. The Sabbath day is also a particularly good time to practice gratitude as you contemplate the blessings you share with those you love. Studies also reveal that those who regularly observe a weekly holy day tend to score higher in areas of optimism, stress management, and general well-being.

Fasting is another spiritual practice that is also healing. Not only can fasting have a cleansing effect on the body, eliminating toxins while giving the organs of digestion and assimilation a rest, it can also elicit a heightened feeling of spirituality and result in the healing of old emotional wounds. In his book *Live Better Longer,* Joseph Dispenza, director of the Parcells Center in Santa Fe, New Mexico, points out that fasting can purge the emotional body of old, toxic feelings, facilitate the release of psychological patterns that no longer work for you, and "open your mind and heart to new emotional, psychological, and spiritual sustenance." (The Parcells Center is based on the work of Hazel Parcells, Ph.D., a scientist and naturopathic physician who, at 41, cured herself of terminal tuberculosis using fasts and other natural methods. She went on to live a life of vibrant, robust health until she died peacefully in her sleep at age 106.)

If you are new to fasting, try a 24-hour fast, selecting a day when work and other responsibilities are limited and you won't be too active. Plan for some quiet time alone, and during the final two hours of the fast, drink six to eight glasses of water to help cleanse your body of toxins.

Gabriel Cousens, M.D., director of the Tree of Life Rejuvenation Center in Patagonia, Arizona, has had great success in treating a variety of diseases, including arthritis, diabetes, alcoholism, and asthma, with fasting and meditation.

The potential that spiritual practices have to heal is illustrated in the case of my friend and colleague Dr. Bob Anderson's patient, a 64-year-old woman named Lois, who had undergone the surgical removal of a very large, aggressive ovarian cancer. The procedure left her with a colostomy, and part of the original tumor was not removable, leaving hundreds of small metastases throughout her abdominal cavity. On Dr. Anderson's insistence, Lois agreed to consult with an oncologist, only to promptly reject his recommendation of chemotherapy, despite the fact that remnants of her tumor remained in her pelvis and abdomen. She was convinced that her condition would be cured by her own body with God's help, and returned to Dr. Anderson for aid in getting well. Although she undertook many initiatives, central to her program was her faith in the power of prayer and God. Each day she meditated for up to an hour and prayed numerous times.

Four months later Lois was finally able to persuade her surgeon to remove the colostomy to restore her internal bowel function. During the course of a long and tedious surgery, hundreds of small, metastasized tumors appeared as before. Seven of them were biopsied. Three days later the pathology report showed that their cancerous characteristics were gone. Lois fully recovered and resumed an active life focused around the activities she enjoyed and her continued prayers to God. Two years later, an operation to repair an abdominal hernia revealed that her abdomen and pelvis were completely normal, with no residual cancer anywhere. Although he has no way of proving it, Dr. Anderson remains convinced that Lois's daily prayers and meditations were somehow central to her recovery.

Finding Spirit in Nature

Nowhere is the creative power of Spirit more visible than in nature. It is there that we most directly experience life's four elemental forms of energy: earth, water, fire, and air. Earth is matter in its deepest form; water represents the receptive yielding principle; fire is the transformational energy that causes matter to change form; and air is the resultant blend of these other three elements into a subtler vibration of life-force energy. In our bodies, earth is cellular matter, water is blood and circulation, fire is metabolism and energy production, and air is oxygen, the nutrient most essential for our sustenance. By regularly exposing yourself to nature's four elements—ideally on a daily basis—you will expand your awareness of how each of them is uniquely embodied within you. Here are ways for you to do so.

Earth   Spend as much time as possible outdoors in close contact with the earth. Walking is a wonderful way to do this, as are outdoor sports, bike rides in a park, and gardening. When you can, also visit the beach, woods, and mountains, and take time to notice the beauty surrounding you. The more time you spend immersed in nature, the more aware you will become of life's natural rhythms and the ways the earth retains and radiates energy.

Most of us, however, live in urban settings and are relatively detached from the natural world. Making the effort to spend time in nature can go a long way toward restoring more balance in your life while deepening your connection with Spirit at the same time.

Water   One of the most visible forms of Spirit in nature is the flow of water as it follows the contours of the earth. Water is a receptive form of energy and is affected by the forces acting on it. Rivers flow, for example, because of the gravitational pull caused by the gradient of the landscape. The action of water tumbling over rocks also releases a more subtle energy in the form of negative ions, which can contribute to feelings of well-being. Swimming in the ocean, lakes, or rivers provides invaluable exposure to this special form of energy. Soaking in a mineral hot spring can also provide therapeutic benefits for a variety of ailments, as well as being one of life's great pleasures.

A healthy routine that anyone can adopt is bathing in warm water at least once a day. For added benefit, practice conscious breathing while you enjoy a soak in the tub. This is a very effective way to connect with your body's bioenergy field and can help heal mental and emotional upset.

Fire   Throughout the Bible and other sacred scriptures, the dominant symbols of the divine essence in human beings is fire and light, such as the tale of Moses speaking to God in the burning bush, or the transfiguration of Jesus on the mountaintop before his closest apostles. Candlelight is also common as a tool for spiritual focus in most religions. Anyone who has experienced the pleasures of an open campfire can attest to the healing properties of fire. According to Leonard Orr, the founder of Rebirthing, spending time before an open fire, including a fireplace, cleanses the bioenergy field of negative energies and can be a powerful aid in curing physical disease. Orr recommends spending a few hours each day before fire for people who want to experience such benefits.

Fire is also an important component of the vision quests employed by Native Americans as a means of connecting to Spirit and discerning their life purpose. The ultimate source of fire energy is the sun, which provides healing and creative energy that directly or indirectly gives life to all living organisms. Regular exposure to sunlight has been linked to a variety of mental and emotional benefits, while depression, anxiety, and other mental dis-ease can occur when we are deprived of the sun's healing rays. Time spent daily in the sun is a very healthy practice, as long as appropriate precautions are taken, including sunscreen, hats, and long sleeves and pants when needed.

Air Of the four elements, air is perhaps the closest expression of Spirit, so much so that the ancient Greeks equated Spirit (*pneuma*) with the wind. The most potent method of imbuing yourself with the life-force energy of air is through meditation and other forms of conscious breathing. A daily practice of these methods can significantly energize you, open you up to new levels of creativity and productivity, and make you more aware of Spirit's guidance and power flowing through you.

SOCIAL HEALTH

COMPONENTS OF OPTIMAL SOCIAL HEALTH
Intimacy with a spouse, partner, relative, or close friend
Commitment to relationship
Forgiveness
Sense of belonging to a support group or community
Touch and/or physical intimacy on a daily basis
Selflessness and altruism

Our relationship with others is the crucible that most determines how spiritually healthy we are. Optimal *social health* consists of a strong positive connection to others in community and family, and intimacy with one or more people. It is often much easier to feel our connection with Spirit during moments of solitude than it is to express that connection through our interactions with others. At the same time our relationships offer us the greatest opportunities for spiritual growth and for learning how to receive and impart unconditional love. *True spiritual health is a balance between the autonomy of the self and intimacy with others.*

The importance of social relationships with respect to health is documented in a growing number of studies demonstrating the benefits of the diversity and depth of connection to community, family, and spouse. Lack of healthy social relationships is a common denominator among patients with heart disease, particularly when accompanied by feelings of hostility and a sense of isolation. Conversely, the longevity of terminal cancer patients with long-term survival rates has been attributed to a relatively high degree of social involvement. One of the most convincing studies highlighting the importance of community showed that Hispanics, despite poverty, lack of health insurance, and poor access to medical care, are surprisingly less likely than whites to die of major chronic diseases, including all forms of cancer, heart disease, and respiratory ailments. Further, with the exception of diabetes, liver disease, and homicide, their overall health outlook is significantly better than for whites. Some health experts, including former Surgeon General Coello Novello, the first Latina to serve in that post, postulate that the reason for this stems from Hispanic culture, which promotes strong family values and frowns on health risks such as drinking and smoking. Based on a growing number of relationship studies, researchers have concluded that *social isolation is statistically just as dangerous as smoking, high blood pressure, high cholesterol, obesity, or lack of exercise.*

The primary opportunities available to each of us for improving our social health include forgiveness, friendships, selfless acts and altruism, support groups, and especially marriage, committed relationships, and parenting.

Forgiveness

Intimate relationships and unconditional love cannot exist without forgiveness. How often do you blame yourself for your past actions and mistakes? How often do you blame others for your own problems, stress, or slights (both real and imagined) against you? Forgiveness cancels the demands that you or others *should* have done things differently. Hanging on to these demands changes nothing but keeps us under stress. Refusing to forgive yourself or others keeps you locked into limiting patterns from your past, unable to mobilize the creative power in your life here and now.

The next time you find yourself blaming others, physically point your index finger at them or their images and take a look at where the other three fingers of your hand are pointed. Right back at you! Forgiveness, therefore, begins with accepting responsibility for the role you play in shaping your life's experiences. Only after you begin to forgive yourself can you truly forgive others.

A key first step in your journey of forgiveness is the recognition that you are always doing the best you can at any given moment, in accordance with your awareness at the time. This is true of everyone else as well. All of us make mistakes, and all of us ideally learn from them. You may even choose to believe that there are no mistakes, only lessons. In that moment your action or behavior was based on past experience, environment, and heredity. You can, however, consciously choose to be different in the future. To continue to blame yourself or someone else for something that occurred in the past is energy depleting and keeps you from moving forward with your life.

Forgiving yourself may be your greatest challenge. No doubt there are a number of things in your past that you regret or for which you feel shame. But wouldn't it be healthier to look at what you can learn from your mistake or painful lesson so that it's not repeated; forgive yourself unconditionally for not knowing more or not performing well enough; and be grateful for this opportunity to learn to do better or change your behavior? A tennis player who misses a shot he thinks he should have made will lose his confidence and ultimately his match if he doesn't quickly recognize what he did wrong, forgive himself, and move on to play the next point. Similarly we lose the ability to focus and to do as well as we know we are capable of in the present if we do not forgive ourselves and let go of the past.

The more you are able to do this for yourself, the better you will be able to forgive others. *Remember that you are forgiving the actor, not the action.* You are not condoning cruelty, insensitivity, or incompetence; you are forgiving the offending person. By doing so, you are freeing yourself to move out of the past into the healing present. Anger is the problem, forgiveness is the solution.

Bear in mind that the people you decide to forgive may not choose to accept your forgiveness. Although their refusal to do so can be hurtful, their choice should be respected. What matters is that you are taking the step to heal the relationship. The act of forgiveness takes place within your own psyche, and the person you are forgiving may therefore be totally unaware of your action. Or you may be forgiving someone who is deceased. Be realistic and don't set your sights too high: Begin with someone who has been critical of you or guilty of another relatively minor offense. Forgiving others does not necessarily mean that your relationship with them will change, but forgiving them will enable you to feel a greater sense of wholeness. Your relationship with the people you forgive may remain the same on the surface, but it doesn't mean that healing hasn't taken place. You will know it when you feel it.

Friendship

A 1997 study conducted at Carnegie Mellon University in Pittsburgh found that people with a greater diversity of relationships were less likely to get colds. Those with six or more social ties (family, friends, coworkers, neighbors, etc.) were four times *less* susceptible to colds than those with one to three types of relationships. Researchers found that it was not the number of people in the social network that was the important factor, but the diversity. To varying degrees, most of these types of relationships can be called *friendships.*

As children and teenagers, most of us had a number of friends with whom we enjoyed sharing the day's adventures. Our friends helped us meet such challenges as each new year at school, sports, puberty, dating, family problems, and the existential concerns through which all of us passed during our journey into adulthood. Between kindergarten and college, sustaining friendships was made easier by the fact that our friends provided us with a sense of belonging, a feeling of "being in this together," and offered us a forum in which to mutually discuss the problems and issues we faced at the time. Because of such friendships, many people regard the times they spent in high school and college as the happiest days of their lives. Once past college, as they have entered the workforce, got married, and juggled the responsibilities of their careers and families, a large segment of people in our society have lost track of their friends from the past and have not replaced them with new friends.

While most adults enjoy the company of neighbors, coworkers, and other acquaintances, by the time we reach our thirties, studies reveal, those of us who still have a best friend in whom we can confide are exceptionally rare. This is particularly true of men, who, because of this lack of a confidant, experience feelings of isolation and absence of support, no matter how fulfilled they may otherwise be in their personal lives and careers.

If you find yourself in need of a good friend, realize that it's never too late to rekindle old friendships or to make new ones. All that is required is a willingness to take risks and make the effort. Having a close friend you can talk to from your heart can provide many additional blessings in your life and deepen your connection with Spirit.

Selfless Acts and Altruism

Remember a time when you stopped to spontaneously help someone, either a friend or total stranger? Such selfless acts of giving go to the essence of Spirit, which is always with us supporting our lives while asking for nothing in return. Sharing with others your time, help, and special gifts and talents in ways that benefit them provides you with perhaps the most powerful means of engaging and expressing Spirit and enhancing social health. The opportunities for sharing are abundant and may include donating clothes or money to worthy charities, volunteering time at a homeless shelter, soup kitchen, or afterschool tutoring program, or simply setting aside our own tasks and concerns to address the needs of our spouses or children. (There is a great deal of truth in the adage "Charity begins at home.") Another form of sharing that is regaining popularity is *tithing*. Dating back to biblical times, tithing is the practice of donating a certain percentage (usually 5 to 10 percent) of one's yearly income to charity. Interestingly, many people who adopt the practice of tithing also find that their incomes actually begin to increase, although that should not be your motivation for doing so. However you choose to perform selfless acts, remember that the truest form of giving is one that does not call attention to the giver. As Jesus instructed in the Gospel of Matthew, "When you give to the needy, do not announce it with trumpets." The purpose of sharing is *to share,* not to acquire praise or honors. Sharing selflessly will deepen your awareness of how abundantly Spirit is giving to you.

The late Hans Selye, a pioneer in modern stress research, thought that by helping people you earn their gratitude and affection and that the warmth that results protects against stress. Today, Selye's belief is borne out by mounting evidence that selfless acts not only feel good but are healthy. Epidemiologist James House and his colleagues at the University of Michigan's Survey Research Center studied more than 2,700 men in Tecumseh, Michigan, for almost fourteen years to see how social relationships affected mortality rates. Those who did regular volunteer work had death rates two and one half times lower than those who didn't. It may well be that the highest form of selfishness is selflessness. When we freely choose to help others, we seem to get as much, or more, than what we give.

The closer our contact with those we help, the greater the benefits seem to be. Most of us need to feel that we matter to someone, a need that volunteer work can fulfill. There are a growing number of people requiring help in our society, including the homeless, the elderly, the hungry, runaways, orphans, and the illiterate, and there are many ways to help them. Choose to do so in the way that most compels you, but recognize that altruism works best when it comes from the heart and is not calculated as a means to receive something in return.

Support Groups

As a society we are plagued by social ills, most notably divorce rates that top 50 percent, a general sentiment of feeling overworked, dual-career marriages, an increasing number of single-parent families, and a generation of children more adrift and alone than any that has preceded them. At the same time a movement is afoot in America toward a greater sense of community in response to the silent epidemic of isolation that affects so many of us; there has been a significant increase in support groups for those sharing common values, experiences, and goals. Support groups for couples, divorcées, single parents, men, women, people with an illness in common (especially cancer), and a large number of people recovering from alcohol and drug addiction—and other addictions—are gathering all over the country. Many of them are affiliated with a church or synagogue, with the added purpose of enhancing spiritual growth. They meet regularly—every week, every other week, or every month—and the participants by and large report that they benefit from the social connection they find there. If you would like to participate in such a group, most likely you can find them in your local Yellow Pages, or you can contact organizations such as your local United Way, Catholic Charities, or AA group. Many communities also have support groups devoted to specific diseases. Such groups can also be found on the Internet.

Recent research also verifies that support groups can play an important role in helping people with chronic disease. David Spiegel, M.D., conducted a study at Stanford University School of Medicine on women with metastatic breast cancer. All the women received chemotherapy or radiation therapy. Half of them were in a support group that met weekly for one year. These women lived twice as long as those who were not in a support group, and three of them were still alive ten years later.

Committed Relationships and Marriage

Healthy committed relationships promote physical, emotional, and especially spiritual well-being through the experience of unconditional love. The model for all committed relationships is marriage, usually the most challenging as well as most rewarding of all interpersonal relationships. It is potentially our most powerful spiritual practice. If humanity's fundamental moral principle is to "love thy neighbor as thyself," its practice begins not with the person living next door but with the neighbor with whom we share our bed.

Regardless of who your partner may be or how long you have been involved with him or her, the key to all committed relationships is *intimacy.* Think of intimacy as *into-me-see.* As you develop the skills for seeing into, and learning to appreciate, yourself, you have the opportunity to also "see into" your partner and to allow your partner to see into you. Once a commitment is made, the relationship becomes greater than the sum of its parts, allowing both partners to flourish and realize their full potential as human beings. The transformation that can occur in marriage and other committed relationships is primarily a result of letting go of judgment. As you do so, you will realize that in giving more to the relationship you are ultimately giving to yourself. Studies have shown that you might otherwise be contributing to making yourself and your partner sick. Marital conflict lowers immune function, especially in women, according to researchers at Ohio State University.

Hallmarks of a healthy committed relationship include having a shared vision, attentive listening to each other, the freedom to make requests so that both partners can better ensure that their needs are met, and regular intervals of fun and recreation together. Discussion of these practices follows. If you are interested in making a deeper commitment to your relationship, you might also consider working with a good marriage counselor or other relationship teacher.

Shared vision   A vision that you share with your partner is a way of defining your mutual goals and focusing your energy on their attainment. Lack of a vision can cause your relationship to lose direction or become stagnant. One simple but effective way to create a shared vision with your spouse or partner is to take time to individually list your relationship goals (keep them positive, short, descriptive, specific), prioritizing them in numerical order. Then begin combining lists, starting with the goals that have the highest value and alternating between the two lists to form a composite vision that you and your partner are both comfortable with. The resulting *mutual relationship vision* can help keep you and your partner working together toward your common goals, while reducing conflict and enhancing your relationship.

Attentive listening   Most of us are poor listeners. We *hear* what is being said, but we don't always *listen* to it. This is because hearing can be unconscious while listening requires conscious effort. Since communication is the foundation of any relationship, and listening is a critical aspect of effective communication, it is important to get in the habit of consciously paying attention to what your partner tells you *without responding immediately.* This type of listening can be practiced as a "listening exercise." Schedule an uninterrupted 40-minute block of time in which both you and your partner speak for 20 minutes while the other person listens *without responding.* Talk only about yourself and how you're feeling, without blaming or talking about your relationship issues. There is no discussion following the exercise.

Attentive listening makes it possible for both partners to be able to talk freely and express thoughts and feelings without worrying about judgment or criticism. Focusing on what your partner is saying requires you to empty your mind of your own thoughts and concerns as you listen, thereby minimizing negative reactions. This exercise allows for a balance between intimacy and autonomy, a critical component of healthy relationships. Cultivating the habit of attentive listening will help you and your partner create a safe environment for expressing your feelings, allowing you to be more vulnerable and open with each other, which is extremely valuable for building trust, understanding, and deeper, even exhilarating, feelings of intimacy.

Requests By committing to another person, you enter into a relationship in which you have promised to give and receive love. But since each of us is different, what feels like love to one person may not even be noticed by another. Most of us attempt to love our partners in ways that feel like love to *us* and are surprised when they do not react as we would. A good method for eliminating this problem is simply to tell each other what feels good to you and what you want.

It can be quite a revelation when someone you thought you knew well tells you what they really *need* from you. We often expect our partners to be able to read our minds, but we really can't know what each other wants unless we are told. Refrain from general statements such as "Love me" or "Be nice to me." Making specific requests like "I would like you to buy me flowers once a week" or "I would like you to cook dinner once a week" will significantly improve the likelihood that you will get what you need. When you do, be sure to thank your partner for complying with your request. This is extremely important, since your request is usually not an easy or natural thing for your partner to do. Otherwise you probably wouldn't have had to ask for it in the first place.

Having fun together Life's daily pressures and responsibilities make it difficult to remember to have fun. For many couples, the glue that reinforces their relationship is the memory of the enjoyment they shared during their courtship and early years together. Setting aside time that you and your partner can spend in recreation together is an important way to *re-create* the joy and spontaneity that first brought you together. To rekindle some of that excitement and minimize the risk of boring routines, it helps to schedule fun activities together on a regular basis. Plan to spend at least half a day each week together away from home, taking turns each time to choose your activity. Getting out of the house, alone together, can help you focus attention on each other. Although this is more difficult to do if you have young children, it is still possible to plan an exciting evening at home after they go to bed. Choose something neither of you has tried before to add another dimension of adventure to your play, and if you can manage it, plan several weekends per year out of town. This can be especially rewarding if a real vacation isn't feasible. Having fun regularly with the person you love is refreshing and invigorating and can help ensure that your relationship remains healthy and fulfilling.

Sex

Of all the major world religions, the Judeo-Christian tradition is the only one that does not commonly recognize the potential that sex has as a pathway to Spirit. Other religions, including Hinduism, Buddhism, Islam, and Taoism, as well as the spiritual traditions of Africa and the Amerindians, freely acknowledge that sex, properly entered into, can be a powerful spiritual experience capable of transforming consciousness and enhancing physical and emotional health. In the West, perhaps the most well-known of these teachings on sex is *tantra*. This is an ancient system of sexual and sensual techniques for consciously controlling the mind, increasing life-force energy, and tapping into Spirit. Tantra's erotic practices include specific positions, breath, and visualization to heighten sexual energy and move it upward along the spine in order to create rapturous waves of blissful energy that can ultimately lead to enlightenment. Many mystic writings, such as the verse of the Sufi poet–saint Rumi, also refer to the Divine using the language of sex and romantic love, often equating God with the Beloved while yearning to experience union with the Absolute.

To experience sex from this exalted perspective requires expanding your focus beyond physical gratification and genital orgasm into an experience of yourself and your spouse or lover as expressions of Spirit-in-the-flesh. Adopting this attitude leaves you extremely vulnerable and simultaneously in touch with your own divine power. Lovemaking in this state is free of the machinations of ego and proceeds slowly, gently, and consciously, ensuring that the needs of both partners are always met before moving on to the next cycle of pleasure and awareness. Couples who master this approach are able to remain in a state of heightened excitation for several hours, prolong and intensify orgasm, and experience total body orgasms. Among the experiences they report are a continuous flow of energy throughout their bodies, a joined climax of body and soul, the sensation of being united with the cosmos, and afterward being refreshed and revitalized. The primary goal of "spiritual sex" isn't prolonged orgasm, however, but an experience of being more deeply connected with the person you love, and through that connectedness, an awareness of your integral role within the whole of creation. Not everyone will feel the need to master, or even explore, a tantric approach to sex, yet all of us can benefit from more conscious lovemaking. Of all the spiritual practices, it is certainly the most pleasurable. (To learn more about the tantric approach to sex, see *The Art of Sexual Ecstasy* by Margo Anand.)

Parenting

Parenting is easily one of life's most enriching experiences, and at the same time one of our most challenging jobs. Through their children, parents have the opportunity to reconnect with play, to feel more in touch with their own "inner child," to experience selflessness, and to learn how to love unconditionally. Those of us who are parents are also provided with a wonderful forum for practicing forgiveness, trust, acceptance of ourselves and others, self-awareness, and, most of all, patience (as any parent of a teenager well knows). Perhaps the greatest human expression of love is that of parents for their children.

Unfortunately, in our society parenting isn't always consciously approached. If you are already a parent, however, it is not too late to meet your parental obligations more consciously than you may currently be doing. One useful guideline is to regularly ask yourself: *Will this (action, response, activity, demand) of mine help my child's self-esteem?* The same principle holds true in parenting as it does in marriage: *To love another is to help that person better love him- or herself.* This commitment not only will affect your child's happiness in the present but will significantly impact his or her future health. In the landmark Harvard Mastery of Stress Study, college students rated their parents on their level of parental caring. Thirty-five years later, 87 percent of those who rated both parents low on parental love suffered from a chronic illness, whereas only 25 percent of those who rated both parents high in caring had a disease.

In the field of family therapy, the family is usually seen as a "system." This view holds that if a family member's behavior is harmful to himself or others, the problem and the solution lie not only within the individual but within the entire family system. This perspective encourages parents to examine their roles and the responsibility they share with their child for his or her problem. Often a child's crisis serves as a mirror reflecting an imbalance in his or her individual system as well as in the family system as a whole. One of the significant advantages of family therapy is that change often occurs more rapidly than in individual psychotherapy. In much the same way that holistic medicine treats the entire person, not simply physical symptoms, the family systems approach recognizes the need for family therapy when any family member is suffering. If this is a situation that applies to your family, family counseling is strongly recommended. The family systems approach is practiced predominantly by social workers.

Good parenting requires both *time and consistency* in order to impart to your children the values you would like to instill in them. Putting in time as a parent includes being with them on a regular basis and making an effort to get to know them better. What are their talents? What do they enjoy doing? What are they thinking about and how do they feel? Learning the answers to such questions can pay big dividends for both you and your children. In fostering their growth as individuals, it is essential to give them greater power and responsibility by allowing them to make some of their own decisions. By doing so, you will also help them gain confidence and trust, both in themselves and in you.

Other helpful ways to spend time as a family are to worship together each week at church or synagogue and to designate a regularly scheduled time during the weekend for a fun activity. Take turns allowing each member to choose the activity for the day. The value of such play cannot be overemphasized. Having fun together as a family strengthens the bonds of love between each family member and defuses whatever stress or other problems may have built up during the week. Even if you cannot be with your children daily (due to being away on business or divorce, for instance), spending consistent time with them on a regular basis will help them experience the world and live their lives with the security, confidence, and caring that comes from their knowing that you love them. Despite all of its inherent struggles and perils, parenting is first and foremost an incredible gift. Appreciating that gift by regularly interacting with your children is one of the most potent means for creating community and fostering both spiritual and social healing that you will ever have.

SUMMARY

Your spiritual well-being is ultimately the most important aspect of your ability to care for yourself. It is also the dimension of holistic medicine that is most often neglected in our society. Becoming spiritually healthy is a process of *diminishing fear and increasing love while developing an awareness of soul and Spirit and allowing it to guide you to a deeper connection to other human beings.*

This infinite source of compassionate and forgiving transcendent power is the essence of all life on earth and is the spark of life-force energy within each of us. The most direct path to becoming spiritually healthy is learning to love yourself. As you do, you will appreciate the greater meaning and purpose of your life, experience gratitude for your many blessings, and become highly attuned to and trusting of your intuition. As you move beyond the confining restraints of your ego, you will become a more loving friend, spouse or committed partner, parent, and member of your community. In short, you will achieve the goal of holistic medicine—*to become whole.*

Chapter 9

SINUS SURVIVAL SUCCESS STORIES

After twelve years of working with individuals, teaching seminars and workshops, and receiving thousands of phone calls and letters from grateful readers of the book, I'm very pleased to present the following stories. This new chapter of *Sinus Survival* will enable you to read about people whose sinus disease was ruining their lives. You'll learn how their commitment to the Sinus Survival Program instilled hope, restored their energy and vitality, and eventually cured their chronic sinusitis. Although I've worked with each one of these people personally, the testimonials at the beginning of this book (all but one) come from readers of earlier editions whom I've never met.

Whenever I rate symptoms with a numeric value, they range from 1 (worst/incapacitating) to 10 (best/normal).

Dee G. is a 33-year-old Denver real estate appraiser, married with two daughters, ages 6 and 4. She'd been perfectly healthy until four years prior to coming to see me in 1994. In 1990 she developed hay fever for the first time and has had to varying degrees what seemed like one continuous sinus infection since the first one four and a half years earlier. This situation occurred in spite of undergoing one sinus surgery in 1992 and taking approximately 35 two-week courses of antibiotics during the four-year span. She had compiled a list of thirty different antibiotics that she stated were "completely ineffective." The frequency of the antibiotics and duration and intensity of the infections increased dramatically during the latter two years (following the surgery). She had a multitude of diagnostic tests during this period—CAT scans, EKG's, allergy skin tests, and blood tests. "I continued this way for the next two years, going from doctor to doctor, specialist to specialist, and even trying nonconventional treatments, where available." During the year prior to beginning the Program, she had been seeing a physician at Denver's National Jewish Medical and Research Center, an internationally recognized hospital for treatment of respiratory disease.

Her condition was nearly incapacitating as she rated her energy level and overall health as a 3. "I was physically unable to get off of the couch and mentally I was discouraged, depressed, and saddened about my condition at such a young age." Her most uncomfortable symptoms were headaches, fatigue, and profuse yellow/green postnasal mucus drainage. She also mentioned shortness of breath and wheezing, although she had never been diagnosed with asthma. In spite of her condition, she would push herself to exercise as regularly as possible. She was hard on herself in almost every realm of her life—an independent, high-achieving woman.

Dee had classic Type 1 chronic sinusitis. From her history and symptoms (this was before I began using Dr. Crook's Candida Questionnaire and Score Sheet), I thought that the diagnosis of candidiasis was highly likely. So I began the candida treatment program, including the prescription antifungal drug Nizoral, along with the rest of the Physical and Environmental Components of the Sinus Survival Program. I also had her reduce the intensity of her exercise and listen more attentively to her body. "After coming to see you and getting started on the program, **it took only 3 days for me to start feeling better.** After a couple of weeks my energy returned, my sinuses began to clear, my headaches became less severe and frequent. I had hope for the first time in years." During the first week on Nizoral she described lots of white material, "like snow," coming from her nose. Nearly two months into the Program, and again around four months, she had sinus infections. However, she was not nearly as sick as she'd been with previous infections. They didn't last as long, and she was able to treat them effectively without taking an antibiotic. To me, her most valuable lesson with these infections was that she was able to clearly see how her anger had contributed to causing them. Another helpful factor for Dee was that throughout those first five months on the Program, her husband was extremely supportive of her commitment to healing herself.

Today, more than five years after our fifth and final session together, **Dee has cured her chronic sinusitis and is also free of allergies and candida.** She describes her experience with the Sinus Survival Program as follows: "I believe that the component that helped the most was my diet. Eating healthier, taking vitamins, drinking eight glasses of water a day, and avoiding wheat, dairy, sugar, and caffeine. The healthy habits I've incorporated are:

(1) A healthy diet, avoiding those foods that give me sinus infections
(2) A good regimen of vitamins to keep my immune system strong and efficient, and to avoid getting ill
(3) Drinking at least eight 8-ounce glasses of water a day
(4) Keeping my environment as pollution-free as possible
(5) Exercising whenever possible—great for physical and mental health
(6) Using affirmations to keep me mentally healthy and confident
(7) Taking time for reflection, meditation, and relaxation

"The most significant change in my life is the control I now have over it. It is empowering to make yourself healthy when sick, or even better, to prevent sickness. The belief that you control your world by how you react and live is wonderful. It gives you the freedom and confidence to do anything. It's all possible.

"The most challenging aspect of the Program was the diet. Most grocery stores don't stock 'natural' foods and you have to take the time to become a label reader and familiar with what foods are best for you. I learned how to extract the good foods from the stores and for specialty items I went to health food stores. Restaurants posed a problem also. Look for items with vegetables, choose appetizers that are healthy instead of eating a main course, and avoid sauces whenever possible. I also read lots and lots of books on nutrition and how our body uses the food we eat. This allows you to make the right choices.

"If someone were considering making a commitment to this program, I would stress that it is not a quick fix. It takes dedication and life-altering changes to succeed. Once you do feel better, it's impossible to go back to unhealthy habits. You now have the knowledge and experience to know better.

"I am happy to say that five years later, I am still using the Program. I have made a lifelong commitment to this program and it is now my way of life. Since adopting this program, my health problems in general have vanished. I rarely even have the common cold. As a side benefit, I lost weight and can control it better than I ever could before. And my medical costs have decreased tremendously. On a scale of 1 to 10, my health and happiness are a 9. This program gave me a new lease on life and I am enjoying it. In the past five years I've had my share of stress and hardship, including family sickness, closing a family business, six months without any income, and almost losing my home. Through all this I concentrated even harder on all aspects of the Program. I believe that this is what got me through the hard times and will help me when they come again."

Syd H. is a 49-year-old health and physical education teacher in Westchester County near the New York City metropolitan area. He had been a police officer for twenty years prior to his current teaching position. He's been single for ten years following a divorce, and has no children. The other significant personal history is that he'd been regularly attending AA meetings since

1991 and hadn't had any alcohol since then. I had five sessions with him (the first one in person and the others over the phone) over a four-month period in late 1995 and early 1996.

Syd had been in relatively good health until he had his first sinus infection diagnosed in 1990, and had been sick to some degree since then, in spite of averaging about three to four two-week courses of antibiotics a year. His most uncomfortable symptoms were severe headaches, fatigue, muscle aches, and depression. When the sinusitis began, he was also treated with antidepressant medication. After seeing multiple physicians, he had sinus surgery in 1993, which did not help. Following the unsuccessful surgery, "more doctors followed, none of whom were any help. I was starting to question my sanity, because they all told me that there was nothing wrong with me." He'd also been diagnosed with allergies and was under the care of an allergist. He was taking Seldane-D (antihistamine/decongestant now called Allegra) and Entex (decongestant) regularly but stopped just prior to our first session. He was also drinking eight to ten cups of coffee a day to try to restore his lack of energy.

Syd is the kind of guy who sets challenging goals for himself and pushes himself hard to attain them. He had enjoyed running marathons prior to the sinusitis, but hadn't been physically capable of running one in over five years. That became a primary goal of his in working with the Sinus Survival Program. He not only wanted to cure his chronic sinusitis, but he was determined to run marathons again. A big part of his challenge was to overcome the belief that "I'm not able to run a marathon." He had others, such as "It's winter and this has always been the worst time for my sinuses. I'm still waiting for the shoe to drop." He continued to hear these limiting messages even though his sinuses were feeling much better and he was running again, although more moderately. Another goal was to marry again, but he hadn't dated in several years and he had to change the message "I'll never meet the right woman." Within two months of beginning the Program, he was affirming daily, "I am meeting the ideal woman"; he was dating three different women; he bought a treadmill to help him train; and he had registered for the Long Island Marathon in May (four months hence). He had also stopped the coffee, improved his diet, and strictly adhered to the rest of the Program. One day during the first month of being on the diet, he ate a lot of cheese and was very congested and had a severe sinus headache the next day. He felt as if this episode was very helpful in strengthening his motivation to stay with the diet. After two months of adhering closely to the entire regimen, his chronic sinusitis was gone and he rated his energy level between 8 and 9.

After nearly four months on the Program, Syd got his first sinus infection. We determined the causes to be: too much exercise, stress (having to choose between the three women he was seeing), and not enough sleep. He realized how hard he is on himself, and he eased up on having to make a decision on the women and on meeting the marathon deadline. He decided to do a half-marathon instead. The infection was not nearly as severe as those he'd had in the past, nor did it last as long. And that was without filling the prescription for an antibiotic.

Syd described his experience with the Sinus Survival Program as transformational. "I followed the Program conscientiously, making the following important changes in particular:

- I run a HEPA air purifier in my bedroom 24 hours a day.
- I inhale steam and irrigate my nose on a regular basis.
- I dramatically removed most dairy products from my diet.
- I receive allergy shots on a regular basis and use prescription antihistamines and decongestants on an as-needed basis.
- I try to keep a positive attitude, regardless of circumstances.
- I attend church every Sunday.
- I exercise regularly.
- I use the *Sinus Survival* book as a reference, when I feel a need to. (I have loaned it to and purchased it for a number of friends and relatives.)

"I am a 53-year-old health and physical education teacher who went from barely getting through the day, only to come home and immediately go back to bed in the middle of the afternoon, to the following level of activity:

- I now have more energy than I have had in years.
- I am rarely sick.
- I have not needed one single course of antibiotics since first meeting Dr. Ivker.
- I still receive monthly allergy injections, but thanks to the Sinus Survival Program, my environmental allergies are much more mild and I'm better able to deal with them.
- I have successfully completed the last two New York City Marathons.
- I am a very active Volunteer Firefighter/EMT for a very busy metropolitan area fire department.
- I have been in a monogamous relationship with a woman for the past two and a half years.

"On a scale of 1 to 10, I have gone from being a 1 to being a 9. Dr. Ivker and his Sinus Survival Program have forever changed my life for the better. God bless him for that. You don't really appreciate your health until you don't have it. I was so miserable, I was willing to try anything, and thank God this approach worked. If you are in doubt, try it. You have nothing to lose except your infections, headaches, and fatigue."

Gloria S. is a 55-year-old first-grade teacher from a town north of Denver who attended a weekend Sinus Survival Workshop in early 1996. She's married and has two grown children. Prior to attending, each member of the group took the Candida Questionnaire and Score Sheet in Chapter 6. Gloria's score was 182, which placed her in the "Almost Certainly Candida" category. She was also having six to seven sinus infections per year accompanied by a two- to three-week course of antibiotics with each infection. She was nearly incapacitated by extreme fatigue (energy level of 2), headaches and head congestion, and persistent yellow/green postnasal mucus drainage. Sinus surgery had been recommended by her physician. She also suffered from seasonal hay fever and had taken allergy shots. When she came to the Workshop she was also using a cortisone nasal spray on a daily basis year-round, which she stopped as she began the Program. She adhered to the entire Program, including candida treatment, quite well. However, she preferred using a homeopathic, Mycocan Combo, for the candida rather than an antifungal medication such as Nizoral or Diflucan.

Gloria's condition improved dramatically, but since I did not work closely with her following the weekend Workshop, I'll let her tell her own story. "I started having sinus infections in my twenties, which worked well for many years, as I would have one or two infections yearly. As the years progressed the number of infections increased and I continued to take antibiotics for these infections, but they weren't working very well. I would barely complete the antibiotics and I would have another infection. By this time, I was having six to seven infections a year and still taking antibiotics. My overall health was marginal due to my constant battle with sinus infections. I had severe headaches, sore throats, nausea, and no energy for work or free time. My doctor suggested sinus surgery, but I was terrified of the procedure and also felt it was not the answer. My children had for many years suggested finding another answer for my sinus problems. I always said, 'Sure, next time.' I always wanted the quick fix and yet, I knew I was at the end of the road and badly needed a new approach. After my last visit to my doctor I knew I had no choice but to take control of my own health. He told me that he could not help me any more and I would just have to learn to be more patient and get used to feeling rotten the rest of my life. I said, 'No way!' and left his office and drove directly to my favorite bookstore. Sitting on the shelf, facing out, was *Sinus Survival*. I thumbed through the book and purchased it immediately. I thought this book was written just for me. What a chance to change my health! Little did I know how much this book would change my life.

"I started the Sinus Survival Program on February 16, 1996, and within four to five weeks I started feeling better. My headaches, sore throats, and tiredness started to lessen. What an amazing feeling! I will tell you, I followed the Program very closely and each week I felt better and better. It is now June 1999 and I am feeling great. I still try to watch my diet. Since February 16, 1996, I have had **only one sinus infection** and I treated that myself with the help of the book and **no antibiotics.** I now feel confident that I can treat my allergies and sinus infections with the aid of the information I've learned from *Sinus Survival.* The Program is holistic. I've learned how I allowed stress and other factors to dominate my emotional and mental life, thus causing my physical well-being to suffer. I continue to work daily on affirmations and attitude because I know how important both aspects are for my health. Needless to say, Dr. Rob Ivker is my hero. He has helped me become a healthy, energetic total person. Thanks, Dr. Ivker.

"I would encourage anyone that has sinus, allergies, or asthma to give the Sinus Survival Program a try. Make your commitment and go for it. I wish you luck and a long happy healthy life."

Sam M. is a 35-year-old plant manager from Seattle, Washington, married, with a son from a previous marriage. He came to Littleton to see me for the first session in May 1996 and we had three subsequent sessions by phone over the next four months. Sam had one of the most severe cases of chronic sinusitis and among the worst sinus stories I'd ever heard.

He was in perfect health until 1990, when he got his first sinus infection. Since then he's averaged between ten and fifteen courses of antibiotics per year and has had five sinus surgeries. (For the fourteen years prior to 1990, he'd been on tetracycline, an antibiotic, to treat acne.) Some of the antibiotics would give him a short period of relief before he'd develop another infection. Each surgery also provided him with a few weeks reprieve before the infection and antibiotic cycle began again. He was told by a naturopathic physician in 1994 that he had candidiasis but he did not follow through on the recommended treatment. He did not score the Candida Questionnaire in *Sinus Survival* but he says he had *every symptom* mentioned on the list.

His work environment in the plant was awful—filled with wood dust. He felt better on the weekends when he was away from the plant. I also learned during our first session that Sam loves to play basketball. He would often finish his ten-day course of antibiotic on a Saturday by going all out and playing full-court basketball for a couple of hours. Invariably the infection was back by Sunday morning. Sam is an intense, hardworking, high-achieving man who moves in every realm of his life at only one pace—full speed ahead. It was very difficult for him to slow down, give up his basketball for a few months, and allow his body to heal. (I mentioned in Chapter 6 that strenuous exercise with an already weakened immune system can be devastating and almost guaranteed to trigger another infection.)

I also had him begin a very aggressive candida treatment program with the prescription antifungal medication Diflucan, 200 mg, along with a strict diet, Latero Flora, and Intestinalis. His wife, an RN who had accompanied him to my office, likes to cook and began using recipes from a candida cookbook. After five weeks of strict adherence to this regimen, along with the remainder of the Sinus Survival Program, he felt much better. Every one of his symptoms had improved and he lost fourteen pounds (not uncommon during the first month of candida treatment). He had complied with every recommendation, even coming home for lunch to steam and irrigate. After beginning the Diflucan, he noticed white cottage cheese–like material covering his stools, which had gradually diminished but was not completely gone. (This, no doubt, was the remains of millions of dead yeast organisms.) I decided to keep him on the entire regimen, including daily Diflucan, for another three weeks. He had been able to drastically reduce his exercise to just walking. Since this had been the longest period of time he'd been off antibiotics in six years, he was very pleased with the results and motivated to continue.

After eight weeks of Diflucan, several of his symptoms—especially headache and head congestion—returned during the first week he was off of the medication. I resumed the Diflucan, but every other day for another month. By September, Sam was doing great. He was still on Diflucan every other day, playing basketball once a week without getting sick afterward, his energy level was up to an 8, and he was thrilled with his condition. He was also beginning to realize the extent of his anger. He had been adopted and had experienced serious emotional abuse as a child. At our fourth and final session he had nearly corrected the severe physical imbalance that had been wreaking havoc with his health for six years. And even more importantly he was ready to do the more difficult emotional work that would deepen his healing and heighten his state of well-being.

It is nearly three and a half years since our last consultation. Sam offered the following comments: "The Sinus Survival Program has changed my life. My medical condition prior to working with Dr. Ivker could best be described as miserable. I have had five sinus surgeries and taken sixty to eighty courses of antibiotics. I suffered from flu-like symptoms constantly. I was examined by countless physicians and given a wide range of different diagnoses. My life was absolute hell! My wife and I were desperate when we came across Dr. Ivker's *Sinus Survival* book and made the plane trip that would begin the healing process in every aspect of my life. At first we were skeptical because his concepts worked on restoring health in every aspect of my life. It seemed like a lot of work to fix a sinus condition. The first year after starting the program I experienced remarkable results. My overall health improved by 75 percent. Unfortunately, I became complacent. I drifted off of the diet on business trips and decided all of the soft science work that I had discussed with Dr. Ivker could be postponed. My overall health began to slip. It seemed like all of my work had been for nothing! Finally, with the loving support of my wife and the help of Dr. Ivker, I got back on track. I have had several different setbacks but I am now scheduled to leave my corporate job (a major source of both physical and mental toxicity) and get my master's degree in teaching. My recommendations are as follows:

- Men, don't let your ego get in the way of good health.
- Combine Dr. Ivker's approach with traditional medicine and you will get the most benefits.

"Dr. Ivker is a man on the cutting edge of science. I can tell you from personal experience his intentions are pure and his program works! God bless you, Dr. Ivker. I really appreciate all you have done for me!"

Pat W. is a 58-year-old secretary for a district judge in Shreveport, Louisiana. She's married with three grown children from her two previous marriages. I worked with her for five sessions from August to December 1994. The first session took place in my office in Littleton and the rest were over the phone. She'd suffered with sinus infections for more than twenty years and had averaged about two infections per year until her second husband's suicide in 1987 (they'd been married for 25 years), but then her condition became progressively worse. During the two years prior to our first session, she'd been on almost continuous antibiotics along with steroid injections, "just to keep going." In addition to the sinus infections, she complained most of fatigue (energy level 3), bronchitis, headaches, nasal and head congestion, sore throat, lots of thick colored postnasal mucus, frequent indigestion, and aching joints. She "felt generally bad all the time." When she first came to see me, she rated her "overall level of health as a 2 because the four prior years I had been ill constantly and had no hopes of getting any better. Conventional medicine did not take care of it." During the previous seven years, she'd also had several bouts of pneumonia in addition to bronchitis.

I treated Pat for candidiasis with Nizoral, 200 mg daily, for one month; Latero Flora; Intestinalis; and the candida diet. She experienced a prolonged die-off of the candida, and it took her almost the first full month to begin to turn the comer. By our second session in late September, she rated her energy level as an 8. She adhered very well to the entire Sinus Survival Program in spite of the fact that the vitamins caused her to experience nausea even though she took them following her meals. By the third session, about two months into the Program, she was doing quite well. She was excited to report that she'd had a sinus infection and got over it without taking an antibiotic. Even more importantly, she was getting in touch with and becoming more accepting of her anger. "I'm full of anger. . . . I always thought I was a nice person, and nice people aren't angry." She agreed to start seeing a psychotherapist. By the fourth session she was amazed with her progress, how much more control she had in her life, and how much different the world seemed with this new perspective. She was beginning to realize how powerful she'd become in creating a life that felt so good to her. After seeing a therapist only three times, she was much more aware of the depth of both her anger and grief over her second husband's death, and relieved that she was finally dealing with it after seven years. Her initial reaction to the Social Health recommendations during this fourth session was that "the listening exercise will be the hardest homework you've given me so far. My husband doesn't express feelings and I'm just starting to." By the next month, at our final session, she had not yet done a listening exercise but was feeling great and quite proud of herself. Everyone at work was sick, but she continued to maintain her excellent health. As we completed our work together, four months into the Program, her final comment to me was, "I love my life."

Now, five years later, Pat's review of her experience is as follows:

"After beginning the Sinus Survival Program in August, 1994:

- I had significant results in about sixty days. No prescribed antibiotic since that date.
- Specific symptoms changed: more energy, felt better emotionally, fewer headaches and sinus stuffiness, less drainage, felt alive again.

- Components of the program that helped me most were vitamins, minerals, herbs, echinacea with goldenseal, Neti Pot.
- The most important factor of the whole program was your gift to me: **AWARENESS!** You taught me that my mind, body, and spirit all work together and that it takes all three to make a whole person, and that listening to my body was my responsibility. It opened up a whole new world for me.

"The healthy habits that I've incorporated into my daily life:

(1) Use vitamins (especially C) on a regular basis and echinacea/goldenseal at first sign of possible infection. Discontinue sinus medications and instead use Neti Pot irrigation and saline spray, and drink hot tea.
(2) Use ion generators constantly in den and bedroom, humidifiers as needed; have fireplace, ductwork and carpets cleaned on a regular basis.
(3) Drink water all day.
(4) Changed diet to include more vegetables and fruits and less meat. Use lots less sugar and fats. (Sometimes ice cream is a must to survive.)
(5) Have had counseling when needed to keep my emotional health, which thank goodness you recommended. Life can surely get tedious.
(6) Began a spiritual journey that has opened my heart to God.

"What a difference you have made in my life. I had been ill for several years, with the year prior to seeing you being the worst year as far as sinus infections, bronchitis, lack of energy, and general despondency due to the above. I found your book by accident in the bookstore, and put it down and came back to it three times before deciding to purchase it. I feel my guardian angel was watching over me that day, and I was meant to buy your book when I went into the store. May I also mention it was the last copy they had in the store. Coincidence??

"After meeting with you in our first session, I was excited and optimistic that I had made the right decision and felt very dedicated to following your Program. The most challenging aspects for me were taking supplements on a regular basis, journaling, and listening to my body for warning signs. The diet was completely new and different, and really had to be dealt with on a daily, almost hourly basis. My withdrawal from sweets was especially hard for me. *It was a matter of being determined to get well,* and I trusted you and had enough faith in the Program to discipline myself to do the things you suggested. Not always easy, but better than being ill.

"The most dramatic change in my physical condition has been the minimal sinus symptoms and no bronchitis. My immune system is an asset, again. The most dramatic change in my life has been that I now search within for my answers. Your program started me searching for health and happiness, with one including the other. Today I would rate both my health and happiness a 9. I need to exercise more and I am still growing spiritually and emotionally (that journey will never be over). Your holistic approach was very new to me, but after experiencing your program I realize there is no other way to really be healthy. You have given me a new insight into my whole self, and I have started on a journey that is changing my entire life. There is still a lot of exploring and discovery ahead for me, but with your guidance I have improved my physical health first, which made the rest of it fall into place. This is a very rewarding time in my life, thanks to you. I would urge anyone with upper respiratory problems to enter your program, as it was the best thing I have ever done for my body, my soul, my mind, and my emotions. You gave me the tools I needed to manage all of them."

Chapter 10

MOST COMMONLY ASKED QUESTIONS

Do you still see patients?
I have continued to see patients, but due to my writing commitments—I will have written eight books between 1995 and 2001—I've had to greatly limit the number of people I can work with. I see individuals in private consultation for treatment of chronic illness and/or optimal health counseling. The life-changing holistic medical program that I teach consists of the following:

- Five sessions, two to three hours in length, are conducted over a period of one year.
- The first three sessions will be scheduled during the first six months, and the last two over the second half of the year.
- The first and final sessions must be in person, and for those living outside of Colorado the other sessions may be done over the phone.
- Session number 1—*Healing Your Body*—consists of a review of your medical history and the Wellness Self-Test, along with the introduction of the components of *Physical and Environmental Health*.
- Session number 2—*Healing Your Mind*—involves the components of *Mental and Emotional Health*.
- Session number 3—*Healing Your Spirit*—involves the components of *Spiritual and Social Health*.

- Sessions number 4 and number 5 consist of review and reinforcement of the first three sessions and a reassessment of the Wellness Self-Test.
- Each of the five consultations will include a Reiki/healing touch treatment; phone consultations will be followed by a long-distance Reiki session.

For additional information or to schedule an appointment, please call Sinus Survival at (888) 434-0033.

Where can I find a local doctor who is familiar with the Sinus Survival Program?
Beginning in 2000, there are several physicians throughout the U.S. who are considering establishing "Sinus Survival Centers," or who know the Sinus Survival Program. The list of physicians familiar with the program is continually updated and is available on the Internet at http://www.sinussurvival.com or phone (888) 434-0033. They include the following physicians:

American Whole Health
Centers
Littleton, CO
(393) 694-2626
Chicago
(743) 296-6700

Craig Anderson, M.D.
Sandy, UT (outside SLC)
(801) 572-0041

Benjamin Asher, M.D.
Berlin, VT
(802) 371-4585

Paul Berger, M.D.
Boulder, CO
(303) 443-2544

Gabriel Cousens, M.D.
Patagonia, AZ
(520) 394-2520

Karl Diehn, M.D.
Baltimore, MD
(410) 821-5151

Deborah Glasser Green, M.D.
Canby, OR (outside Portland)
(503) 266-7933

Mary Hardy, M.D.
Los Angeles, CA
(310) 423-9700

Katherine Roth, M.D.
Traverse City, MI
(616) 922-0400

Mark Hoch, M.D.
New York, NY
(212) 988-9665

Nancy Russell, M.D.
Kansas City, MO
(816) 453-5545

Karen Lawson, M.D.
Grand Rapids, MI
(616) 752-9623

Amy Saltzman, M.D.
San Francisco, CA
(415) 925-3503

E.J. Linkner, M.D.
Ann Arbor, MI
(734) 973-1010

William Silvers, M.D.
Denver, CO
(303) 794-0908

Steve Morris, N.D.
Mukilteo, WA (outside Seattle)
(425) 347-1951

Jacqueline Stoken. D.O.
West Des Moines, IA
(515) 327-0046

Todd Nelson, N.D.
Denver, CO
(303) 744-7858

Alan Warshowsky, M.D.
New York, NY
(516) 488-2877

Carol Roberts M.D.
Brandon, FL (outside Tampa)
(813) 661-3662

I've had chronic sinusitis for many months (or years) and my doctor is recommending sinus surgery. Do you think it's necessary?
Although I would need to do a thorough evaluation of your history before rendering a definitive opinion, the answer to this question is usually no. However, there are instances where surgery can be quite helpful, especially in people with large nasal polyps. If your sinuses are filled with polyps or cysts that are blocking the ostia, then I would recommend surgery. But

then to prevent them from recurring, which often occurs, begin the Sinus Survival Program following the surgery.

Sinus surgery should always be considered a last resort, when all else has failed. But unfortunately, for many ENT physicians (sinus surgeons), "all else" usually refers to multiple courses of antibiotics. The reason most often given to justify nasal/sinus surgery is a deviated nasal septum, the "dividing wall" between the two nostrils. The majority of people in our society have a deviated septum to some degree, but most of them do not have sinus problems. It is important to realize that if you have a deviated septum, it has been that way for most of your life; but most likely you've had sinus infections only in recent years. The septum is therefore not usually the cause of your problem. It is the swollen and inflamed mucous membranes covering the septum and the other sides of your nostrils (the turbinates) that are responsible for preventing your sinuses from draining. If a deviated septum is the reason given for surgery, I'd postpone the surgery and diligently follow the Program, especially Chapter 6 and the table on pages 183–186. An aggressive approach to treating candida would be extremely helpful if you consider yourself a candidate. After treating yourself for one to two months, if your condition is unchanged (which is highly unlikely), you can then choose the surgical option, knowing that you've "given it your best shot."

Do I still need to take antibiotics for every sinus infection?
No. Sinus infections can be treated effectively without antibiotics, if you strictly adhere to the Sinus Survival Program. I would especially recommend getting as much sleep as possible; steaming while adding V-VAX eucalyptus oil and tea tree oil, followed by irrigation three or four times a day; taking the maximum dosages of the vitamin and herbal regimen (a natural "antibiotic") prescribed in Chapter 6; and addressing the emotional causes of your infection. It may take about two weeks to feel 100 percent normal and have consistently clear or white mucus. Recovery time will be shorter if you can identify and treat all the causes of the sinus infection, especially releasing your anger.

However, if you do all of the above for ten days or two weeks and notice no improvement with your infection, e.g., the mucus is still a thick yellow-green and you've still got a headache, are very congested, feverish, and very tired, then I would suggest seeing your physician and taking an antibiotic. This situation may also be an indication of a yeast overgrowth, especially if you're someone who's had candidiasis in the past. Consider adding candida treatment (see p. 18) to the rest of the Sinus Survival Program after two unsuccessful weeks of treatment, or begin it after you've finished your course of antibiotic.

For most of the patients whom I've treated for chronic sinusitis, repeated use of antibiotics has been a primary cause of their sinus disease (see p. 78). If you're someone with Type 1 or 2 chronic sinusitis, taking three or more courses of antibiotics within a six-month period, then I would avoid any additional antibiotics in treating your sinus infection. If you have one or two infections per year, then it's probably okay to take an antibiotic; but there's no assurance that it will work any faster than the natural regimen I prescribe in this book. I'd recommend you try another way and take the "risk." However, if your experience has you convinced that you can get better only by taking the prescription drug, then do so in addition to steaming, irrigation, more sleep, and the vitamin/herbal regimen. Follow the antibiotic by a two- to three-week course of acidophilus (see p. 251).

What vitamin, herb, and supplement dosages do you recommend for children?
Please refer to the charts in Chapter 1 and at the end of Chapter 6.

What are the best air cleaners, ion generators, and humidifiers, and where can I find them?
See Chapter 6 and the Product Index for my recommendations. For information and purchasing most of these products, you can contact Sinus Survival at (888) 434-0033 or (303) 771-0033, or http://www.sinussurvival.com.

How can I prevent sinus infections when I travel?

This problem seems to be increasingly common. It's probably a result of a combination of factors—extremely unhealthy cabin air in addition to a weakened immune system. Prolonged exposure to the air in aircraft is becoming one of our most significant health risk factors. Fortunately, most flights are now smoke-free, but the air is still dry, filled with the viruses and bacteria of our fellow travelers, and very low—nearly devoid—of negative ions (see p. 111). When you combine this factor with extreme dryness, which is an irritant to the mucous membrane, it's easy to see why prolonged exposure to the infections of the other travelers poses a challenge to our defense systems. The lining of the mucous membrane is our chief protection against upper respiratory infections—colds and sinus infections. Secondarily we are protected by the immune system. However, the stress of travel, often coupled by the lack of sleep, can significantly weaken our resistance to infection.

To prevent illness while traveling you should focus on minimizing both risk factors. To strengthen your immune system, I would recommend the following:

- Get a good night's sleep before and after your flight.
- Arrive at the airport at least an hour before your scheduled departure to minimize stress.
- Have something to eat before leaving for the airport and request a vegetarian meal for the flight.
- Take grape-seed extract (100 mg) at least 20 minutes before the preflight meal.
- Following your meal take several antioxidants, herbs, and supplements: vitamin C (2,000 mg), vitamin E (400 IU), alpha lipoic acid (100 mg), garlic (200 mg), grape-seed extract (100 mg), and a multivitamin. If your flight is two hours or longer and you are served a meal in-flight, then take the same dosage of vitamin C and garlic following that meal. Take another capsule of grape-seed extract on an empty stomach either during or following the flight. Following your first meal

after the flight take all of the above antioxidants and supplements in the same dosage as above.

- Minimize stress as much as possible upon arrival at your destination, e.g., make reservations for lodging, arrange transportation (taxis and hotel shuttles are less stressful than renting a car and driving yourself around a new city), and give yourself plenty of time to make your first appointment.

To help maintain optimal function of your mucous membranes:

(1) Drink lots of bottled water before, during, and after the flight. The only liability with this practice is frequent trips to the rest room. Try to get an aisle seat on the plane.

(2) Avoid caffeine and alcohol, since they are both diuretics.

(3) Use a saline nasal spray frequently, both during and after the flight. I would recommend the Sinus Survival Spray, which contains three medicinal herbs (see p. 136). I also spray V-VAX eucalyptus oil on a tissue, hold it close to my nose, and breathe it in for 10–15 minutes shortly after a flight. If the trip is longer than three hours, I'll also do this during the flight.

(4) As soon as you're settled in your room, give yourself a Steam Inhaler treatment with V-VAX added to the Inhaler, or take a hot shower and spray V-VAX in the shower.

(5) Using a negative-ion generator by your bed in the hotel room or wherever you're staying after the flight can also be quite helpful for cleaning the air and preventing infection.

I'm very pleased to report that after twelve years of being free of chronic sinusitis, I recently put my sinus and the Sinus Survival Program to its greatest challenge ever: For nine weeks, during October and November 1999, I took 26 flights en route to 20 of the first 35 cities of a media tour in conjunction with my newly published book, *The Complete Self-Care Guide to Holistic Medicine.* At the conclusion of this marathon on November

30, I was just as healthy and full of vitality as I was when I left Denver on September 29. I've just described a significant portion of the holistic preventive program that I followed during the book tour.

I've been reluctant to try irrigation. How important is it?
Nasal irrigation can potentially be the most therapeutic measure in completely eliminating a sinus infection (see p. 137). It can help quickly and dramatically. I've heard from people who have had an infection for months, and within two days of beginning irrigation, the infection was gone and did not return, even if irrigation was not continued beyond a few days.

If the problem is chronic sinusitis, your mucous membranes may have been inflamed and irritated for years, with the cilia badly damaged. In this case, daily irrigation is an essential part of the Program used to heal the membranes and prevent further infection. The bathing of the membranes with salt water keeps them moist and eliminates pollutants and particles usually removed by the cilia. While irrigation in this instance helps temporarily (just while you're doing it), it also has the long-term benefit of helping the membranes return to normal.

Are there any studies proving the effectiveness of the Sinus Survival Program?
In March 2000, the first Sinus Survival Study was completed. Working in collaboration with William Silvers, M.D., a Denver allergist, we invited eleven of his most challenging patients with chronic sinusitis to make a four-month commitment to the Sinus Survival Program. These were all people who had been suffering with sinusitis for many years, had been on multiple courses of antibiotics, and in three instances had had sinus surgery. One woman had undergone four surgeries. We met as a group in five two-hour sessions approximately one month apart. One person dropped out of the study after attending the first two sessions.

Each of the participants began the study by subjectively assessing their health status using the Rhinitis Quality of Life Questionnaire, the Wellness Self-Test (see Chapter 2), the Symptom Chart (see Chapter 6), and the Candida Questionnaire and Score Sheet (see Chapter 6). A physical (nasal cavity) and rhinoprobe exam (evaluates the nasal mucosa histology) was performed by Dr. Silvers at the beginning and at the end of the study. All but one of the participants scored high (above 180) on the Candida Questionnaire. The lone exception was a woman who scored 93 and who also suffered with asthma in addition to sinusitis. At the second session, all were prescribed a six-week course of Diflucan, 200 mg daily for four weeks and every other day for two weeks, along with the candida diet and the remainder of the Sinus Survival Program. However, the Program was limited to less than thirty distinct therapies. In addition to Diflucan, these modalities included: negative-ion generator, warm-mist humidifier, air duct cleaning, Steam Inhaler, nasal irrigation, V-VAX eucalyptus spray, Sinus Survival Nasal Spray, diet (elimination of dairy products, sugar, alcohol, wheat), increased water (bottled or filtered) intake, vitamins C (Ester C) and E, a multivitamin, grape-seed extract (Masquelier's Original OPC Grape Seed), garlic, flaxseed oil, echinacea and grapefruit-seed extract (for acute infection—with yellow/green mucus), light aerobic exercise, affirmation/ goal list, anger release, acidophilus (after six weeks of Diflucan), meditation or prayer, listening exercise, and recreation (a date night per week).

One person dropped out after attending only two of the sessions. In spite of the fact that the study took place during the height of the "sinusitis season"—October to March—all but one of the ten remaining participants experienced a dramatic improvement in their sinus conditions and in their overall general health, and had a far better season than the previous year. Nearly everyone rated their general health and energy level a 9 or 9.5, with 10 being optimum. The one man who did not improve had to take a course of prednisone and antibiotics for severe asthma and acute sinusitis while on the Diflucan. The woman who scored lowest on the Candida Questionnaire experienced a significant change in both her sinusitis and asthma following the combination of Diflucan and the candida diet. Three of the participants had a marked improvement after the first month, before starting the Diflucan. Four people had sinus infections during the study, and all but one (the severe asthmatic) were able to resolve without an antibiotic. They also mentioned feeling not nearly as sick with their infection as they had in the past. By the end of their four-month commitment, almost all of the participants were practicing most of the Sinus Survival Program on a regular basis. Many of the components of the Program had already been incorporated into their lives as healthy habits. In doing so, *they had in fact broken the cycle of chronic and recurrent sinus infections that had been making their lives miserable for many years. They were well on the way to curing chronic sinusitis.*

After a thorough evaluation by a biostatistician, the results of the first Sinus Survival Study will be published in a medical journal, and I will personally present them at the Annual Conference of the American Academy of Otolaryngology in September 2000.

PRODUCT INDEX

The following are all currently available through *Sinus Survival Products* (toll free at (888) 434-0033 or the Web site: www. sinussurvival.com). Some of these products are also available at health food stores, pharmacies, department stores, and bookstores.

Vitamins/Herbs/Homeopathics

Sinus Survival Ester C
Sinus Survival Masquelier's OPC Grape Seed
Sinus Survival V-VAX Eucalyptus Spray
Sinus Survival Elderberry Cough Syrup
Sinus Survival Zinc Cold Lozenges
Sinus Survival EchinOsha Blend
Professional Health Products Mycocan Combo
Life Center Intestinals
International Bio-Tech Latero-Flora

Nasal Hygiene—Moisture/Stream/Irrigation

Sinus Survival Nasal Spray
Kaz TheraSteam Personal Steam Inhaler
RST Respiratory Steam Inhaler
SinuCleanse Irrigation System
SinuCleanse Saline Refills
SinuCleanse Video
Grossan Nasal Irrigator
Water Pik

Ionizers/Air Cleaners/Humidifiers

Sinus Survival "Air Vitalizer" Ionizer
Bionaire ULPA Filter Air Cleaners
Bionaire ULPA Filter Replacements
Bionaire Warm Mist Humidifiers
Bionaire Climate Check (Temperature/Humidity Gauge)
Sinus Survival Pleated Furnace Filters

Cleaning Products

DuPont Vacuum Bags
Wizard Dust Cloths

Books

Sinus Survival: The Holistic Medical Treatment for Sinusitis, Allergies, and Colds by Robert S. Ivker, D.O., New York: Tarcher/ Putnam, 2000.

The Self-Care Guide to Holistic Medicine: Creating Optimal Health by Robert S. Ivker, D.O., Robert A. Anderson, M.D., and Larry Trivieri, Jr., New York: Tarcher/Putnam, 1999.

Thriving: The Holistic Guide to Optimal Health for Men by Robert S. Ivker, D.O., and Ed Zorensky, New York: Three Rivers Press, 1998.

Starting Points for a Healthy Habitat by Carl Grimes, Denver: GMC Media, 1999.

RESOURCE GUIDE

SinusSurvival.com, accessible on the Internet or by calling (888) 434-0033, is the most comprehensive resource for:

- Information about the Sinus Survival Program
- Referrals to a Sinus Survival Center in or near your city
- Making appointments with Dr. Ivker
- Location and dates of Sinus Survival Seminars
- Obtaining Sinus Survival Products

The following organizations offer additional information about various aspects of the Sinus Survival Program and provide referrals to practitioners of the many therapies that contribute to this holistic approach for treating, preventing, and curing sinusitis, allergies, and asthma.

Holistic Medicine

American Board of Holistic Medicine (ABHM)
PO Box 5388
Lynnwood, WA 98043

Phone (425) 741–2996   Fax (425) 787–8040
Email blh@halcyon.com
The ABHM is the first organization to certify physicians in Holistic Medicine (December 2000 will be the first certification examination) and to create the standard of care for holistic medical practice. Provides a referral list of board-certified holistic physicians.

American Holistic Medical Association (AHMA)
6728 Old McLean Village Drive
McLean, VA 22101–3906
Phone (703) 556–9728   Fax (703) 556–8729
www.holisticmedicine.org (A physician referral directory is available.)
The nation's oldest advocacy group (founded in 1978) devoted to promoting, teaching, and researching holistic medicine. Provides a list of referrals nationwide of holistic physicians (M.D.'s and D.O.'s) (also available on the Web site).

Osteopathic Medicine

American Academy of Osteopathy
3500 DePauw Blvd, Suite 1080
Indianapolis, IN 46268
(317) 879–1881
Affiliate organization representing D.O.'s who provide osteopathic manipulative treatments and/or cranial osteopathy as part of their practice.

Craniosacral Therapy

Cranial Academy
8606 Allisonville Road, Suite 130
Indianapolis, IN 46268
Phone (317) 594–0411   Fax (317) 594–0411 and (317) 594–9299
Provides information and a referral list of craniosacral therapists.

Upledger Institute
11211 Prosperity Farms Road
Palm Beach Gardens, FL 33410
Phone (407) 622-4706   Fax (407) 622-4771
Offers training, information, and referrals.

Acupuncture/Traditional Chinese Medicine

American Academy of Medical Acupuncture
58200 Wilshire Blvd., Suite 500
Los Angeles, CA 90036
(213) 937-5514
Professional association of physician acupuncturists (M.D.'s and D.O.'s). Provides educational materials, postgraduate courses, and a membership directory of members nationwide.

American Association for Oriental Medicine
433 Front Street
Catasauqua, PA 18032
Phone (610) 266-1433   Fax (610) 264-2768
Professional association for non-M.D. acupuncturists. Offers publications and a referral directory of members nationwide.

National Acupuncture Detoxification Association
3115 Broadway, Suite 51
New York, NY 10027
(212) 993-3100
Leading organization of its kind. Conducts research on, and provides training in the use of acupuncture to treat addiction, including alcoholism.

National Commission for the Certification of Acupuncturists
1424 16th NW, Suite 601
Washington, DC 20036
(202) 232-1404
Provides information about acupuncture and offers a test used by various states to determine competency of acupuncture practitioners.

Qigong Institute/East-West Academy of Healing Arts
450 Sutter, Suite 916
San Francisco, CA 94108
(415) 788-2227
Provides education, training, and research about qigong in relation to health and healing.

Behavioral Medicine/Mind-Body Medicine

Association for Humanistic Psychology
45 Franklin Street, Suite 315
San Francisco, CA 94102
(415) 864-8850
Provides publications about humanistic psychology and a list of referrals.

Center for Mind–Body Medicine
5225 Connecticut Avenue NW, Suite 414
Washington, DC 20015
(202) 966-7338
An educational program for health and mental health professionals as well as laypeople interested in exploring their own capacities for self-knowledge and self-care. Provides educational and support groups for people with chronic illness, stress management groups, and training and programs in mind/body health care.

Mind/Body Medical Institute
New Deaconess Hospital
185 Pilgrim Road
Boston, MA 02215
(617) 632-9530
Provides research, training, and conferences related to behavioral medicine, stress reduction, yoga, and meditation.

National Institute for the Clinical Application of Behavioral
   Medicine
PO Box 523
Mansfield Center, CT 06250

Phone (860) 456-1153   Fax (860) 423-4512
Provides conferences and information for practitioners.

Bodywork/Massage Therapies

American Massage Therapy Association
820 Davis Street, Suite 100
Evanston, IL 60201
(312) 761-2682
Provides comprehensive information on most areas of bodywork and massage, including an extensive review of the latest scientific research. Also publishes Massage Therapy Journal, *available at most health food stores and many newsstands nationwide.*

Associated Bodywork and Massage Professionals
PO Box 489
Evergreen, CO 80439
(303) 674-8478
Provides information and referrals.

Rolfing

International Rolf Institute
302 Pearl Street
Boulder, CO 80306
(303) 449-5903
Provides information, training, and referral directory.

Reflexology

International Institute of Reflexology
PO Box 12462
St. Petersburg, FL 33733
(813) 343-4811
Provides information, training, and referrals.

Chiropractic

American Chiropractic Association
1701 Clarendon Blvd.
Arlington, VA 22209
(703) 276-8800
*Professional association offering education and research into chiropractic.
Also offers publications.*

International Chiropractors Association
1110 North Glebe Road, Suite 1000
Arlington, VA 22201
(800) 423-4690 and (703) 528-5000
*Professional association offering education and research into chiropractic.
Also offers publications.*

Diet and Nutrition

American College for Advancement in Medicine (ACAM)
23121 Verdugo Drive, Suite 204
Laguna Hills, CA 92653
(800) 532-3688
*ACAM provides information about the use of nutritional supplements
and a referral directory of physicians worldwide who have been trained in
nutritional medicine.*

American College of Nutrition
722 Robert E. Lee Drive
Wilmington, NC 28480
(919) 452-1222
Information resource for nutrition research.

American Dietetic Association
216 West Jackson, Suite 800
Chicago, IL 60606
(312) 899-0040
Provides information and certification.

Center for Science in the Public Interest
1875 Connecticut Avenue NW, Suite 300
Washington, DC 20009
Phone (202) 332-9110   Fax (202) 265-4954
Provides a directory of organic mail order suppliers, hormone-free beef suppliers, and general information on diet and nutrition.

International Association of Professional Natural Hygienists
Regency Health Resort and Spa
2000 South Ocean Drive
Hallandale, FL 33009
(305) 454-2220
Professional organization of physicians who specialize in therapeutic fasting.

Diagnostic Laboratory

Great Smokies Diagnostic Laboratory
63 Zillicoa Street
Asheville, NC 28801-4762
(800) 522-4762
Offers fully certified advanced assessments using over 100 diagnostic tests of digestive, immune, endocrine, nutritional, and metabolic function—supported by a comprehensive network of educational and scientific resources.

Energy Medicine

International Society for the Study of Subtle Energies and Energy Medicine (ISSSEEM)
356 Goldco Circle
Golden, CO 80401
Phone (303) 278-2228   Fax (303) 279-3539
Research organization; provides education and information, as well as publications.

Resource Guide

Therapeutic Touch

Nurse Healers Professional Associates, Inc.
1211 Locust Street
Philadelphia, PA 19107
(215) 545-8079
Provides information on training, conferences, and referrals of TT practitioners. Also publishes a newsletter.

Healing Touch

Colorado Center for Healing Touch, Inc.
198 Union Blvd., Suite 204
Lakewood, CO 80228
Phone (303) 989-0581   Fax (303) 985-9702
Email ccheal@aol.com
Provides information and referrals.

Reiki

Reiki Alliance
PO Box 41
Cataldo, ID 83810
(208) 682-3535
Provides information and referrals.

Energy Devices

Tools for Exploration
9755 Independence Avenue
Chatsworth, CA 91311
(888) 748-6657
Provides nonmedical energy machines and other devices. Free catalog available by request.

Environmental Medicine

Human Ecology Action League (HEAL)
PO Box 49126
Atlanta, GA 30359
(404) 248-1898
Provides referrals to support groups that assist people suffering from environmental illness.

Immuno Labs
1620 West Oakland Park Blvd., Suite 300
Fort Lauderdale, FL 33311
(800) 321-9197
A lab specializing in allergy testing. Also provides referrals to environmental physicians worldwide.

Herbal Medicine

American Botanical Council
PO Box 201660
Austin, TX 78720
(512) 331-8868
A nonprofit research organization and education council that serves as a clearinghouse of information for professionals and laypeople alike.

Herb Research Foundation
1007 Pearl Street
Boulder, CO 80302
(303) 449-2265
Provides research information and referrals to resources on botanical medicine worldwide. Also publishes HerbalGram.

Homeopathy

International Foundation for Homeopathy
2366 Eastlake Avenue East, Suite 301
Seattle, WA 98102
(206) 324-8230
Provides training in homeopathy and offers referrals.

National Center for Homeopathy
801 North Fairfax, Suite 306
Alexandria, VA 22314
(703) 548-7790
Offers training in homeopathy and provides referrals.

Naturopathic Medicine

American Association of Naturopathic Physicians
2366 Eastlake Avenue East, Suite 322
Seattle, WA 98102
(206) 323-7610
Provides information, publications, and a referral directory of naturo-
pathic physicians. Also in the forefront in licensing of naturopaths
throughout the U.S.

The Institute for Naturopathic Medicine
66½ North State Street
Concord, NH 03301
(603) 255-8844
A nonprofit organization promoting research about naturopathy. Offers
information to professional and laypeople, along with the general media.

Medical Astrology
Jonathan Keyes
(503) 231-9146
Email jonkeyes@qwest.net

BIBLIOGRAPHY

Anand, Margo. *The Art of Sexual Ecstasy.* Los Angeles: Tarcher, 1989.

Anderson, Robert A. *Wellness Medicine.* New Canaan, CT: Keats, 1990.

Bandler, Richard. *Using Your Brain for a Change.* Moab, UT: Real People Press, 1985.

Bauer, Cathryn. *Acupressure for Everybody.* New York: Holt, 1991.

Benedict, Martha S. "Holistic Approaches to Colds and Flu." *Body Mind Spirit,* February/March 1995.

Byrd, Randolph C. "Positive Therapeutic Effects of Intercessory Prayer in a Coronary Care Unit Population." *Southern Medical Journal,* July 1988.

Carey, Benedict. "A Jog in the Smog." *Hippocrates,* May/June 1989.

Carper, Jean. *Food—Your Miracle Medicine.* New York: HarperCollins, 1993.

Challem, Jack. "Defend Yourself Against Supergerms." *Natural Health,* March/April 1995.

Cherry, Rona. "The Best News of the Year." *Longevity,* May 1991.

Chopra, Deepak. *Ageless Body, Timeless Mind.* New York: Harmony, 1993.

Clerico, Dean M., and David W. Kennedy. "Chronic Sinusitis: Diagnostic and Treatment Advances." *Hospital Medicine,* July 1994.

Cooper, Robert K. *Health and Fitness Excellence*. New York: Houghton Mifflin, 1989.

Cotton, Paul. "'Best Data Yet' Say Air Pollution Kills Below Levels Currently Considered Safe." *Journal of the American Medical Association,* June 23/30, 1993.

Crerand, Joanne. "Home Remedy: Insomnia." *Natural Health,* March/April 1992.

Crook, William. *The Yeast Connection*. New York: Vintage, 1986.

Crowther, Richard L. *Indoor Air: Risks and Remedies*. Denver: Directions Publishing, 1989.

Cutler, Ellen W. *Winning the War Against Asthma and Allergies*. Albany, NY: Delmar Publishers, 1998.

Dadd, Debra L. *Nontoxic, Natural, & Earthwise*. Los Angeles: Tarcher, 1982.

Dockery, Douglas W., C. Arden Pope III, Xiphing Xu, John D. Spengler, James H. Ware, Martha E. Fay, Benjamin G. Ferris, Jr., and Frank E. Speizer. "An Association Between Air Pollution and Mortality in Six U.S. Cities." *The New England Journal of Medicine,* December 9, 1993.

Dossey, Larry. *Healing Words*. San Francisco: Harper, 1993.

Dreher, Henry. "Why Did the People of Roseto Live So Long?" *Natural Health,* September/October 1993.

Eisenberg, D. M., et. al. "Use of Alternative Medicine in the U.S." *Journal of the American Medical Association,* November 11, 1998.

Feltman, John, ed. *Hands-on Healing: Massage Remedies for Hundreds of Health Problems*. Emmaus, PA: Rodale, 1989.

Gaby, Alan R. "Human Canaries and Silent Spring." *Holistic Medicine: Magazine of the American Holistic Medical Association,* Fall/Winter 1992.

Gantz, Nelson M., Donald Kaye, C. Wayne Weart. "Antibiotics '95: Back to Basics." *Patient Care,* January 15, 1995.

Georgitis, J. W. "Nasal Hyperthermia and Simple Saline Irrigation for Perennial Rhinitis, Changes in Inflammatory Mediators." *Chest* 106 (1994) 1482–87.

Golan, Ralph. *Optimal Wellness*. New York: Ballantine, 1995.

Gray, Henry. *Anatomy of the Human Body*. 8th ed. Edited by Charles Mayo Goss. Philadelphia: Lea and Febiger, 1967.

Grimes, Carl E. *Starting Points for a Healthy Habitat*. Denver: GMC Media, 1999.

Growald, Eileen Rockefeller, and Allan Luks. "The Healing Power of Doing Good." *American Health,* March 1988.

Guyton, Arthur C. *Textbook of Medical Physiology.* Philadelphia: W. B. Saunders Company, 1968.

Hay, Louise L. *You Can Heal Your Life.* Santa Monica: Hay House, 1984.

Hendeles, Leslie, Miles Weinberger, and Lai Wong. "Medical Management of Noninfectious Rhinitis." *American Journal of Hospital Pharmacy,* November 1980.

Hendrix, Harville. *Getting the Love You Want: A Guide for Couples.* New York: Harper & Row, 1988.

Hersch, Patricia. "The Resounding Silence." *The Family Therapy Networker,* July/August 1990.

Josephson, Jordan S., and Seth I. Rosenberg. "Sinusitis." *Clinical Symposia, Ciba,* 1994.

Joy, W. Brugh. *Joy's Way: A Map for the Transformational Journey.* Los Angeles: Tarcher, 1979.

Kozora, E. J. *American Holistic Medical Association's Nutritional Guidelines.* Seattle: American Holistic Medical Association, 1987.

Krakovitz, Rob. *High Energy: How to Overcome Fatigue and Maintain Your Peak Vitality.* New York: Ballantine, 1986.

Langs, Robert. "Understanding Your Dreams." *New Age Journal,* July/August 1988.

LaPerriere, Arthur, Gail Ironson, Michael H. Antoni, Neil Schneiderman, Nancy Kilmas, and Mary Ann Fletcher. "Exercise and Psychoneuroimmunology." *American College of Sports Medicine,* 1994.

Laskow, Leonard. *Healing with Love.* San Francisco: HarperSanFrancisco, 1992.

Levine, Stephen. *Healing into Life and Death.* New York: Anchor/Doubleday, 1987.

Maharishi Ayur-Veda Newsletter. "Sleep Like a Baby: The Ayurvedic Approach to Insomnia." September 1992.

Myss, Caroyln. *Anatomy of the Spirit.* New York: Harmony, 1996.

National Institute of Allergy and Infectious Diseases. "Sinusitis." Bethesda, MD, 1989.

Neile, Caren. "Banish Allergies Forever!" Globe Communications Corp., 1991.

Ophir, Dov, and Yigal Elad. "Effects of Steam Inhalation on Nasal Patency and Nasal Symptoms in Patients with the Common Cold." *American Journal of Otolaryngology,* 1987.

Ophir, Dov, Yigal Elad, Zvi Dolev, and Carmi Geller-Bernstein. "Effects of Inhaled Humidified Warm Air on Nasal Patency and Nasal Symptoms in Allergy Rhinitis." *Annals of Allergy,* March 1988.

Ornish, Dean. *Love and Survival: The Scientific Basis for the Healing Power of Intimacy.* New York: HarperCollins, 1998.

Ornstein, Robert, and David Sobel. *Healthy Pleasures.* New York: Addison-Wesley, 1989.

Parker, Sharon. "Drugs vs. the Bug." *Utne Reader,* March/April 1995.

Patent, Arnold. *You Can Have It All.* Great Neck, NY: Money Mastery, 1984.

Peck, M. Scott. *The Road Less Traveled.* New York: Simon & Schuster, 1978.

Pert, Candace B. *Molecules of Emotion: Why You Feel the Way You Feel.* New York: Scribners, 1997.

Ponika, J. V., D. A. Sherris, and E. B. Kern, et al. "The Diagnosis and Incidence of Allergic Fungal Sinusitis." *Mayo Clinic Proceedings* 74 (1999): 877–884.

Rapp, Doris. *Allergies and Your Family.* Buffalo, NY: Practical Allergy, 1990.

Reid, Clyde. *Celebrate the Temporary.* New York: Harper & Row, 1972.

Ruddy, John R. "Diagnosing and Treating Sleep Disorders." *National Jewish Center for Immunology and Respiratory Medicine Medical/Scientific Update,* April 1993.

Scraf, Maggie. *Intimate Partners.* New York: Random House, 1987.

Siegel, Bernie S. *Love, Medicine and Miracles.* New York: Harper & Row, 1986.

South Coast Air Quality Management District. *Where Does It Hurt?: Answers to Questions about Smog and Health.* El Monte, CA, 1988.

Spangler, Tina. "The Solution for Indoor Pollution." *Natural Health,* January/February 1995.

Togias, Alkis G., Robert M. Nacierio, and David Proud. "Nasal Challenge with Dry Cold Air in Release of Inflammatory Mediators: Possible Mast Cell Involvement." The American Society for Clinical Investigation, October 1985.

United States Environmental Protection Agency, Office of Air Quality Planning and Standards Technical Support Division. *National Air Quality and Emissions Trend Report,* 1993. Research Triangle Park, NC, 1994.

Vital and Health Statistics, from the Centers for Disease Control and Prevention/National Center for Health Statistics. "Current Estimates From the National Health Interview Survey," 1995.

Warga, Claire. "You Are What You Think." *Psychology Today,* September 1988.

Yerushalmi, Aharon, Sergiu Karman, and Andre Lwoff. "Treatment of Perennial Allergic Rhinitis by Local Hyperthermia." *Proceedings of National Academy of Science USA,* August 1982.

INDEX

Index

Index

Index

Index

Index

Index

Index

Reflexology, 201–202, 203 fig.
Reid, Clyde, 279
Relaxation, 172–173
Relaxation response, 301
REM sleep, 171
Remembrance technique, 273–274
Resource guide, 355–364
Respiratory epithelium, 32
Respiratory tract, 32, 32 fig., 100
Rhinorrhea, 64
Rice, recipes, 239–242
Riverside, CA, 42
Robitussin, 84
Room humidifiers, 120
Rumi, 322

Sabbath, 308
Saline irrigation, 136–138, 137 fig.
Saline nasal spray, 135–136, 181
Salt, 144
San Bernardino, CA, 42
The Science of Mind (Holmes), 262
Screaming, 287
Seasonal symptoms, 71
Secondhand smoke, 38, 96
Selenium, 156, 176
Selfless acts, 316–318
Selye, Hans, 317
Septra, 79
Setliff, Reuben, Dr., 91
Sex, 322–323
Shared vision, 320
Sick-building syndrome, 47–50, 105
Siegel, Bernie, Dr., 263, 269–270
Silvers, William, Dr., 5, 166, 207, 349
Simonton, O. Carl, Dr., 271
Sinobronchitis, 66
SinuCleanse, 137
Sinus:
    infection, 57–66
    pain, 59 fig., 59–60
    surgery, 89–92, 344–345
Sinus drainage and lymphatic pump
        techniques, 194–195
Sinus Survival Air Vitalizer, 113
Sinus Survival Centers, 343–344
Sinus Survival Grape-Seed Extract,
    160

Sinus Survival Program:
    Allergy Treatment, 16 tab.
    Candida Treatment Program, 18 tab.
    Cold Treatment Program, 17 tab.
    as healing process, 1–7, 102
    Natural Quick-Fix Symptom Treat-
        ments, 19–21 tab., 182, 187–189
        tab., 189–190
    Physical and Environmental Health
        components, 13 tab., 183 tab.
    primary objective of, 9
    success stories, 327–341
    Vitamins and Supplements for, 14–15
        tab., 184–185 tab.
Sinus Survival Spray, 136
Sinus Survival Study, 207–208, 349–351
Sinuses:
    anatomy of, 31–33, 32 fig.
    functions of, 33–34
    lining of, 33 fig.
    malformations of, 55
Sinusitis, 57
    diagnosing
        acute, 57–66
        chronic, 67–70
    prevalence and causes of, 34–35
    quick-fix for, 13–15 tab.
    treating
        acute, 77–92
        chronic, 77–92
Skin tests, 73
Skullcap, 172
Slant/Fin GF-200, 134
Sleep, 170–172
Smoking, 37–39
Sobel, David, Dr., 276–277
Social health, 25, 312–325
Socrates, 262
Soil depletion, 150
Sore throat, 64–65
Southern California, 107
Spiegel, David, Dr., 318–319
Spiritual:
    counselors, 307–308
    health, 25, 296–312
    practices, 308–310
Spontaneous imagery, 274–275
Sporanox, 224–225, 253

Index

Sport utility vehicles (SUVs), 46
Stanford University School of Medicine, 318–319
Staphylococcus aureus, 78–79
Steam inhaler, 134–135, 135 fig.
Still, Andrew Taylor, Dr., 191
Stinging nettles, 176
Strength conditioning, 167
Streptococcus pneumoniae, 78
Stress, 282
Stretching, 168
Sturdivant, John, 47
Success stories, 327–341
Sudafed, 84
Sugar, 140–141, 209
Sulfur dioxide, 42
Supergerms, 81
Support groups, 318–319
Suppressor T-cells, 212
Sutherland, William Garner, Dr., 193
Swollen mucosa, 55
Symptom treatment, 122–124
    natural quick-fix, 19–21 tab.
    symptom chart, 125–126

Tai chi, 169
Tai Pan (Clavell), 287
Tantra, 322
Tea, 143
Technology, 100
Teculescu, Dan, Dr., 51
Temperature:
    inversion, 39
    regulation, 34
Texas Gulf Coast, 107
Thayer, Robert, Dr., 166
Thich Nhat Hanh, 303
Thought distortions, 280–281
Thymus gland, 140
Tithing, 317
Titrating to bowel tolerance, 153
TMP/SMX, 79
Toothache, 59
Toxins, 101, 209, 211–213
Traditional Chinese medicine, 197–202, 200 fig., 203 fig.
Travel and prevention, 347–349

Treatment, 76
    allergic rhinitis, 92–95, 94 tab.
    allergies, 92–95, 94 tab.
    Candida albicans, 224–254
    otitis media, 95–98
    sinusitis, acute and chronic, 77–92
Triggers, 173
Triglycerides, 141
Truss, C. Orian, Dr., 222
Tryptophan, 172
Turbinate hypertrophy, 55
Twerski, Mordecai, Rabbi, 305
Tympanostomy tube, 97

UCLA School of Medicine, 46
ULPA filters, 112
Ultra Clear, 253
Unconditional love, 30, 296
University of Michigan Survey Research Center, 317
University of Minnesota School of Public Health, 162–163
Upper respiratory infection, 178
Urine, 130–131

Vacuum cleaners, 115
Valerian, 172
Vegetables, 229
    carbohydrate classifications of, 235 tab.
Ventilation, 116–118
Virus, 179
Visualization, 271–275
Vitamin A, 154–156, 176, 181
Vitamin B complex, 171
Vitamin B_6, 153, 176
Vitamin C, 152–154, 176, 180–181
Vitamin E, 155–156, 176
V-VAX, 161

Walford, Roy, Dr., 146
Walking meditation, 303
Warm-mist humidifier, 127
Water, 129–133, 311
    filtration, 132–133
    leaks, 110
Weight training, 167
Weisburger, John, 143

Index

ABOUT THE AUTHOR

Dr. Robert Ivker is a holistic family physician and healer. He began practicing family medicine in Denver in 1972, after graduating from the Philadelphia College of Osteopathic Medicine. For the past thirteen years his holistic medical practice has focused on the treatment of chronic disease and the creation of optimal health. He is an Assistant Clinical Professor in the Department of Family Medicine and a Clinical Instructor in the Department of Otolaryngology at the University of Colorado School of Medicine, and was the President of the American Holistic Medical Association from 1996 to 1999. As one of the directors of the American Board of Holistic Medicine, he is helping to create board certification in holistic medicine, which will set a new standard for quality health care in America. Along with the four editions of the best-selling *Sinus Survival,* Dr. Ivker is the co-author of *The Self-Care Guide to Holistic Medicine* and *Thriving: The Holistic Guide to Optimal Health for Men.* In 2001, Tarcher/Putnam will publish his Survival Guide series: *Arthritis Survival, Backache Survival, Headache Survival,* and *Asthma Survival.* He has been married for thirty-two years to Harriet, a psychiatric social worker; they have two daughters, Julie and Carin, and live in Littleton, Colorado.